Essential OS Topics for Medical and Surgical Finals

Kaji Sritharan BSc (Hons), MBBS, MRCS
Specialist Registrar in General Surgery
North West Thames Rotation, London

Vivian A Elwell BA (Hons), MA (Cantab),
MBBS, MRCS
Specialist Registrar in Neurosurgery, London

Sachi Sivananthan BSc (Hons)
Final-Year Medical Student, Guy's, King's and
St Thomas' School of Medicine, London

Radcliffe Publishing
Oxford ● New York

Radcliffe Publishing Ltd
18 Marcham Road
Abingdon
Oxon OX14 1AA
United Kingdom

www.radcliffe-oxford.com
Electronic catalogue and worldwide online ordering facility.

British Library Cataloguing in Publication Data

A catalogue record for this book is available from the British Library.

ISBN-13: 978 1 84619 218 0

Typeset by Advance Typesetting Ltd, Oxford
Printed and bound by TJI Digital, Padstow, Cornwall

In memory of Dr S Sritharan.
1946–2006

Contents

Foreword

Medical education has undergone a massive transformation in the past decade. Gone are the didactic lectures, replaced by problem-based and e-learning. Gone are the old-style clinical exams in which chance played a major role in terms of both patients seen and the way in which performance was marked. Now we have Objective Structured Clinical Examinations (OSCEs) and other standardised assessment tools.

This book is a comprehensive attempt to help medical students prepare for these modern tests of knowledge. The first section is devoted to structured history-taking for common symptoms such as cough, shortness of breath and chest pain and has useful text boxes included giving common differential diagnoses. The next section focuses on clinical examination, and between them these early chapters will help prepare the student for the clinical examination. Obviously, they are not a substitute for hands-on experience of history-taking and examination, but they are a useful and thorough aide memoir.

The third section is about clinical skills and how to describe them in an examination environment. Once again the syllabus covered is impressive, ranging from how to take a wound swab, how to mix baby formula milk, to lumbar puncture. There are clear text boxes of indications and complications, making it easy to dip into and revise.

The rest of the book is given over to softer aspects of medical practice which were never really broached in my halcyon days as a medical student: how to write a form or a fluid chart, how to take informed consent, and extensive tips on communication skills. I was particularly impressed by the section on cross-cultural communication and the final chapter on ethics and law, and the multicultural aspects of death and dying – something I have never read about but often found puzzling as a junior doctor when called to Patient Affairs to complete forms for a recently deceased.

The style of the book is very much bullet point/notes, making it easy to read and navigate. Both Kaji Sritharan and Vivian Elwell were outstanding medical students within my own Institution and have gone on to be successful junior doctors with an interest in teaching. Their clear, well-structured thought processes come through in this book. They have involved a final year medical student in Sachi Sivananthan who I am sure is destined for an equally successful career, and she has provided the necessary balance from someone still facing the challenges of these modern assessment methods. They are to be congratulated on this revision text which I am sure will have a place on the book shelf of every medical student, and probably every examiner! I could certainly have done with this book the night before I was asked to examine an orthopaedics station during a recent OSCE examination.

Justin Vale
**Consultant Urological Surgeon and
Honorary Clinical Senior Lecturer
Imperial College School of Medicine**
August 2007

About the authors

Kaji Sritharan BSc (Hons), MBBS, MRCS

Kaji trained at St Mary's Hospital Medical School, London, completed her basic surgical training in London, and is currently a Specialist Registrar in General Surgery on the North West Thames Rotation in London.

She has extensive teaching experience and has held posts as an anatomy demonstrator and tutor in anatomy and embryology at Christ Church College, Oxford University. In addition, she has taught on numerous revision courses at the Royal Society of Medicine, and has experience of organising the final-year surgical and third-year OSCE examinations at Imperial College School of Medicine.

Kaji was awarded a BSc in physiology from University College London, and has recently completed an MD with the Department of Vascular Surgery, Charing Cross Hospital and the Kennedy Institute of Rheumatology, Imperial College London.

Vivian A Elwell BA (Hons), MA (Cantab), MBBS, MRCS

Vivian is currently working as a Specialist Registrar in Neurosurgery, and has held posts in accident and emergency, orthopaedics, neurosurgery, and general surgery with the Surgical Rotation at St Mary's Hospital, London.

She has taught clinical skills to medical students and doctors, and was an anatomy demonstrator at the Imperial College School of Medicine, London. She served on the Imperial College School of Medicine Curriculum Development Committee.

Vivian's awards include the Swinford Edward Silver Medal Prize for her OSCE Examination, the Columbia University Research Fellowship at Columbia College of Physicians and Surgeons in New York City, the Columbia University King's Crown Gold and Silver Medal Awards, the Kathrine Dulin Folger Cancer Research Fellowship, and the 'Who's Who of Young Scientists Prize.'

Vivian was awarded a BA in biological sciences at Columbia College, Columbia University, and an MA from the University of Cambridge. She earned a Bachelor of Medicine and Bachelor of Surgery from the Imperial College School of Medicine, and is a member of the Royal College of Surgeons.

Sachi Sivananthan BSc (Hons)

Sachi Sivananthan is currently a final-year medical student at Guy's, King's and St Thomas' School of Medicine, King's College London. Prior to this she graduated with a BSc from Guy's, King's and St Thomas' School of Biomedical Sciences. She has an avid interest in clinical anatomy, and has given presentations at international meetings in the field of surgery. At present she is a Council member of the Clinical Section and Student's Section of the Royal Society of Medicine. Her past responsibilities include being chairperson of the Student's Group of the International Campaign to Revitalise Academic Medicine (ICRAM).

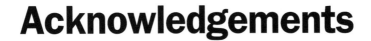

Acknowledgements

This book would not have been possible without support from the following people: Carole D Elwell; TGV Sritharan; Dr Richard Phillips, King's College London; Dr James Dennison, Conquest Hospital, East Sussex Hospital NHS Trust; and Dr Ahmed Abbas, GP Registrar, Bexhill.

History taking

History-taking model

Personal details

Name, age, occupation and ethnic origin.

Presenting complaint (PC)

Reason for presentation to the doctor (in patient's own words).

History of presenting complaint (HPC)

- System-specific questions related to PC.
- Risk factors for PC.
- Investigations and treatment to date.

Past medical, surgical and anaesthetic history

Thyroid dysfunction, hypertension, rheumatic fever, epilepsy, asthma, diabetes, stroke, myocardial infarction, jaundice (THREADS MIJ)

Medication, allergies and immunisations

Family history

First-degree relatives with relevant familial diseases

Social history

- Marital status.
- Occupation.
- Exposure to industrial toxins.
- Smoking habits (number of pack years).

- Alcohol intake (units/week).
- Recreational drug use.
- Living accommodation (i.e. house or flat, including access).
- Independence with regard to activities of daily living (ADL).
- Recent travel history.
- Household pets (if relevant).

Review of systems

Cardiovascular system

Chest pain, dyspnoea (shortness of breath, SOB), orthopnoea (SOB when lying flat), palpitations, dizziness, ankle swelling.

Respiratory system

Dyspnoea (SOB), exercise tolerance, paroxysmal nocturnal dyspnoea (SOB at night which disrupts sleep) (paroxysmal nocturnal dyspnoea), wheeze, chest pain, cough (productive or non-productive), haemoptysis (coughing up blood), hoarseness, fever.

Gastrointestinal system

Change in appetite, diet regime, weight loss (amount and duration), dysphagia (difficulty with swallowing), odynophagia (pain on swallowing), regurgitation of food/liquids, indigestion, nausea, vomiting, haematemesis (vomiting of blood), abdominal pain, abdominal distension, change in bowel habit (frequency, colour, size, specific gravity and/or odour of stools), PR bleeding, flatulence, jaundice.

Urogenital system

Abdominal pain, frequency of micturition, dysuria (pain on micturition), urgency, polyuria, colour of urine, haematuria (blood in the urine), nocturia, impotence, sensation of incomplete voiding.

Central and peripheral nervous system

Fits, faints or funny turns, headache, loss of consciousness, tremor, muscle weakness, paralysis, sensory disturbances, paraesthesiae (pins and needles), alteration in senses (smell, vision or hearing), change in behaviour or personality.

Musculoskeletal system

Muscle, bone or joint pain, deformity, swelling, stiffness, limb weakness, decreased range of movement, functional loss.

Metabolic system

Change in weight (BMI) and appetite, alteration of build and appearance.

Thank the patient. Turn to the examiner and present your history.

1 Chest pain

Introduction and consent

- Introduce yourself to the patient and establish a rapport.
- Be ready to be sympathetic, listen to the patient, and allow the history to flow uninterrupted.
- Explain to the patient that you are going to take their history.
- Sit opposite the patient in order to allow good eye contact.

Personal details

Confirm name, age, occupation and ethnic origin.

Presenting complaint (PC)

History of presenting complaint (HPC)

- Direct question related to the chest pain (**SOCRATES**)
  Site of pain
  Onset of pain
  Character
  Radiation
  Associations
  Timing and duration
  Exacerbating and relieving factors
  Severity
- Associated cardiovascular symptoms:
  - shortness of breath, (orthopnoea (ask how many pillows they use at night), paroxysmal nocturnal dyspnoea)
  - exercise tolerance (as how far they can walk before they get SOB)
  - palpitations
  - dizziness and syncopal episodes
  - ankle swelling.
- Risk factors for ischaemic heart disease:
  - hypertension
  - hypercholesterolaemia
  - diabetes
  - smoking
  - family history of diabetes, previous MI (before the age of 50 years)
- Questions related to the respiratory system:
  - cough – productive or non-productive

- – sputum – colour and consistency (e.g. mucoid, purulent, muco-purulent, bloodstained)
  - – haemoptysis.
  - – hoarseness.
  - – wheeze.
- Investigations to date (chest X-ray, ECG, exercise ECG, Echo, thallium scan or angiogram).
- Treatment to date: medical, interventional or surgical.

Past medical, surgical, radiological and anaesthetic history

- THREADS MIJ.
- Past history of cardiovascular and respiratory disease.

Medication and allergies

These include aspirin, statins, ACE inhibitors, β-blockers, etc.

Family history

First-degree relatives with a history of cardiovascular or respiratory disease.

Social history

- Marital status.
- Living accommodation.
- Occupational exposure.
- Smoking habits and alcohol intake.
- Use of recreational drugs (e.g. cocaine).
- Recent long-haul travel flights.

Review of systems (see history-taking model)

- Gastrointestinal system.
- Urogenital system.
- Central and peripheral nervous system.
- Musculoskeletal system.
- Metabolic system.

Thank the patient. Turn to the examiner and present your history.

Differential diagnosis of chest pain by anatomical location

- **Heart:** angina (ischaemic heart disease [IHD], left ventricular hypertrophy [LVH]/hypertrophic obstructive cardiomyopathy [HOCM]), acute myocardial infarction (MI), pericarditis, myocarditis, post-MI Dressler's syndrome.
- **Lungs/pleura:** pulmonary embolus (PE), pneumothorax, pleurisy, pneumonia.
- **Aorta:** dissection, aneurysm.
- **Gastrointestinal system:** oesophageal spasm, oesophagitis, gastritis, pancreatitis, cholecystitis, peptic ulcer disease.
- **Other:** shingles, costochondritis, rib/vertebral collapse.

Causes of sudden-onset central chest pain

Exacerbation of IHD, MI, oesophageal spasm, PE, dissecting aneurysm, pneumothorax, pneumonia, rib fracture.

2 Shortness of breath

Introduction and consent

- Introduce yourself to the patient and establish a rapport.
- Be ready to be sympathetic, listen to the patient, and allow the history to flow uninterrupted.
- Explain to the patient that you are going to take their history.
- Sit opposite the patient in order to allow good eye contact.

Personal details

Confirm name, age, occupation and ethnic origin.

Presenting complaint (PC)

History of presenting complaint (HPC)

- Onset of symptoms (acute or chronic), duration, progression, persistence (worsening or resolving) and variability (i.e. paroxysmal nocturnal dyspnoea, diurnal fluctuation or orthopnoea).
- Predisposing events.

- Aggravating and relieving factors.
- Functional assessment:
  - exercise tolerance: impact on ADL and lifestyle
  - what the patient's breathlessness prevents them from doing
  - whether washing or dressing causes breathlessness
  - whether breathlessness disrupts normal conversation
  - whether breathlessness occurs at rest
  - exercise tolerance: how far the patient can walk on the flat before stopping, and how many stairs they can climb before stopping
- Associated symptoms:
  - chest pain (i.e. pleuritic)
  - cough
  - sputum
  - haemoptysis
  - wheeze
  - hoarseness.
- Smoking history (past and present tobacco consumption).
- Systemic symptoms:
  - fever, rigors or night sweats
  - malaise
  - loss of appetite or weight loss (suggestive of malignancy).
- Investigations and treatment to date.

Past medical and surgical history surgical history

- Past history of atopy (hay fever, eczema and allergy) and cardiac or respiratory disease.
- THREADS MIJ.

Medication and allergies

These include:

- inhaled or nebulised bronchodilators
- steroids (inhaled or oral)
- oxygen therapy.

Family history

- First-degree relatives with a history of cardiovascular or respiratory disease.

- History of inherited disorders (e.g. α-1-antitrypsin deficiency, cystic fibrosis).

Social history

- Occupational exposure to dust, pollen, coal, asbestos and other chemicals, and animals.

Number of 'sick days' taken due to illness.

- Exposure to pets and other animals (e.g. pigeons).
- Alcohol consumption.
- Marital status.
- Living accommodation.
- Recent travel abroad (TB).
- Ethnic origin (if black, consider sarcoidosis).

Review of systems (see history-taking model)

- Gastrointestinal system.
- Urogenital system.
- Central and peripheral nervous system.
- Musculoskeletal system.
- Metabolic system.

Thank the patient. Turn to the examiner and present your history.

Differential diagnosis of shortness of breath

- **Cardiac disorders:** mitral stenosis, left ventricular failure (LVF).
- **Respiratory disorders:** asthma, chronic obstructive pulmonary disease (COPD), chronic bronchitis, emphysema, pulmonary fibrosis, extrinsic allergic alveolitis.
- **Anatomical disorders:** diseases of the chest wall, muscles or pleura (e.g. ankylosing spondylitis, respiratory muscle paralysis, kyphoscoliosis)
- **Other:** thyrotoxicosis, ketoacidosis, pharmacological disorders (e.g. aspirin poisoning), anaemia, psychological disorders (e.g. hyperventilation, anxiety, panic disorder), physiological disorders (e.g. due to exercise and/or high altitude).

Speed of onset

Acute	*Subacute*	*Chronic*
Foreign body	Asthma	COPD
Pneumothorax	Parenchymal disease (alveolitis)	Chronic parenchymal disease
Acute asthma	Pneumonia	Non-respiratory cause
Pulmonary embolus	(cardiac failure, anaemia)	
Acute pulmonary oedema		

3 Cough

Introduction and consent

- Introduce yourself to the patient and establish a rapport.
- Be ready to be sympathetic, listen to the patient, and allow the history to flow uninterrupted.
- Explain to the patient that you are going to take their history.
- Sit opposite the patient in order to allow good eye contact.

Personal details

Confirm name, age, occupation and ethnic origin.

Presenting complaint (PC)

History of presenting complaint (HPC)

- Onset of symptoms (acute or chronic).
- Nature of symptoms (continuous or episodic).
- Duration of symptoms.
- Character (wet, dry, bovine).
- Predisposing events.
- Precipitating events (e.g. emotion, exercise, infection).
- Persisting factors.
- Severity.
- Progression (worsening, constant or improving).
- Variability (diurnal).

- Aggravating and relieving factors.
- Exercise tolerance: impact on ADL and lifestyle.
- Associated symptoms:
  - pleuritic chest pain
  - SOB
  - PND
  - sputum production (quantity, colour, odour)
  - haemoptysis
  - wheeze
  - hoarseness.
- Systemic symptoms:
  - fever, rigors and night sweats
  - malaise
  - loss of appetite and weight loss.
- Investigations and treatment to date.

Past medical and surgical history surgical history

- History of allergic, cardiac or respiratory disease.
- History of congenital disease (e.g. cystic fibrosis, Kartagener's syndrome).

Medication and allergies

These include:

- bronchodilators
- steroids (inhaled or oral)
- ACE inhibitors, β-blockers and NSAIDs (these can precipitate a cough).

Family history

- First-degree relatives with a history of cardiovascular or respiratory disease.
- History of inherited disorders (i.e. α-1-antitrypsin deficiency, cystic fibrosis).

Social history

- Smoking history.
- Occupational exposure to dust, pollen, radiation or asbestos.

- Number of 'sick days' taken due to illness.
- Exposure to pets and other animals (e.g. pigeons).
- Alcohol consumption.
- Marital status.
- Living accommodation.
- Recent travel abroad (TB).

Review of systems (see history-taking model)

- Gastrointestinal system.
- Urogenital system.
- Central and peripheral nervous system.
- Musculoskeletal system.
- Metabolic system.

Thank the patient. Turn to the examiner and present your history.

Differential diagnosis of the common cough

Site	Cause
Pharynx	Post nasal drip
Larynx	Laryngitis, tumour, croup
Trachea	Tracheitis
Bronchi	Bronchitis, asthma, pneumonia, bronchiectasis, pulmonary oedema, interstitial fibrosis

---

4 Abdominal pain

Introduction and consent

- Introduce yourself to the patient and establish a rapport.
- Be ready to be sympathetic, listen to the patient, and allow the history to flow uninterrupted.
- Explain to the patient that you are going to take their history.
- Sit opposite the patient in order to allow good eye contact.

Personal details

Confirm name, age, occupation and ethnic origin.

Presenting complaint (PC)

History of presenting complaint (HPC)

- Abdominal pain: SOCRATES.
- Associated symptoms:
  - loss of appetite
  - change in diet
  - weight loss
  - nausea
  - vomiting (frequency, composition of vomitus, haematemesis)
  - abdominal distension
  - bowel habit (frequency, colour, size, specific gravity and odour)
  - rectal bleeding
  - flatulence
  - dysphagia and odynophagia
  - regurgitation
  - indigestion/dyspepsia
  - jaundice.
- Investigations and treatment to date.

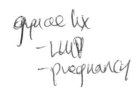

Past medical and surgical history surgical history

- THREADS MIJ.

Medication and allergies

These include current analgesia requirement.

Family history

First-degree relatives with a history of inheritable gastrointestinal disease.

Social history

- Occupation.
- Smoking history.
- Alcohol consumption.
- Marital status.
- Living accommodation.

Review of systems (see history-taking model)
- Cardiovascular system.
- Respiratory system.
- Urogenital system.
- Central and peripheral nervous system.
- Musculoskeletal system.
- Metabolic system.

Thank the patient. Turn to the examiner and present your history.

Differential diagnosis of abdominal pain

- **Right upper quadrant (RUQ):** cholecystitis, duodenal ulcer, hepatitis, congestive hepatomegaly, pyelonephritis, appendicitis, right-sided pneumonia.
- **Left upper quadrant (LUQ):** ruptured spleen, gastric ulcer, aortic aneurysm, perforated colon, pyelonephritis, left-sided pneumonia.
- **Right lower quadrant (RLQ):** appenditis, gynaecological causes (cyst, abscess, ectopic pregnancy), renal stone, hernia, mesenteric adenitis, Meckel's diverticulitis, inflammatory bowel disease (IBD), perforated bowel (caecum), psoas abscess.
- **Left lower quadrant (LLQ):** diverticulitis, gynaecological causes (cyst, abscess, ectopic pregnancy), renal stone, hernia, inflammatory bowel disease (IBD), perforated bowel (sigmoid).
- **Epigastrium:** myocardial infarct (MI), peptic ulcer, cholecystitis, perforated oesophagus.; pancreatitis

---

5 Weight loss

Introduction and consent
- Introduce yourself to the patient and establish a rapport.
- Be ready to be sympathetic, listen to the patient, and allow the history to flow uninterrupted.
- Explain to the patient that you are going to take their history.
- Sit opposite the patient in order to allow good eye contact.

Personal details

Confirm name, age, occupation and ethnic origin.

Presenting complaint (PC)

History of presenting complaint (HPC)

- How much weight loss
- How quickly weight loss has occurred.
- Fluid balance (intake/output).
- Onset (acute or chronic)
- Duration and persistence of weight loss.
- Predisposing events (e.g. increased activity, stress).
- Aggravating and relieving factors.
- Associated symptoms:
  - loss of appetite.
  - change in diet (e.g. change in calorie intake)
  - dysphagia, odynophagia
  - regurgitation, indigestion
  - nausea
  - vomiting and haematemesis
  - abdominal pain or distension
  - flatulence
  - change in bowel habit (frequency, colour, size, specific gravity and/or odour).
  - rectal bleeding
  - jaundice.
- Questions related to metabolic system:
  - alteration in build and appearance.
- Investigations and treatment to date.

Past medical and surgical history surgical history

THREADS MIJ.

Medication and allergies

These include:

- diuretics
- over-the-counter or prescription diet medication.

Family history

First-degree relatives with a history of inheritable gastrointestinal disease.

Social history

- Occupation.
- Smoking history.
- Alcohol intake or abuse.
- Exercise habits.
- Change in lifestyle (family, job, major life events).
- Psychological or social stresses.
- Marital status.
- Living accommodation.

Review of systems (see history-taking model)

- Cardiovascular system.
- Respiratory system.
- Urogenital system.
- Central and peripheral nervous system.
- Musculoskeletal system.
- Metabolic system.

Thank the patient. Turn to the examiner and present your history.

Differential diagnosis of weight loss

Cause	Symptoms
Anorexia nervosa, gastric cancer	Vomiting
Cardiac failure, bronchitis, lung cancer	Shortness of breath
Infections (HIV, TB)	Fever
Malabsorption syndromes, inflammatory bowel disease	Diarrhoea
Diabetes, Addison's disease	Polyuria

6 Dysphagia

Introduction and consent

- Introduce yourself to the patient and establish a rapport.
- Be ready to be sympathetic, listen to the patient, and allow the history to flow uninterrupted.
- Explain to the patient that you are going to take their history.
- Sit opposite the patient in order to allow good eye contact.

Personal details

Confirm name, age, occupation and ethnic origin.

Presenting complaint (PC)

History of presenting complaint (HPC)

- Time and onset of symptoms (sudden or gradual).
- Duration.
- Progression.
- Nature of symptoms (intermittent or constant).
- Variability.
- Predisposing events.
- Aggravating and relieving factors.
- Specific questions:
  - Is there difficulty swallowing liquids, solids or both?
  - Determine whether there is difficulty in initiating swallowing, or in swallowing itself.
  - Has the patient noticed a bulge in the neck or gurgling sounds on swallowing liquids?
  - Is there regurgitation of food?
  - Can the patient eat a complete meal? If not, at what level does the food stick (throat, neck or chest)?
  - Is swallowing painful (odynophagia), or is the patient pain free during swallowing and at rest?
- History of fever, chest infection or trauma.
- Associated gastrointestinal symptoms:
  - loss of appetite
  - weight loss
  - change in diet (e.g. change in calorie intake)
  - nausea

- vomiting and haematemesis
- abdominal pain or distension
- flatulence
- change in bowel habit (frequency, colour, size, specific gravity and/or odour).
- rectal bleeding
- jaundice.
- Investigations and treatment to date.

Past medical, interventional and surgical history

THREADS MIJ, including:

- anaemia (iron deficiency)
- neurological diseases (e.g. myasthenia gravis).

Medication and allergies

Family history

First-degree relatives with a history of inheritable gastrointestinal disease.

Social history

- Occupational exposure (e.g. to corrosive agents).
- Smoking history.
- Alcohol consumption.
- Dietary history (e.g. spicy food).
- Marital status.
- Living accommodation.

Review of systems (see history-taking model)

- Cardiovascular system.
- Respiratory system.
- Urogenital system.
- Central and peripheral nervous system.
- Musculoskeletal system.
- Metabolic system.

Thank the patient. Turn to the examiner and present your history.

Differential diagnosis of dysphagia

Mechanical block

- **Painful mouth or throat:** aphthous ulceration, tonsillitis, glandular fever.
- **Luminal obstruction:** peptic stricture, oesophageal web, pharyngeal cancer, oesophageal carcinoma, gastric cancer.
- **Extrinic pressure:** lung cancer, retrosternal goitre, mediastinal cancers.

Motility disorders

- **Neurological disorders:** pseudobulbar palsy, bulbar palsy, syringomyelia.
- **Neuromuscular disorders:** achalasia, myasthenia gravis.

Other

- Oesophagitis (infection, reflux oesophagitis).

7 Jaundice

Introduction and consent

- Introduce yourself to the patient and establish a rapport.
- Be ready to be sympathetic, listen to the patient, and allow the history to flow uninterrupted.
- Explain to the patient that you are going to take their history.
- Sit opposite the patient in order to allow good eye contact.

Personal details

Confirm name, age, occupation and ethnic origin.

Presenting complaint (PC)

History of presenting complaint (HPC)

- Onset of symptoms (gradual or sudden).
- Who noticed the changes (i.e. yellow skin, sclera or mucosal membranes).
- Duration of symptoms (acute or chronic).
- Progression (worsening, constant or improving).
- Predisposing events (e.g. increased activity, stress) or precipitating factors.

- Associated symptoms:
  - pruritus (itchiness)
  - dark urine
  - steatorrhoea (pale floating stools, often difficult to flush away)
  - fever and rigors
  - lethargy
  - bruising.
- Gastrointestinal symptoms:
  - loss of appetite
  - change in diet
  - weight loss (total amount and over how long)
  - nausea
  - vomiting (frequency and nature of vomitus, including haematemesis)
  - abdominal pain or distension
  - altered bowel habit (frequency, colour, size, specific gravity and/or odour)
  - rectal bleeding
  - flatulence
  - dysphagia or odynophagia
  - regurgitation of food
  - indigestion/dyspepsia.
- Investigations and treatment to date:
  - imaging (e.g. ultrasound, CT scanning)
  - upper GI endoscopy
  - ERCP/MRCP.

Past medical and surgical history surgical history

THREADS MIJ, including:

- previous jaundice or hepatitis
- autoimmune diseases (chronic active hepatitis)
- emphysema
- bleeding tendency (Budd–Chiari syndrome)
- previous blood transfusions.

Medication and allergies

These include:

- immunisations
- statins

- paracetamol overdose
- anti-TB medication
- sodium valproate
- MAO inhibitors
- halothane
- antibotics (flucloxacillin, co-amoxiclav, fusidic acid, nitrofurantoin)
- steroids
- oral contraceptive pill
- chlorpromazine
- sulphonylureas
- gold.

Family history

First-degree relatives with a history of inheritable gastrointestinal disease, including α-1-antitrypsin deficiency, haemochromatosis and Wilson's disease.

Social history

- Sexual and contact history.
- Travel history.
- Tattoos and piercing.
- Occupation (e.g. health workers).
- Recreational drug use.
- Alcohol consumption.
- Smoking history.
- Marital status.
- Living accommodation.

Review of systems (see history-taking model)

- Cardiovascular system.
- Respiratory system.
- Urogenital system.
- Central and peripheral nervous system.
- Musculoskeletal system.
- Metabolic system.

Thank the patient. Turn to the examiner and present your history.

Differential diagnosis of jaundice

- Pre-hepatic jaundice: haemolysis, ineffective erythropoiesis, Crigler–Najjar syndrome, Gilbert syndrome.
- Hepatocellular jaundice: viruses (hepatitis A, B, C and E, Epstein–Barr virus), chemical (alcohol) leptospirosis, autoimmune diseases, chronic hepatitis, rare syndromes (Rotor syndrome, Dubin–Johnson syndrome, Wilson's disease), cirrhosis.
- Post-obstructive jaundice:
  - intrahepatic – primary biliary cirrhosis, primary sclerosing cholangitis, cholangiocarcinoma, sepsis, hepatocellular disease
  - extrahepatic – gallstones, bile duct, head of pancreas or periampullary carcinoma, benign stricture of common bile duct, enlarged porta hepatis (lymphoma).

8 Constipation

Introduction and consent

- Introduce yourself to the patient and establish a rapport.
- Be ready to be sympathetic, listen to the patient, and allow the history to flow uninterrupted.
- Explain to the patient that you are going to take their history.
- Sit opposite the patient in order to allow good eye contact.

Personal details

Confirm name, age, occupation and ethnic origin.

Presenting complaint (PC)

History of presenting complaint (HPC)

- Time and onset of symptoms.
- Duration (acute or chronic).
- Progression (improving or worsening).
- Aggravating and relieving factors.
- Frequency of bowel opening.
- Colour of stool, including associated blood, mucus or pus.

- Consistency of stool (soft, watery, unformed or semi-solid).
- Quantity of stool (large or small volume).
- Flatulence.
- Tenesmus.
- Straining during defecation.
- Urgency or faecal incontinence.
- Abdominal, rectal or anal pain.
- Abdominal distension, lumps or masses.
- Associated gastrointestinal symptoms:
  - dysphagia or odynophagia
  - regurgitation of liquids or solids
  - indigestion or dyspepsia
  - haematemesis
  - jaundice.
- Associated systemic symptoms:
  - thirst
  - weight loss
  - loss of appetite
  - nausea or vomiting.
- Investigations and treatment to date.

Past medical and surgical history

THREADS MIJ, including:

- history of gastrointestinal and neurological diseases and surgery
- childhood diseases, such as Hirschsprung's disease.

Medication and allergies

These include:

- over-the-counter and prescription medication
- opiate analgesia
- iron tablets
- anticholinergics (tricyclic antidepressants).

Family history

First-degree relatives with a history of inheritable gastrointestinal disease.

Social history

- Occupation.
- Smoking history.
- Alcohol consumption.
- Exercise (e.g. immobility).
- Dietary habits (e.g. low fluid, solid or fibre intake).
- Living accommodation.
- Marital status.

Review of systems (see history-taking model)

- Cardiovascular system.
- Respiratory system.
- Urogenital system.
- Central and peripheral nervous system.
- Musculoskeletal system.
- Metabolic system.
- Dermatological system.

Thank the patient. Turn to the examiner and present your history.

Differential diagnosis of constipation

- **Organic:** bowel obstruction, paralytic ileus, colorectal cancer, diverticular disease.
- **Painful anal conditions:** fissure in ano, prolapsed piles.
- **Adynamic bowel:** Hirschsprung's disease, senility, spinal cord injury and disease, myxoedema, Parkinson's disease.
- **Drugs:** aspirin, opiates, analgesics, anticholinergics, ganglion blockers.
- **Habit and diet:** dyschezia, dehydration, starvation, lack of dietary bulk.

---

9 Diarrhoea

Introduction and consent

- Introduce yourself to the patient and establish a rapport.
- Be ready to be sympathetic, listen to the patient, and allow the history to flow uninterrupted.

- Explain to the patient that you are going to take their history.
- Sit opposite the patient in order to allow good eye contact.

Personal details

Confirm name, age, occupation and ethnic origin.

Presenting complaint (PC)

History of presenting complaint (HPC)

- Time and onset of symptoms.
- Duration (acute or chronic).
- Progression (improving or worsening).
- Aggravating and relieving factors.
- Frequency of bowel opening.
- Colour of stool, including associated blood, mucus or pus.
- Consistency of stool (soft, watery, unformed or semi-solid).
- Quantity of stool (large or small volume).
- Flatulence.
- Tenesmus.
- Straining during defecation.
- Urgency or faecal incontinence.
- Abdominal, rectal or anal pain.
- Abdominal distension, lumps or masses.
- Associated gastrointestinal symptoms:
  - dysphagia or odynophagia
  - regurgitation of liquids or solids
  - indigestion or dyspepsia
  - haematemesis
  - jaundice.
- Associated systemic symptoms:
  - thirst
  - weight loss
  - loss of appetite
  - nausea or vomiting.
- Investigations and treatment to date.

Past medical and surgical history

THREADS MIJ, including:

- previous history of gastrointestinal diseases, surgery or radiotherapy.

Medication and allergies

These include:

- over-the-counter and prescription medication
- laxatives
- antibiotics
- cimetidine
- propranolol
- cytotoxics
- digoxin.

Family history

First-degree relatives with a history of inheritable gastrointestinal disorders, including:

- gluten enteropathy (coeliac disease)
- inflammatory bowel disease (Crohn's disease and ulcerative colitis)
- colorectal cancers, familial adenomatous polyposis (FAP), hereditary non-polyposis colorectal cancer (HNPCC).

Social history

- Occupation.
- Smoking history.
- Alcohol consumption.
- Recreational drug use.
- Dietary habits.
- Travel and contact history with individuals with diarrhoea.
- Sexual history.
- Living accommodation.
- Marital status.

Review of systems (see history-taking model)

- Cardiovascular system.
- Respiratory system.
- Urogenital system.
- Central and peripheral nervous system.
- Musculoskeletal system.
- Metabolic system.

Thank the patient. Turn to the examiner and present your history.

Differential diagnosis of diarrhoea

- **Intestinal disorders:** enteritis, inflammatory bowel disease (IBD), tumour, faecal impaction, topical spruce.
- **Gastric disorders:** gastrocolic fistula, Post gastrectomy or vagotomy.
- **Pancreatic disorders:** pancreatitis, tumour.
- **Pelvic disorders:** fluid collection, abscess.
- **Drugs:** digoxin, antibiotics, laxatives.
- **Endocrine disorders:** uraemia, thyrotoxicosis, thyroid cancer (medullary), hypothyroidism, carcinoid syndrome, Zollinger–Ellison syndrome.

10 Haematemesis

Introduction and consent

- Introduce yourself to the patient and establish a rapport.
- Be ready to be sympathetic, listen to the patient, and allow the history to flow uninterrupted.
- Explain to the patient that you are going to take their history.
- Sit opposite the patient in order to allow good eye contact.

Personal details

Confirm name, age, occupation and ethnic origin.

Presenting complaint (PC)

History of presenting complaint (HPC)

- Onset of symptoms (sudden or gradual).
- Duration (acute or chronic).
- Progression (worsening or improving).
- Nature of symptoms (intermittent or constant).
- Preceding events (e.g. violent retching).
- Predisposing events (e.g. trauma).
- Aggravating factors (e.g. NSAID use, alcohol) and relieving factors.

- Colour and volume of vomitus (e.g. coffee grounds or frank blood).
- Colour and volume of stools (e.g. melaena (black tarry stools) or fresh per rectal blood).
- Associated symptoms:
  - fainting
  - fever
  - weight loss and loss of appetite.
- Gastrointestinal symptoms:
  - loss of appetite
  - change in diet
  - weight loss
  - nausea
  - vomiting
  - abdominal pain and distension
  - dysphagia
  - flatulence
  - indigestion and dyspepsia
  - jaundice.
- Factors associated with high risk (Rockall scoring system) include:
  - age < 60 years
  - melaena
  - hypotension
  - severe bleed, and re-bleed during same admission
  - concurrent anticoagulation treatment
  - coexisting cardiac, respiratory or renal failure
  - known oesophageal varices or cirrhosis.
- Investigations and treatment to date.

Past medical, endoscopic and surgical history

THREADS MIJ, including history of:

- haematemesis
- melaena
- peptic ulcer
- jaundice
- haematological disorders
- liver disease.

Medication and allergies

These include:

- analgesics
- anticoagulation
- non-steroidal anti-inflammatory drugs (NSAIDs).

Family history

First-degree relatives with a history of inheritable gastrointestinal disorders.

Social history

- Occupational exposure (e.g. to corrosive substances).
- Smoking history.
- Alcohol consumption.
- Marital status.
- Living accommodation.

Review of systems (see history-taking model)

- Cardiovascular system.
- Respiratory system.
- Urogenital system.
- Central and peripheral nervous system.
- Musculoskeletal system.
- Metabolic system.

Thank the patient. Turn to the examiner and present your history.

Differential diagnosis of haematemesis

General causes

- Haemophilia.
- Leukaemia.
- Thrombocytopenia.
- Hereditary haemorrhagic telangiectasia.
- Medication (NSAIDS, steroids, thrombolytic agents, anticoagulants).

Local causes by anatomical site

- Oesophagus: peptic oesophagitis, oesophageal varices.
- Stomach: gastritis, gastric ulcer, erosions, Mallory–Weiss syndrome, tumours (benign and malignant).
- Duodenum: duodenal ulcer, erosions.
- Small intestine: tumours, Meckel's diverticulum.
- Large bowel: tumours, angiodysplasia, diverticulitis, angiodysplasia, colitis (ulcerative, ischaemic, infective or radiation induced).

11 Per rectal bleeding

Introduction and consent

- Introduce yourself to the patient and establish a rapport.
- Be ready to be sympathetic, listen to the patient, and allow the history to flow uninterrupted.
- Explain to the patient that you are going to take their history.
- Sit opposite the patient in order to allow good eye contact.

Personal details

Confirm name, age, occupation and ethnic origin.

Presenting complaint (PC)

History of presenting complaint (HPC)

- Onset of symptoms (sudden or gradual).
- Duration of symptoms (acute or chronic).
- Nature of symptoms (constant or episodic).
- Progression (worsening, constant or improving).
- Predisposing events (e.g. history of trauma).
- Aggravating and relieving factors.
- Colour of blood (black tarry stool (melaena), bright red or dark blood).
- Quantity of blood.
- Relationship of blood to stool:
  - mixed with stool

- – on the surface
- – after passing stool (seen on toilet paper or dripping into the pan).
- Bowel habit:
  - – frequency of motion
  - – consistency of stool (hard, soft or watery)
  - – size (bulky, pellet or string-like)
  - – specific gravity (floats or sinks)
  - – malodorous mucus or pus
  - – urgency, incontinence or tenesmus.
- Gastrointestinal symptoms:
  - – abdominal pain (beginning before, during or after defecation, or unrelated to defecation)
  - – masses, lumps or abdominal distension
  - – dysphagia or odynophagia
  - – regurgitation of fluids or solids
  - – indigestion and dyspepsia
  - – haematemesis
  - – jaundice
  - – diet (e.g. beetroot).
- Associated symptoms:
  - – dizziness
  - – shortness of breath
  - – rashes
  - – fever, rigors and night sweats
  - – weight loss
  - – loss of appetite
  - – nausea or vomiting.
- Investigations and treatment to date.

Past medical and surgical history

THREADS MIJ, including:

- history of anaemia
- previous blood transfusions
- history of colorectal cancers, inflammatory bowel disease (ulcerative colitis, Crohn's disease), infective colitis, diverticular disease or anal fissures.

Medication and allergies

These include:

- anticoagulants (aspirin, warfarin)
- over-the-counter and prescription medication.

Family history

First-degree relatives with a history of inheritable gastrointestinal disorders, including:

- colorectal cancers
- familial adenomatous polyposis (FAP)
- hereditary non-polyposis colorectal cancer (HNPCC).

Social history

- Occupational exposure to industrial hazards (e.g. asbestos, dyes, rubber, paint).
- Smoking history.
- Alcohol consumption.
- Geographical location (climate).
- Living accommodation.
- Sexual history.

Review of systems (see history-taking model)

- Cardiovascular system.
- Respiratory system.
- Urogenital system.
- Central and peripheral nervous system.
- Musculoskeletal system.
- Metabolic system.

Thank the patient. Turn to the examiner and present your history.

Differential diagnosis of per rectal bleeding

General causes

- Bleeding diatheses.
- Medication (NSAIDS, steroids, thrombolytic agents, antico-agulants).

Local causes

- Haemorrhoids.
- Fissure in ano.
- Tumours of colon and rectum (benign and malignant).
- Diverticulitis.
- Colitis (inflammatory, infective, radiation induced).
- Trauma.
- Angiodysplasia.

---

12 Per vaginal bleeding

Introduction and consent

- Introduce yourself to the patient and establish a rapport.
- Be ready to be sympathetic, listen to the patient, and allow the history to flow uninterrupted.
- Explain to the patient that you are going to take their history.
- Sit opposite the patient in order to allow good eye contact.

Personal details

Confirm name, age, occupation and ethnic origin.

Presenting complaint (PC)

History of presenting complaint (HPC)

- Onset (sudden or gradual).
- Duration (acute or chronic).
- Amount of bleeding and timing (e.g. intermenstrual, post-coital).
- Quantity of blood (include clots).
- Progression (worsening, constant or improving).
- Nature (continuous or gradual).

- Predisposing events.
- Aggravating and relieving factors.
- Symptoms associated with hypotension:
  - fits, faints or funny turns
  - headache
  - loss of consciousness
  - muscle weakness, paralysis, sensory disturbances, paraesthesiae
  - changes in senses (smell, vision or hearing)
  - changes in behaviour or personality.
- Symptoms associated with blood loss:
  - anaemia
  - fatigue
  - dyspnoea
  - palpations.
- Symptoms associated with infection:
  - fever and rigors
  - pelvic pain
  - diarrhoea (pelvic collection).
- Symptoms associated with malignancy:
  - weight loss and loss of appetite.
- Investigations and treatment to date.

Gynaecological history

- Menstruation:
  - date of last menstrual period (LMP).
  - if the patient is post-menopausal, age of menopause
  - post-menopausal bleeding (PMB)
  - regular/irregular periods (dysmenorrhoea)
  - frequency and duration of menses
  - heavy (menorrhagia) or light menses (estimated by number of pads or tampons used, or number of clots)
  - associated pain
  - history of premenstrual tension (PMT).
- Intermenstrual bleeding (IMB).
- Post-coital bleeding (PCB).
- Vaginal discharge, including nature of discharge (clear, white, purulent, bloodstained).
- Sexual history, including contraception:
  - sexual activity
  - single or multiple sexual partners

  – dyspareunia – painful intercourse (superficial or deep)
  – contraception used currently and previously.
- Cervical smear history:
  – last smear
  – results of previous smear tests
  – abnormal smears and treatment.

Genito-urinary history

- Urinary frequency,
- Nocturia (waking at night to micturate).
- Urgency.
- Enuresis.
- Incontinence (stress or urge incontinence).
- Dysuria (discomfort when passing urine).
- Haematuria.
- Vaginal prolapse.

Obstetric history

- Number of pregnancies.
- Dates in chronological order.
- Mode of delivery.
- Complications in pregnancy and labour.

Past medical and surgical history

THREADS MIJ, including:

- previous gynaecological operations
- major illness
- blood transfusions and hospital admissions for current problem
- thyroid disease
- haematological disorders.

Medication and allergies

These include:

- anticoagulants
- hormone therapy (e.g. HRT).

Family history

First-degree relatives with a history of breast, ovarian or endometrial cancer.

Social history

- Smoking history.
- Alcohol consumption.
- Marital status.
- Occupation.
- Living accommodation.
- Independence with regard to activities of daily living.

Review of systems (see history-taking model)

- Cardiovascular system.
- Respiratory system.
- Urogenital system.
- Central and peripheral nervous system.
- Musculoskeletal system.
- Metabolic system.

Thank the patient. Turn to the examiner and present your history.

Differential diagnosis of per vaginal bleeding

- **General causes:** thyroid disease, coagulopathy, anticoagulation.
- **Local causes:** fibroids, polyps, adenomyosis, endometriosis, infection, tumours (ovarian, endometrial and cervical).
- **Dysfunctional uterine bleeding:** no anatomical or systemic cause is found.

---

13 Haematuria

Introduction and consent

- Introduce yourself to the patient and establish a rapport.
- Be ready to be sympathetic, listen to the patient, and allow the history to flow uninterrupted.

- Explain to the patient that you are going to take their history.
- Sit opposite the patient in order to allow good eye contact.

Personal details

Confirm name, age, occupation and ethnic origin.

Presenting complaint (PC)

History of presenting complaint (HPC)

- Microscopic or macroscopic.
- When first noticed (e.g. incidental finding on dipstick).
- Onset of symptoms (sudden or resolving).
- Duration (acute or chronic).
- Progression (worsening, constant or improving).
- Predisposing events (e.g. trauma).
- Aggravating and relieving factors.
- Painless, or associated with loin, abdominal or urethral pain.
- Haematuria at the start, throughout or at the end of the urinary stream.
- Associated masses or lumps.
- Irritative urogenital symptoms:
  - frequency
  - dysuria
  - nocturia
  - urgency
  - incontinence
  - suprapubic pain.
- Obstructive or lower urinary tract symptoms (LUTS):
  - hesitancy (problems initiating the stream)
  - reduced flow pressure
  - terminal dribbling
  - intermittent flow
  - sensation of incomplete emptying.
- Pneumaturia (air in the urine).
- Faecaluria (faeces in the urine).
- Associated gastrointestinal symptoms:
  - change in appetite
  - diet (e.g. beetroot)
  - weight loss
  - dysphagia or odynophagia

- regurgitation of liquids or solids
- indigestion or dyspepsia
- nausea, vomiting and haematemesis
- abdominal distension and flatulence
- change in bowel habits (frequency, colour, size, specific gravity and/or odour)
- rectal bleeding
- jaundice.
- Associated systemic symptoms:
  - shortness of breath
  - fever, night sweats and weight loss
  - loss of appetite.
- Investigations and treatment to date.

Past medical and surgical history

THREADS MIJ, including:

- congenital disorders (e.g. polycystic kidney or horseshoe kidney, von Hippel–Lindau disease)
- haematological disorders (e.g. bleeding diathesis and sickle-cell disease).

Medication and allergies

These include:

- anticoagulants (e.g. aspirin, warfarin)
- all over-the-counter or prescription medication.

Family history

First-degree relatives with a history of urological cancers.

Social history

- Occupational exposure to industrial hazards (e.g. asbestos, dyes such as aniline (which cause bladder cancers), rubber, paint).
- Smoking history.
- Alcohol consumption.
- Geographical location (climate) (e.g. schistosomiasis and bladder stone formation).
- Living accommodation.
- Sexual activity.

Review of systems (see history-taking model)

- Cardiovascular system.
- Respiratory system.
- Central and peripheral nervous system.
- Musculoskeletal system.
- Metabolic system.

Thank the patient. Turn to the examiner and present your history.

Differential diagnosis of haematuria

- **Renal tract disorders:** UTI, trauma (e.g. due to catheter, surgery), calculi, prostatic disease, tumours, bladder inflammation (e.g. due to infection, recent surgery, chemotherapy).
- **Parenchymal disease:** acute glomerulonephritis, cystic disease, tumour, analgesic nephropathy, TB.
- **Extra-renal disorders:** bleeding diathesis, vasculitis (systemic lupus erythematosus), malignant hypertension, emboli, sickle-cell disease.

---

14 Headache

Introduction and consent

- Introduce yourself to the patient and establish a rapport.
- Be ready to be sympathetic, listen to the patient, and allow the history to flow uninterrupted.
- Explain to the patient that you are going to take their history.
- Sit opposite the patient in order to allow good eye contact.

Personal details

Confirm name, age, occupation and hand dominance.

Presenting complaint (PC)

- Pain: SOCRATES.
- History of trauma (e.g. road traffic accident, falls).

- Neurological symptoms:
  - nausea and vomiting
  - fits, faints or funny turns
  - loss of consciousness
  - tremor
  - muscle weakness, paralysis
  - sensory disturbances, paraesthesiae
  - changes in senses of smell, vision (blurring, spots, flashing lights) or hearing
  - changes in behaviour or personality.
- Associated symptoms:
  - fever, photophobia, neck stiffness and rash
  - weight loss and loss of appetite.
- Investigations and treatment to date.

Past medical and surgical history

THREADS MIJ.

Medication and allergies

These include:

- corticosteroids
- antibiotics (tetracycline)
- hormonal supplementation (oral contraceptive pill)
- anticoagulation.

Family history

First-degree relatives with a history of malignancy.

Social history

- Occupation.
- Smoking history.
- Alcohol consumption.
- Change in lifestyle (family, job, major life events).
- Psychological or social stresses.
- Diet (calorie intake).
- Marital status.

- Living accommodation.
- Lifestyle (stress, lack of sleep).

Review of systems (see history-taking model)

- Cardiovascular system.
- Respiratory system.
- Gastrointestinal system.
- Urogenital system.
- Peripheral nervous system.
- Musculoskeletal system.
- Metabolic system.

Thank the patient. Turn to the examiner and present your history.

Differential diagnosis of headache

- Intracranial disorders: migraine, infections (including meningitis), tumour, stroke, haemorrhage, hydrocephalus.
- Extracranial disorders: arthritis (e.g. neck, temporomandibular joint), cervical spondylosis, glaucoma, dental sepsis, ear and sinus infections, temporal arteritis.

---

15 Expressive dysphasia

Introduction and consent

- Introduce yourself to the patient and establish a rapport.
- Be ready to be sympathetic, listen to the patient, and allow the history to flow uninterrupted.
- Explain to the patient that you are going to take their history.
- Sit opposite the patient in order to allow good eye contact.

Personal details

Confirm name, age, occupation and hand dominance.

Presenting complaint (PC)

History of presenting complaint (HPC)

- Onset of symptoms (sudden or gradual).
- Duration (acute or chronic).
- Progression (deteriorating or improving).
- Frequency (continuous or episodic).
- Predisposing events.
- Aggravating and relieving factors.
- Specific questions:
  - speech – assess fluency, grammar and content
  - comprehension – ask the patient to follow a three-step command (e.g. 'Take the paper in your right hand, fold it in half and put it on the floor')
  - repetition – ask the patient to repeat a sentence
  - writing skills (these may also be impaired).
- Associated symptoms:
  - fits, faints or funny turns
  - headache
  - loss of consciousness
  - tremor
  - muscle weakness, paralysis
  - sensory disturbances, paraesthesiae
  - changes in senses (smell, vision or hearing)
  - changes in behaviour or personality.
- Investigations and treatment to date.

Past medical and surgical history

THREADS MIJ, including:

- CNS abnormalities
- previous strokes and transient ischaemic attack
- history of atrial fibrillation, hypertension, hyperlipidaemia or diabetes.

Medication and allergies

These include:

- anticoagulation (aspirin, warfarin)
- anti-hypertension medication
- over-the-counter or prescription medication.

Family history

First-degree relatives with a history of malignancy and vascular disease.

Social history

- Occupation.
- Smoking history.
- Alcohol consumption.
- Living accommodation (type, level, modification, home help, aids).
- Marital status.
- Support (family, friends).

Review of systems (see history-taking model)

- Cardiovascular system.
- Respiratory system.
- Gastrointestinal system.
- Urogenital system.
- Musculoskeletal system.
- Metabolic system.

Thank the patient. Turn to the examiner and present your history.

Differential diagnosis of dysphasia

- **Broca's (expressive) dysphasia:** Broca's area is the area of the cerebral motor cortex that is responsible for the initiation of speech. Expressive dysphagia results in a reduction in the number of words used, non-fluent speech, and errors in grammar and syntax.
- **Wernicke's (receptive) dysphasia:** this results in fluent speech with abnormal content, incorrect words, incorrect letters and nonsense words.
- **Conductive dysphasia:** this results in the inability of the patient to repeat phrases or words.
- **Global dysphasia:** this results in both Broca's and Wernicke's dysphasias.

16 Fits, faints and funny turns

Introduction and consent

- Introduce yourself to the patient and establish a rapport.
- Be ready to be sympathetic, listen to the patient, and allow the history to flow uninterrupted.
- Explain to the patient that you are going to take their history.
- Sit opposite the patient in order to allow good eye contact.

Personal details

Confirm name, age, occupation and hand dominance.

Presenting complaint (PC)

History of presenting complaint (HPC)

- Onset of symptoms (sudden or gradual).
- Duration (acute or chronic).
- Progression (deteriorating or improving).
- Frequency (continuous or episodic).
- Predisposing events.
- Aggravating and relieving factors.

Specific questions

Fits

- What happens during the fit?
  - Lack of movement.
  - Jerking.
  - Tongue biting.
  - Urinary incontinence.
  - Eyewitness account.
- What happens before the fit?
  - Warning (aura).
- What happens after the fit?
  - Drowsiness or sleeping (post-ictal)
  - Changes in senses (smell, vision and hearing).
  - Motor and sensory weakness in limbs.
  - Change in mental state.

Falls (faints and funny turns)

- Factors influencing accidental fall:
  - recall of events, tripping or slipping
  - walking surface
  - footwear
  - lighting and visual acuity.
- Factors affecting spontaneous fall:
  - preceding events (e.g. sitting or standing up)
  - associated symptoms (e.g. vertigo, deafness, tinnitus, associated chest pain, shortness of breath, palpations)
  - awareness of hitting the ground
  - eyewitness account
  - resulting injuries
  - incontinence
  - recall of events (retrograde and anterograde amnesia)
  - ability to regain original position
  - history of dementia, confusion or parkinsonism
  - history of hypertension, blackouts or epilepsy
  - medication (e.g. antidepressants).
- Other neurological symptoms:
  - headache
  - loss of consciousness
  - tremor
  - muscle weakness, paralysis
  - sensory disturbances, paraesthesiae
  - changes in senses (smell, vision or hearing).
- Investigations and treatment to date.

Past medical and surgical history

THREADS MIJ, including CNS, cardiac or musculoskeletal disorders.

Medication and allergies

These include:

- medication linked to postural hypertension
- sedation
- over-the-counter or prescription medication.

Family history

First-degree relatives with a history of neurological diseases (e.g. Huntington's disease).

Social history

- Occupation.
- Smoking history.
- Alcohol consumption.
- Marital status.
- Living accommodation.
- Ability to perform activities of daily living.

Review of systems (see history-taking model)

- Cardiovascular system.
- Respiratory system.
- Gastrointestinal system.
- Urogenital system.
- Metabolic system.

Thank the patient. Turn to the examiner and present your history.

Differential diagnosis of fits, faints and funny turns

Fits

- Physical causes: trauma, space-occupying lesions, stroke, hypertension, tuberous sclerosis, systemic lupus erythematosus, PAN, sarcoid and vascular malformations.
- Metabolic disorders: alcohol intoxication and withdrawal, hypoglycaemia, hyperglycaemia, hypoxia, uraemia, hyponatraemia, hypernatraemia, hypocalcaemia, liver disease.
- Drugs: phenothiazines, tricyclic antidepressants, cocaine, withdrawal of benzodiazepines.
- Infections: encephalitis, syphilis, HIV.

Falls (faints and funny turns)

- Vasovagal syncope.
- Situational syncope: postural, cough, effort, micturition, carotid sinus.

- Cardiac syncope :
  - arrhythmias: bradyarrhythmias (Stokes–Adams attacks), tachyarrhythmias
  - Outflow obstruction: aortic, pulmonary, mitral stenosis, hypertrophic cardiomyopathy, atrial myxoma, constrictive pericarditis.
- Epilepsy.
- Vertebrobasilar arterial insufficiency.
- Carotid sinus hypersensitivity.
- Transient ischaemic attack/stroke.
- Hypoglycaemia.
- Orthostatic hypotension.
- Drop attacks.
- Anxiety.
- Ménière's disease.
- Choking.

17 Leg weakness

Introduction and consent

- Introduce yourself to the patient and establish a rapport.
- Be ready to be sympathetic, listen to the patient, and allow the history to flow uninterrupted.
- Explain to the patient that you are going to take their history
- Sit opposite the patient in order to allow good eye contact.

Personal details

Confirm name, age, occupation and hand dominance.

Presenting complaint (PC)

History of presenting complaint (HPC)

- Onset of symptoms (sudden or gradual).
- Duration (acute or chronic).
- Progression (deteriorating or improving).
- Frequency (continuous or episodic).
- Aggravating and relieving factors.
- Pain (e.g. in the back and legs): SOCRATES.
- Predisposing events (e.g. trauma, tumour, stroke, infection).

- Sensory disruption (determine sensory level).
- Sphincter control (bowel and bladder).
- Weakness (partial or total paralysis).
- Paralysis (note whether flaccid or spastic).
- Associated symptoms:
  - pain in muscle, bone or joint
  - deformity
  - swelling
  - stiffness
  - loss of movement
  - loss of function (impact on daily activities, walking distance).
- Investigations and treatment to date.

Past medical and surgical history

THREADS MIJ, including:

- tumours – primary or secondary (breast, lung, prostate)
- infections
- neurological disease
- skeletal deformities
- disc prolapses
- recent surgery (haematoma) and epidural/spinal anaesthesia
- recent radiotherapy in patient with malignancy.

Medication and allergies

These include:

- analgesia
- anticoagulation.

Family history

First-degree relatives with a history of neurological or skeletal diseases (Duchenne's muscular dystrophy).

Social history

- Smoking history.
- Alcohol consumption.

- Marital status.
- Living accommodation (type, modifications and allowances).
- Walking aids (e.g. stick, chair).

Review of systems (see history-taking model)

- Cardiovascular system.
- Respiratory system.
- Gastrointestinal system.
- Urogenital system.
- Metabolic system.

Thank the patient. Turn to the examiner and present your history.

Differential diagnosis of leg weakness

- **Acute spinal cord compression:** secondary malignancy (breast, lung, prostate), infection, disc prolapse, haematoma, intrinsic cord tumour, subluxation.
- **Chronic spastic paresis:** MS, cord compression, syringomyelia, motor neuron disease, subacute degeneration of the cord, syphilis.
- **Chronic flaccid paresis:** tabes dorsalis, peripheral neuropathies, myopathies.
- **Unilateral foot drop:** diabetes mellitus, stroke, prolapsed disc, MS, common peroneal nerve palsy.

---

18 Loss of vision

Introduction and consent

- Introduce yourself to the patient and establish a rapport.
- Be ready to be sympathetic, listen to the patient, and allow the history to flow uninterrupted.
- Explain to the patient that you are going to take their history.
- Sit opposite the patient in order to allow good eye contact.

Personal details

Confirm name, age, occupation and hand dominance.

Presenting complaint (PC)

History of presenting complaint (HPC)

- Onset of symptoms (sudden or gradual).
- Duration (acute or chronic).
- Progression (deteriorating or improving).
- Frequency (continuous or episodic).
- Aggravating and relieving factors.
- Predisposing events (e.g. trauma, tumour, stroke, infection).
- Pain (e.g. sensation of foreign body in the eye, deep severe pain, eye strain, headache).
- Disturbance of vision:
  - blurred vision
  - loss of vision
  - double vision
  - photopia
  - presence of haloes and floaters.
- Investigations and treatment to date.

Past medical and surgical history

THREADS MIJ, including:

- diabetes
- cancer
- stroke.

Medication and allergies

Family history

First-degree relatives with a history of:

- malignancy
- neurological disease
- vascular disease.

Social history

- Smoking history.
- Alcohol consumption.
- Marital status.
- Living accommodation.

- Visual aids (e.g. guide dog, Braille).
- Occupation.

Review of systems (see history-taking model)

- Cardiovascular system.
- Respiratory system.
- Gastrointestinal system.
- Urogenital system.
- Metabolic system.

Thank the patient. Turn to the examiner and present your history.

Differential diagnosis of loss of vision

Sudden loss of vision

- Amaurosis fugax.
- Temporal arteries.
- Retinal artery occlusion.
- Optic neuritis.
- Vitreous haemorrhage.

Gradual loss of vision

- Old age.
- Choroiditis.
- Malignant melanoma.
- Macular degeneration.

---

19 Fever (pyrexia of unknown origin)

Introduction and consent

- Introduce yourself to the patient and establish a rapport.
- Be ready to be sympathetic, listen to the patient, and allow the history to flow uninterrupted.
- Explain to the patient that you are going to take their history.
- Sit opposite the patient in order to allow good eye contact.

Personal details

Confirm name, age, occupation and ethnic origin.

Presenting complaint (PC)

History of presenting complaint (HPC)

- Onset of symptoms (sudden or gradual).
- Duration (acute or chronic).
- Progression (deteriorating or improving).
- Frequency (continuous or episodic).
- Aggravating and relieving factors.
- Predisposing events (e.g. trauma, tumour, infection).
- History of rashes or lumps.
- Systemic systems:
  - sweats/rigors
  - weight loss
  - headache
  - diarrhoea, nausea or vomiting
  - pruritus.
- Investigations and treatment to date.

Past medical and surgical history

THREADS MIJ, including:

- sexual history
- immunosuppressive illnesses.

Medication and allergies

These include antibiotics.

Immunisation history

Family history

First-degree relatives with a history of haematological disease.

Social history

- Smoking history.
- Alcohol consumption.

- History of intravenous drug use.
- Marital status.
- Living accommodation.
- Foreign travel.
- Animal contact or bites (e.g. dogs, cats or other pets, and birds).

Review of systems (see history-taking model)

- Cardiovascular system.
- Respiratory system.
- Gastrointestinal system.
- Urogenital system.
- Central and peripheral nervous system.
- Musculoskeletal system.
- Metabolic system.

Thank the patient. Turn to the examiner and present your history.

Differential diagnosis of pyrexia of unknown origin

- **Infection:** abscess, TB, granulomata, parasites, bacteria, rheumatic fever, fungi, viruses (including HIV).
- **Multisystem diseases:** connective tissue diseases, systemic lupus erythematosus, polyarteritis nodosa, sarcoidosis, cranial arteritis, polymyalgia rheumatica, rheumatoid arthritis, Still's disease, inflammatory bowel disease.
- **Tumours:** lymphomas, solid tumours (gastrointestinal and renal).
- **Drug fever.**

---

20 Swollen legs

Introduction and consent

- Introduce yourself to the patient and establish a rapport.
- Be ready to be sympathetic, listen to the patient, and allow the history to flow uninterrupted.
- Explain to the patient that you are going to take their history.
- Sit opposite the patient in order to allow good eye contact.

Personal details

Confirm name, age and occupation.

Presenting complaint (PC)

History of presenting complaint (HPC)

- Onset of symptoms (sudden or gradual).
- Duration (acute or chronic).
- Progression (deteriorating or improving).
- Frequency (continuous or episodic).
- Aggravating and relieving factors.
- Unilateral/bilateral.
- History of trauma.
- Painful/pain free.
- Oedema (pitting).
- Skin changes.
- Mobility (affecting daily activities and quality of life).
- Exclude the possibility of pregnancy in females.
- Exclude other underlying pathologies.
- Investigations and treatment to date.

Past medical and surgical history

THREADS MIJ, including history of:

- malignancy (including pelvic malignancy)
- pregnancy
- radiation
- venous disease
- lymphoedema.

Medication and allergies

These include:

- analgesics
- antibiotics
- anticoagulation therapy.

Family history

First-degree relatives with a history of malignancy.

Social history

- Smoking history.
- Alcohol consumption.
- Marital status.
- Living accommodation.
- Social assistance (direct nursing).
- Walking aids (e.g. stick, wheelchair).

Review of systems (see history-taking model)

- Cardiovascular system.
- Respiratory system.
- Gastrointestinal system.
- Urogenital system.
- Central and peripheral nervous system.
- Metabolic system.

Thank the patient. Turn to the examiner and present your history.

Differential diagnosis of swollen legs

- **Central causes:** right heart failure, hypoalbinaemia, nephritic syndrome, hypothyroidism.
- **Peripheral causes:** lymphoedema, venous disease (deep vein thrombosis, Klippel–Trenaunay syndrome, chronic venous insufficiency, post-phlebitic limb).
- **Rare causes:** angiooedema, arteriovenous malformations.

---

21 Leg ulcers

Introduction and consent

- Introduce yourself to the patient and establish a rapport.
- Be ready to be sympathetic, listen to the patient, and allow the history to flow uninterrupted.

- Explain to the patient that you are going to take their history.
- Sit opposite the patient in order to allow good eye contact.

Personal details

Confirm name, age and occupation.

Presenting complaint (PC)

History of presenting complaint (HPC)

- When did you first notice it?
- What made you notice it?
- Predisposing events (e.g. trauma).
- Symptoms (e.g. pain, discharge, swelling of surrounding tissue or limb, increased temperature).
- Has it changed?
- Has it ever healed completely?
- Are there any other ulcers?
- Dressing care (frequency, individual responsible for wound care).
- Investigations and treatment to date (including hospital admissions).

Past medical and surgical history

In addition to THREADS MIJ, look for underlying disease:

- venous ulcers associated with varicose veins or deep vein thrombosis
- arterial ulcers associated with atheroma, Beurger's disease, rheumatoid arthritis or polyarteritis nodosa
- elicit risk factors for peripheral vascular disease
- traumatic/neuropathic ulcers associated with alcohol, diabetes, syphilis, bedsores or self-harm
- infective ulcers associated with pyogenic infections, syphilis or TB
- neoplastic ulcers associated with squamous-cell carcinoma (Marjolin's ulcer), basal-cell carcinoma or malignant melanoma.

Medication and allergies

These include requirements for analgesia.

Family history

First-degree relatives with a history of vascular disease.

Social history

- Smoking history.
- Alcohol consumption.
- Marital status.
- Living accommodation.
- Impact on activities of daily living.

Review of systems (see history-taking model)

- Cardiovascular system.
- Respiratory system.
- Gastrointestinal system.
- Urogenital system.
- Central and peripheral nervous system.
- Musculoskeletal system.
- Metabolic system.

Thank the patient. Turn to the examiner and present your history.

Differential diagnosis of leg ulcers

- Venous ulcers.
- Ischaemic (arterial) ulcers.
- Malignancy.
- Infective diabetic ulcers.
- Deliberate self-harm.
- Gummatous ulcers.
- Vasculitis.
- Pyoderma gangrenosum.

---

22 Swollen knee

Introduction and consent

- Introduce yourself to the patient and establish a rapport.

- Be ready to be sympathetic, listen to the patient, and allow the history to flow uninterrupted.
- Explain to the patient that you are going to take their history.
- Sit opposite the patient in order to allow good eye contact.

Personal details

Confirm name, age, occupation and ethnic origin.

Presenting complaint (PC)

History of presenting complaint (HPC)

- Onset of symptoms (sudden or gradual).
- Precipitating factors (e.g. trauma), including their relationship to the onset of symptoms.
- Duration (acute or chronic).
- Progression (deteriorating or improving).
- Frequency (continuous or episodic).
- Aggravating and relieving factors (e.g. walking up or down stairs).
- Associated symptoms:
  - fever
  - pain
  - deformity
  - joint stiffness
  - loss of function or reduced range of movement
  - restriction of activities of daily living.
- Does the knee lock or give way (suggestive of meniscal damage)?
- Investigations and treatment to date.

Past medical and surgical history

THREADS MIJ, including history of:

- trauma and fractures
- infection
- haematological conditions (sickle-cell disease, haemophilia)
- cancer
- previous orthopaedic surgery (arthroscopy, total knee replacement).

Medication and allergies

These include:

- analgesia requirement

- antibiotics
- anticoagulation (may cause haemarthrosis).

Family history

First-degree relatives with a history of malignancy or haematological disease (e.g. haemophilia or sickle-cell anaemia).

Social history

- Smoking history.
- Alcohol consumption.
- Marital status.
- Occupation (e.g. builder, athlete).
- Living accommodation (number of stairs).
- Hobbies (sports).

Review of systems (see history-taking model)

- Cardiovascular system.
- Respiratory system.
- Gastrointestinal system.
- Urogenital system.
- Central and peripheral nervous system.
- Metabolic system.

Thank the patient. Turn to the examiner and present your history.

Differential diagnosis of swollen knees

Knee swelling occurs as a result of the accumulation of fluid (synovial fluid, blood or pus) within the joint cavity.

- Arthritis: osteoarthritis, rheumatoid arthritis, gout, septic arthritis.
- Meniscal cysts.
- Trauma: bone fractures, soft tissue injury, ligamental tears, meniscus lesions, patellar dislocation, loose bodies.
- Osteochondritis dissecans.
- Bursitis.
- Infection.
- Tumours.

23 Rash

Introduction and consent

- Introduce yourself to the patient and establish a rapport.
- Be ready to be sympathetic, listen to the patient, and allow the history to flow uninterrupted.
- Explain to the patient that you are going to take their history.
- Sit opposite the patient in order to allow good eye contact.

Personal details

Confirm name, age, occupation and ethnic origin.

Presenting complaint (PC)

History of presenting complaint (HPC)

- Onset of symptoms (sudden or gradual).
- Precipitating factors:
  - exposure to allergens
  - recent change in diet or medication.
- Appearance of rash and location:
  - blanching or non-blanching
  - raised or flat
  - colour
  - size and shape.
- Duration (acute or chronic).
- Progression (deteriorating or improving) as well as areas of spread.
- Frequency (persistent or episodic).
- Aggravating and relieving factors.
- Associated symptoms:
  - itchiness
  - increased temperature
  - arthralgia.
- Previous similar episodes and their cause.
- Exposure to unwell patients.
- Recent travel.
- Investigations and treatment to date.

Past medical and surgical history

THREADS MIJ, including history of:

- atopy
- asthma
- skin diseases (eczema, psoriasis).

Medication and allergies

These include:

- systemic and topical steroids
- inhalers
- antibotics
- opiate analgesia.

Note all allergies (e.g. nickel, copper, latex).

Family history

First-degree relatives with a history of atopy and skin diseases.

Social history

- Smoking history.
- Alcohol consumption.
- Marital status.
- Occupation and exposure to industrial insults.
- Living accommodation.
- Household pets (cats, dogs, birds, etc.).
- Recent travel (if relevant).

Review of systems (see history-taking model)

- Cardiovascular system.
- Respiratory system.
- Gastrointestinal system.
- Urogenital system.
- Central and peripheral nervous system.
- Musculoskeletal system.
- Metabolic system.

Thank the patient. Turn to the examiner and present your history.

Skin lesions can represent systemic diseases.

Skin lesion	Association	Direct questioning
Erythema nodosum	Sarcoid, drugs, TB, streptococci	Shortness of breath, cough, sputum, drugs
Pyogenic gangrenosum	Ulcerative colitis, Crohn's disease, autoimmune hepatitis, myeloma	Change in bowel habit, joint pain
Dermatitis herpetiformis	Coeliac disease	Change in bowel habit, family history, anaemia
Erythema multiforme	Herpes simplex, viruses, mycoplasma, drugs	Fever, drugs, recent contact, travel

24 Taking a gynaecological history

Introduction and consent

- Introduce yourself to the patient and establish a rapport.
- Be ready to be sympathetic, listen to the patient, and allow the history to flow uninterrupted.
- Explain to the patient that you are going to take their history.
- Sit opposite the patient in order to allow good eye contact.

Personal details

Confirm name, age and occupation.

Presenting complaint (PC)

History of presenting complaint (HPC)

- Onset of symptoms (sudden or gradual).
- Duration (acute or chronic).
- Progression over time (deteriorating or improving).
- Aggravating and relieving factors.
- How do these impact on your life and activities of daily living?
- Investigations and treatment to date.

Gynaecological history

- Menstruation:
  - date of last menstrual period (LMP)

- if the patient is post-menopausal, age of menopause
- post-menopausal bleeding (PMB)
- regular/irregular menstrual periods (dysmenorrhoea)
- frequency and duration of menses
- heavy (menorrhagia) or light menses (estimated by number of pads or tampons used, or number of clots)
- associated pain
- history of premenstrual tension (PMT).
- Intermenstrual bleeding (IMB).
- Post-coital bleeding (PCB).
- Vaginal discharge, including nature of discharge (clear, white, purulent, bloodstained).
- Sexual history, including contraception:
  - sexual activity
  - single or multiple sexual partners
  - dyspareunia – painful intercourse (superficial or deep)
  - contraception used curently and previously
  - history of infertility, including IVF or miscarriages.
- Cervical smear history:
  - last smear
  - results of previous smear tests
  - abnormal smears and treatment.

Genito-urinary history

- Urinary frequency,
- Nocturia (waking at night to micturate).
- Urgency .
- Enuresis.
- Incontinence (stress or urge incontinence).
- Dysuria (discomfort when passing urine).
- Haematuria.
- Vaginal prolapse.

Obstetric history

- Number of pregnancies (including miscarriages or abortions).
- Dates in chronological order.
- Mode of delivery.
- Complications in pregnancy and labour.

Past medical and surgical history

THREADS MIJ, including:

- previous gynaecological operations
- major illness and hospital admissions.

Medication and allergies

These include:

- hormone replacement therapy (HRT)
- contraception (e.g. oral contraceptive pill, depot, Mirena coil).

Family history

First-degree relatives with a history of malignancy (breast, ovarian or endometrial cancer).

Social history

- Smoking history.
- Alcohol consumption.
- Marital status.
- Occupation.
- Living accommodation.

Review of systems (see history-taking model)

- Cardiovascular system.
- Respiratory system.
- Gastrointestinal system.
- Central and peripheral nervous system.
- Musculoskeletal system.
- Metabolic system.

Thank the patient. Turn to the examiner and present your history.

25 Taking a paediatric history

Introduction and consent

- Introduce yourself to the patient and establish a rapport.
- Be ready to be sympathetic, listen to the patient, and allow the history to flow uninterrupted.
- Explain to the patient that you are going to take their history.
- Sit opposite the patient in order to allow good eye contact.

Personal details

Confirm name, age and weight.

Presenting complaint (PC)

- Onset of symptoms (sudden or gradual).
  - When and how did it start?
  - Was the child well beforehand?
- Precipitating factors.
  - Has the child been exposed to unwell individuals (e.g. siblings)?
- Duration (acute or chronic).
- Progression (deteriorating or improving).
- Frequency (continuous or episodic).
- Aggravating and relieving factors (e.g. walking up or down stairs).
- Associated symptoms:
  - loss of appetite
  - growth consistent with age
  - alertness and activity level.
- Investigations and treatment to date.

Past medical and surgical history

THREADS MIJ, including complications:

- during pregnancy (e.g. oligohydramnios)
- at birth:
  - prematurity
  - prolonged labour
  - type of delivery (i.e. vaginal, assisted or Caesarian section)
  - birth weight (over- or underweight)

- as a neonate and in early childhood:
  - jaundice
  - convulsions
  - fevers
  - bleeding
  - feeding problems
  - failure to meet developmental milestones.

Growth and development

Has the child met their growth and developmental milestones? *(see* Topic 47)

Medication and allergies

These include:

- drug intolerances
- adverse drug reactions
- allergies (e.g. to food, pets, etc.).

Immunisations

At birth, 2 months, 3 months, 4 months, 1 year, 3–5 years, 10–14 years, 15–18 years and boosters.

Family history

First-degree relatives with a history of inherited disease (e.g. cystic fibrosis).

Social history

- Activities and behaviour (playing, eating, sleeping).
- Schooling and learning difficulties.
- Living accommodation (location, type, and with whom).

Review of systems (see history-taking model)

- Cardiovascular system.
- Respiratory system.
- Gastrointestinal system.

- Urogenital system.
- Central and peripheral nervous system.
- Musculoskeletal system.
- Metabolic system.
- Ear, nose and throat.

Thank the patient. Turn to the examiner and present your history.

Key topics commonly arising from the paediatric history

Jaundice

Neonatal jaundice can be classified as

- Hyperbilirubinaemia (after the first day of life) and may be physiological
- Jaundice (within 24 hours) is pathological
  - Causes to consider: Resus haemolytic disease, ABO incompatibility; Red Cell anomalies
  - Investigations: FBC, film, blood group, Coomb's test, septic screen, urinalysis
- Prolonged jaundice (not resolved by the 7–10 days)
  - Causes to consider: Hypothyroidism, Biliary atresia, Galactosaemia
  - Investigations: Thyroid function, conjugated/unconjugated bilirubin, urinalysis, galactose-1-phosphate levels
- Kernicterus (brain damage secondary haemolytic disease of the newborn) 4 stages (I: sleepy, reduced suck, lethargy; II: pyrexia, restless, abnormal movements, lid retraction; III: latent phase; IV: results in cerebral palsy, hearing impairments, learning difficulties.

Short stature

This occurs when the child's height falls below the 3rd centile on growth charts. Causes to consider are as follows.

- Physiological causes: short stature in parents.
- Pathological causes.
- Congenital causes: Turner's syndrome, cystic fibrosis.
- Chronic disease.
- Endocrine causes: hypopituitarism (thyroid and growth hormone).
- Drugs: steroids.
- Environment: poor diet and abuse.

Painful hip

When a child complains of a painful hip, examine the hip clinically and radiologically. It is important to have a low threshold for admission and investigation. Treatment includes bed rest and analgesia. Ultrasound examination of the affected joint may be helpful.

Causes according to age

Age	Condition
At birth (0 years)	Congenital dislocation of the hip (CDH)
Childhood (0–5 years)	Irritable hip
Childhood (5–10 years)	Perthes' disease
Adolescence (10–15 years)	Slipped upper femoral epiphysis

- **Congenital dislocation of the hip:** one or both hips are dislocated at birth or in the first few weeks of life. There is a higher incidence in girls and in breech presentations. There is also a familial tendency. CDH is diagnosed during the examination of the neonate (*see* Topic 46). The stability of the hips is assessed by the Ortolani and Barlow tests. Ultrasound is the investigation of choice.
- **Irritable hip:** conditions that are commonly responsible include transient synovitis, acute pyogenic arthritis (due to *Staphylococcus*), Perthes' disease and tuberculosis.
- **Perthes' disease:** There is impairment of the blood supply to the epiphysis of the femoral head, resulting in avascular necrosis. There is a higher incidence in boys.
- **Slipped upper femoral epiphysis:** This condition commonly occurs in adolescence, and is more common in boys. The attachment of the femoral epiphysis loosens, giving rise to a coxa vara deformity. It has been linked to trauma and hormonal imbalance in adolescence. Investigations should include radiographs.

26 Psychiatric assessment

There are five key sections to this assessment:

- history taking
- Mental State Examination
- physical examination
- assessment of risk
- management plan.

History taking

Introduction and consent

- Introduce yourself to the patient and establish a rapport.
- Be ready to be sympathetic, listen to the patient, and allow the history to flow uninterrupted.
- Explain to the patient that you are going to take their history.
- Sit opposite the patient in order to allow good eye contact.
- Ensure that you are safe (e.g. a chaperone may be required).

Personal details

Confirm name, age and occupation.

Presenting complaint (PC)

History of presenting complaint (HPC)

- Onset of symptoms (sudden or gradual).
- Duration (acute or chronic).
- Progression over time (deteriorating or improving).
- Precipitating factors (e.g. life events).
- How do these impact on your life, family and activities of daily living?
- Associated symptoms:
  - suicidal thoughts, plans or actions
  - depression
  - mania
  - psychosis (beliefs, delusions, hallucinations)
  - recreational drug use.
- Risk factors for this HPC in neonates:
  - genetic factors
  - prenatal insults
  - birth trauma.
- Risk factors for this HPC in childhood:
  - delayed development
  - behavioural problems
  - poor peer relationships
  - parental neglect
  - physical and emotional abuse
  - sexual abuse.
- Precipitating factors (e.g. unemployment, divorce, relocation, death).

- Maintaining factors (e.g. poverty, illness, disability, bullying).
- Investigations and treatment to date (including physician responsible for managing mental health).

Past psychiatric history (plus past medical and surgical history)

- Date, duration and nature of all previous episodes.
- Admission to hospital (either voluntary or involuntary under the Mental Health Act).

Medication and allergies

- Type and dose of all medications.
- Duration of treatment.
- Complications.

Family history

First-degree relatives with a history of psychiatric disorders (e.g. depression, schizophrenia).

Personal history

- Gestation and delivery.
- Childhood milestones.
- Family relationships and upbringing.
- Peer relationships.
- Schooling and academic achievements.
- Occupational history.
- Marital and sexual history.

Premorbid personality

- Premorbid character (e.g. criminal behaviour).
- Habits (alcohol, smoking and illicit drugs).
- Interests.

Social circumstances

- Accommodation (type, sharing, living alone).
- Marital status.
- Finances and occupation.

- Social network (friends and family).
- Support structure (social worker, community nurses).

Mental State Examination

This assesses the state of mind of the patient at the time of assessment.

Appearance and behaviour

- Look for signs of self-neglect (unkempt appearance) and inappropriate dress.
- Look at facial expression, posture and movements.
- Document cooperation with the assessment.

Speech

- Rate and volume.

Affect (objective and subjective)

- Emotional state (depression, elation, anxiety or anger).
- Objective (based on appearance, behaviour and speech).
- Subjective (ask the patient how they are feeling).

Thoughts

Note the way that the patient speaks (form) and what they tell you (content).

- Formal thought disorder is characterised by abnormalities of rhythm and flow of thought.
- Delusions are false beliefs that are firmly held by the patient, even in the face of clear evidence that they are not true.
- Obsessional thoughts are repetitive and intrusive thoughts.

Perceptions

- Illusions are distorted perceptions in which a real external object is perceived inaccurately.

- Hallucinations are perceptions that occur in the absence of an external object. They may be auditory, visual, olfactory, gustatory or tactile.

Cognitive state/Mental Status Examination (FOLSTEIN)

Maximum score	Task
5	What time is it? (year, season, month, day and date)
5	Where are we? (state, county, town, hospital, floor)
3	Name three objects. Ask patient to repeat all three. Repeat the names of the three objects until the patient learns them.
5	Serial sevens from 100 to 5 (answers 93, 86, 79, 72, 65), or spell the word 'world' backwards.
3	Ask for the names of the three above-mentioned objects.
2	Point to a pencil and a watch and ask the patient to name them.
1	Ask the patient to repeat the following: 'No ifs, ands or buts.'
3	Ask the patient to follow this three-step command: 'Take the paper in your right hand, fold it in half, and put it on the floor.'
1	Ask the patient to read and obey the following command: 'Close your eyes.'
1	Ask the patient to write a sentence.
1	Ask the patient to copy a design.

Assess the patient's level of consciousness along the following continuum: Alert – Drowsy – Stupor – Coma.

The final score is the sum of 11 evaluations. The possible score ranges from 0 (worst) to 30 (best). A good score is > 20.

Insight

How aware is the patient of their own mental state and need for treatment?

Physical examination

Assessment of risk

- Classify level of risk as low, medium or high.
- High-risk group includes:
  - suicide
  - deliberate self-harm
  - aggressive behaviour
  - neglect and self-neglect.

Factors associated with suicide

- Male
- Old age (>75 years)
- Previous attempts
- Mental illness
- Social isolation
- Divorced, single or widowed
- Bereavement
- Living in city
- Physical illness (chronic, painful and life-threatening illness)
- Unemployment

- The main factor is the patient's safety to him- or herself and others.

Management plan

Diagnosis

- Functional mental illness.
- Organic mental illness.
- Personality disorder.
- Medical disorder.

Treatment (immediate, early and long term)

- **Address:** medical, psychological and social treatment.
- **Settings:** inpatient, outpatient, day hospital.

- **Key players:** community mental health teams, multi-disciplinary team (MDT) consisting of psychiatrists, psychiatric nurses, community psychiatric nurses (CPNs), clinical psychologists, occupational therapists, social workers, psychotherapists, psychoanalysts and counsellors.

Thank the patient. Turn to the examiner and present your history.

Examination

27 Examining the cardiovascular system

Introduction and consent

- Introduce yourself to the patient and ask permission to examine them.
- Ensure that you are in a quiet and private area.
- Position: sit the patient at 45°.
- Expose the chest.

Inspection

- General: shortness of breath, peripheral cyanosis, pallor, scars, ankle oedema.
- Hands: look for clubbing and sphincter haemorrhages.
- Pulses:
  - rate and rhythm
  - test for collapsing pulse
  - radio-radial delay
  - radio-femoral delay
  - brachial pulses.
- Blood pressure.
- Face:
  - skin (malar flush)
  - eye (pale conjunctiva)
  - mouth (central cyanosis).
- Neck:
  - jugular venous pressure (JVP) and hepatojugular reflex (liver pressure)
  - carotid pulses (rate, rhythm and character, and auscultate over carotid area for bruits).
- Precordium:
  - inspection for scars and pulsations

- palpation – apex beat (left fourth intercostal space, mid-clavicular line), left sternal angle, manubrium. Assess for heaves and thrills.
- Auscultation:
  - mitral area (left fourth intercostal space – roll patient to left side)
  - tricuspid area (left fifth intercostal space – ask patient to breathe out)
  - aortic area (right second intercostal space – patient is now sitting up)
  - pulmonary area (left second intercostal space – keep patient sitting up).
- Back of chest:
  - lung bases
  - sacral oedema.
- Ankle oedema.

Complete examination

- Examine the rest of the vascular tree.
- ECG.
- Echocardiography.
- Chest X-ray.

Cover and thank the patient.

Turn to the examiner and summarise your findings.

28 Examining the respiratory system

Introduction and consent

- Introduce yourself to the patient and ask permission to examine them.
- Ensure that you are in a quiet and private area.
- Position: sit the patient up.
- Expose the chest.

Inspection

- General: well, thin, ill looking.
- At rest: comfortable or short of breath.
- Using accessory muscles of respiration.

- Colour: good, pale or cyanotic.
- Surrounding environment: look for antibiotic drip, peak flow meter, oxygen and/or nebulisers.

Hands and arms

- Nails: clubbing, nicotine stains, cyanosis.
- Palms: pallor in palmar creases.
- Skin: thin due to steroid use.
- Systemic diseases: rheumatoid arthritis (fibrosing alveolitis).
- Arms straight out: tremor (salbutamol), CO_2 retention flap.

Pulse

Rate, rhythm and character.

Respiration

Respiratory rate: count over 1 minute.

Face

- Eyes: pale conjunctiva.
- Tongue: central cyanosis.

Neck

- Jugular venous pressure (cor pulmonale).
- Trachea central.
- Assess the lymph nodes for lymphadenopathy.

Chest

- Inspect with patient's arms on hips. Ask them to take two deep breaths.
- Look for scars, radiation burns, abnormal shape or deformity.
- Does the chest move normally and symmetrically with respiration?
- Is the patient using all of the accessory muscles?
- Can you hear an audible wheeze or stridor?
- Palpation:
  - expansion: ask the patient to take a deep breath in and out (below and above level of nipples)

  - percussion: normal, dull, hyper-resonant, stony or dull
  - tactile fremitus: ask the patient to say '99.'
- Auscultation:
  - breath sounds: ask the patient to breathe in and out through their mouth (vesicular, bronchial, absent, crepitations, crackles); start at clavicles and move downward, including the axilla
  - vocal fremitus: ask the patient to say '99.'
- Back of chest:
  - expansion
  - percussion
  - tactile fremitus
  - auscultation of breath sounds and vocal fremitus.
- Sacral oedema.

Complete examination

- Ankle oedema.
- Peak flow.
- Observation chart (temperature, pulse, respiratory rate, blood pressure, saturations).
- Sputum analysis.
- Arterial blood gas (ABG).
- Chest X-ray.

Cover and thank the patient.

Turn to the examiner and summarise your findings.

29 Examining the gastrointestinal system

Introduction and consent

- Introduce yourself to the patient and ask permission to examine them.
- Ensure that you are in a quiet and private area.
- Position: ask the patient to lie flat with their arms by their sides.
- Expose the patient from the nipples to the knees (it is best to cover the external genitalia in the first instance).
- Stand at the end of the bed.
- Ask the patient to cough and to lift their head from the bed – hernia and divarication of recti can be easily seen.

Inspection:

- General appearance: well or unwell (cachexic).
- State of patient: comfortable or in pain.
- Colour: good, pale or jaundiced.
- Surrounding environment: look for IV fluid lines and/or sickness bowl.

Hands and arms

- Nails: clubbing, leukonychia (hypoalbinaemia, chronic liver disease), koilonychias (iron-deficiency anaemia).
- Palms: Dupuytren's contracture, palmar erythema, pale palmar creases.
- Skin: turgor (dehydration), jaundice, scratch marks, purpura (impaired clotting), tattoos (hepatitis).
- Arms straight out: liver flap.

Pulse

Rate and rhythm (tachycardia or atrial fibrillation).

Face

- Conjunctiva: pale (anaemia).
- Sclera: yellow (jaundice).
- Mouth: angular stomatitis (iron-deficiency anaemia), telangiectasia (CREST, Osler–Weber–Rendu syndrome).
- Inside of mouth (use a pen torch): ulcers and Peutz–Jeghers spots.
- Teeth: state of dentition.
- Tongue: smooth red beef tongue (vitamin B_{12} deficiency), blue (cyanosis).
- Mucous membrane: pale (anaemia).
- Smell: hepatic foetor.

Neck

Palpate Virchow's node (left supraclavicular node), also known as Troisier's sign.

Chest

Spider naevi (in SVC distribution), gynaecomastia, scratch marks, axillary hair loss (microgonadism).

Abdomen

Inspection

Distension, swelling, visible peristalsis and pulsations (abdominal aneurysm), distended abdominal veins and scars.

Palpation for masses and organomegaly

Kneel down at the side of the bed and ask the patient whether they have pain in their abdomen. Start with non-tender areas first, and be systematic.

- Superficial (nine quadrants) palpation.
- Deep palpation.
- Organomegaly:
  - AAA (epigastric area above umbilicus)
  - liver (breathe in and out, starting in right iliac fossa)
  - spleen (breathe in and out, starting in right iliac fossa)
  - kidney (ballot).
- Rebound tenderness.
- Shifting dullness (ascites).

Percussion

- Liver (right nipple down to RIF).
- Spleen (left nipple down to LIF).
- Bladder.
- Kidney (both flanks).

Auscultation

- Bowel sounds.
- Aortic renal and liver bruits.

Complete examination

- Examine the groin and external genitalia.

- Rectal examination.
- Assess for peripheral oedema.
- Review the observation chart (temperature, respiratory rate, pulse and blood pressure).
- Urine dipstick and MC&S.

Cover and thank the patient.

Turn to the examiner and summarise your findings.

30 Examining the groin and external genitalia

Introduction and consent

- Introduce yourself to the patient and ask permission to examine them.
- Ensure that you are in a quiet and private area.
- Position: ask the patient to stand if possible.
- Expose the focus area with the patient's pants removed.
- It is best to have a chaperone present.

Inspection

- Look for surgical scars and swelling in both sides of the groin and scrotum.
- Identify the pubic tubercle (PT). Inguinal hernias bulge above and lateral to this landmark. Femoral hernias bulge below and medial to it.
- Ask the patient to cough.
- Does the swelling extend into the scrotum?

Palpation

- With one hand on the pubic tubercle, ask the patient to cough. This helps to discriminate between inguinal and femoral hernias.
- Then identify the anterior superior iliac spine (ASIS) and the pubic tubercle (PT). The line connecting these two points is the inguinal ligament. The point halfway point these two points is the deep ring. Ask the patient whether they can reduce the swelling. If they can, then you can identify the deep ring and apply direct pressure over this point. Once the hernia is reduced and controlled at the deep ring, ask the patient to cough again. If the swelling is controlled at the deep ring, this is the site of the indirect inguinal hernia.

- Next move to the scrotum. There are three questions you must answer (**SAT**).
  - Can you feel the testicle **S**eparately?
  - Can you get **A**bove it? If you can, it is a scrotal swelling. If not, it could be an inguinal scrotal hernia.
  - Does it **T**ransilluminate?
- Move to the side of the patient and examine the lump:
  - position
  - colour
  - texture of overlying skin
  - temperature
  - tenderness
  - shape
  - size
  - surface
  - edge
  - composition
  - consistency
  - compressibility
  - fluctuation
  - fluid thrill
  - translucency
  - resonance
  - pulsatility
  - bruits
  - reducibility
  - relationship to surrounding structures (nerves and vessels)
  - state of the regional lymph nodes.

Auscultation

Check for bowel sounds.

Complete examination

- Examine both groins and external genitalia (including the scrotum, cord and testis).
- Complete an abdominal examination (*see* Topic 29).
- Rectal examination.

Cover and thank the patient.

Turn to the examiner and summarise your findings.

31 Examining the peripheral vascular system (upper and lower limb)

Introduction and consent

- Introduce yourself to the patient and ask permission to examine them.
- Ensure that you are in a quiet and private area.
- Position: ask the patient to sit down for the upper limb examination and to lie down for the lower limb examination.
- Expose the focus area.

Inspection

- At rest: look for obvious signs of cardiovascular disease (e.g. shortness of breath, increased BMI, cyanosis).
- Surgical scars.
- Surrounding environment: look for GTN spray and/or oxygen.

Upper limb

Hands

- Nails: clubbing, nicotine stains, cyanosis, vascular lesions, sphincter haemorrhages.
- Palms: pallor in palmar creases.
- Temperature.
- Capillary refill time: normal value is less than 2 seconds.

Radial pulses

- Look at both sides for synchrony (radial–radial), and radial femoral pulse.
- Rate and rhythm.
- Test for collapsing pulse (raise arm up).

Allen's test

Ask the patient to make a fist. Now occlude both radial and ulnar arteries. Then ask the patient to open the palm, which should be white. Release the pressure on the ulnar artery, and the hand should re-perfuse. Repeat the test (i.e. make a fist, occlude both arteries, open the palm, and then release the radial artery). This test is important for demonstrating collateral circulation.

Brachial pulses

Blood pressure (bilateral)

Axillary artery

Neck

- Feel for a cervical rib.
- Carotid pulses: rate, rhythm and character, and auscultate over carotid area.

Lower limb

Legs

- Colour (white or red), guttering of veins, trophic changes (loss of hair, shiny skin), ulceration.
- Look between the toes, under the heel, malleoli, head of fifth metatarsal, tips of toes and between toes, and ball of the foot) for skin breakdown or ulcers.
- Temperature.
- Capillary refill time: normal value is less than 2 seconds.
- Start by examining the pulses (with palpation and auscultation if appropriate):
  - examination of the aorta (including auscultation) (above the level of the umbilicus)
  - examination of the femoral pulses (including auscultation)
  - examination of the popliteal pulses (best in the extended and flexed position)
  - examination of the posterior tibial and dorsalis pulses.

Buerger's test

Support the patient's heel. Note the angle at which the leg blanches in relation to the bed (Buerger's angle). Note that 50° indicates severe ischaemia, and 25° indicates critical ischaemia. Now sit the patient up and swing the leg over the side of the bed. If the leg becomes engorged and purple, Buerger's test is positive.

Complete examination

- Examine the cardiovascular system.
- Complete a neurological examination of the upper and lower limb.
- Arterial duplex.
- Ankle brachial pressure index (ABPI).
- Angiogram.

Cover and thank the patient.

Turn to the examiner and summarise your findings.

32 Examining the venous system (varicose veins)

Introduction and consent

- Introduce yourself to the patient and ask permission to examine them.
- Ensure that you are in a quiet and private area.
- Position: request the patient to stand, and ask if it would be possible for them to stand on a platform or step.
- Expose the groin and leg.

Inspection (front and back of the legs)

- Look for surgical scars in the groin and leg.
- Look for visible dilated or tortuous veins, venous stars, loss of hair, shiny skin, and venous insufficiency in the gaiter area, above the medial malleolus: oedema, haemosiderin deposits, lipodermatosclerosis, eczema, ulceration.

Palpation

- Ask the patient whether they have any pain.
- Assess the temperature (use the back of your hand).
- Palpate the veins.
- Palpate for pitting oedema.
- Next identify the saphenofemoral junction (SFJ) in the groin (just medial to the femoral pulse). Now test for a cough impulse. While your index finger is over the junction, ask the patient to cough.
- Perform a tap test over the SFJ and over the varicose veins.

There are three tests with which you should be familiar.

Tourniquet and Perthes test

Tourniquet test: Lie the patient down, lift their leg to your shoulder, empty the veins, apply a tourniquet around their upper leg and then ask them to stand up. If the veins do not fill, the varicosities are controlled at the SFJ. If the veins fill, the point of incompetence is lower down the leg, and you will need to repeat this test with the tourniquet applied lower down the affected leg.

Perthes test: The tourniquet should still be on. Ask the patient to stand on the tips of their toes. If the veins enlarge or the patient experiences pain, the deep veins are also involved.

Trendelenburg's test

This test is similar to the tourniquet test. After the vein has been emptied, use your hand (not the tourniquet) to control the SFJ. Place two fingers at the SFJ (find the femoral pulse in the groin and place two fingers medially to occlude the SFJ). While holding the SFJ (this can be awkward), ask the patient to stand up. The same interpretation applies as before.

Doppler ultrasound

Use a hand-held Doppler (with KY Jelly). Identify the femoral artery with the Doppler. Move medially so that the probe is over the SFJ. Then bend down and compress the patient's calf. If there is venous incompetence at the SFJ, you will hear a backflow.

Auscultation

Check for venous bruits.

Complete examination

- Examine the gastrointestinal system and perform a rectal examination.
- Venous duplex.

Cover and thank the patient.

Turn to the examiner and summarise your findings.

33 Examining an ulcer

Introduction and consent

- Introduce yourself to the patient and ask permission to examine them.
- Ensure that you are in a quiet and private area.
- Position: ask the patient to lie down.
- Expose the area.
- Have gloves ready.
- Try to illicit from the examination whether the ulcer is arterial, venous, neuropathic or mixed in origin.

Inspection

- At rest, is the patient comfortable or in pain?
- Surgical scars in the groin and limbs.
- Look for evidence of end-stage disease (gangrene or amputations).
- Examine the ulcer (similar examination to that of the 'lump').
- Position:
  - venous: medial gaiter area
  - arterial: periphery of limbs and pressure areas
  - neuropathic: sites of trauma – sole of foot or heel.
- Colour.
- Tenderness (prior to touching the patient, ask whether they have any pain):
  - if there are painful ulcers, think of arterial causes.
- Temperature.
- Size.
- Shape.
- Surface.
- Edge:
  - venous: flat, sloping edge
  - arterial and neuropathic: squared or punched out.
- Depth – look for tendons or bones.
- Discharge – any evidence of infection (purulent discharge).
- Base – look for granulation tissue and sloughy areas.
- Relationship to surrounding tissue (nerves and vessels):
  - test of neurological status: modalities, fine touch and vibration sense
  - test of vascular integrity: capillary refill time (CRT) and palpation of foot pulses.
- Regional lymph nodes.

Complete examination

- Perform a complete vascular, venous and neurological examination.
- Arterial and venous duplex.
- Ankle brachial pressure index (ABPI).
- Angiogram.
- Blood test to exclude diabetes and infection.

Cover and thank the patient.

Turn to the examiner and summarise your findings.

34 Examining the cranial nerves

Introduction and consent

- Introduce yourself to the patient and ask permission to examine them.
- Ensure that you are in a quiet and private area.
- Position: sit the patient up in bed or in a chair.

Inspection

- Involuntary movements (tremor, fasciculation, choreiform movements).
- Dysphasia (expressive, receptive).
- Abnormal facial expressions (facial weakness, ptosis).

I	Olfactory	Smell
II	Optic	Visual acuity, visual fields, fundoscopic examination of each eye
III, IV, VI	Oculomotor, Trochlear, Abducens	Eyelid opening; extra-ocular movements (IV, superior oblique; VI, lateral rectus; III, all others); direct and consensual papillary light reflex
V	Trigeminal (V1, ophthalmic; V2, maxillary; V3, mandibular)	Corneal reflex, facial sensation, jaw opening, bite strength
VII	Facial	Eyebrow raise, eyelid close, smile, frown, pucker, taste

VIII	Vestibulochlear	Auditory acuity of each ear, Rinne test (air vs. bone conduction) and Weber (lateralising) test, oculocephalic reflex (doll's eye manoeuvre), oculovestibular reflex (ear canal caloric stimulation)
IX, X	Glossopharyngeal, Vagus	Palate elevation, swallow, posterior taste, phonation, gag reflex
XI	Spinal Accessory	Lateral head rotation, neck flexion, shoulder shrug
XII	Hypoglossal	Tongue protrusion and strength on lateral deviation

Thank the patient.

Turn to the examiner and summarise your findings.

35 Examining the peripheral nervous system

Introduction and consent

- Introduce yourself to the patient and ask permission to examine them.
- Ensure that you are in a quiet and private area.
- Position: sit the patient up in bed or in a chair.
- Expose the upper and lower limbs.
- There are five modalities to assess – tone, power, coordination, sensation and reflexes.

Inspection

- Asymmetry, deformities, scars, tremor, muscle wasting, fasciculations, involuntary movement.
- Assess the patient's gait and perform Romberg's test.

Tone

- Ask the patient whether they have any pain.
- Upper limb: roll arm in clockwise and counter clockwise directions.
- Lower limb: roll leg, lift and release knee.
- Upper motor neuron lesions: clasp-knife spasticity and lead-pipe rigidity.
- Parkinson's disease: cogwheel rigidity.

Power

Scoring system:

5	Normal
4	Movement against specific gravity and resistance, but weaker than normal
3	Movement against gravity
2	Movement with gravity eliminated
1	Visible contraction but no movement
0	No contraction

Upper limb

- Shoulder adduction C6,7.
- Shoulder abduction C5,6.
- Forearm flexion C5,6.
- Forearm extension C7,8.
- Median nerve C8,T1. Abductor pollicis brevis (thumb to ceiling).
- Ulnar nerve C8,T1. Interossei (paper between fingers, spread fingers).
- Radial nerve C5,6,7. Finger extension.

Lower limb

- Hip flexion L1,2,3.
- Hip extension L5.
- Knee flexion L5,S1.
- Knee extension L3,4.
- Ankle dorsiflexion L4,5.
- Ankle plantar flexion S1,2.
- Ankle inversion L4.
- Ankle eversion L5, S1.
- Toe extension L5. S1.
- Toe flexion S2,3.

Coordination

- Upper limb: finger–nose test.
- Lower limb: heel–shin test.

Sensation

Fine touch and pin-prick

Dermatomal distribution:

Upper limb
C5 Shoulder
C6 Lateral arm/thumb
C7 Back of hand
C8 Medial hand
T1 Medial arm

Lower limb
L1 Inguinal area
L2,3 Anterior thigh
L4,5 Shin
S1 Lateral foot, sole

Vibration

- Upper limb: sternum, wrist, elbow, shoulder.
- Lower limb: ankle, tibial tuberosity, iliac crest.

Proprioception

- Upper limb: shoulder, elbow, finger.
- Lower limb: hip, knee, toes.

Reflexes

Scoring system:

0	Absent
+	Reduced
++	Normal
+++	Increased

Upper limb
Biceps C5,6
Triceps C6,7
Supinator C5,6

Lower limb
Knee L3,4
Ankle L5, S1
Clonus
Plantar reflex: Babinski (extensor)

Cover and thank the patient.

Turn to the examiner and summarise your findings.

36 Examining the level of consciousness: Glasgow Coma Scale (GCS)

Introduction and consent

- Introduce yourself to the patient and ask permission to examine them.
- Ensure that you are in a quiet and private area.

Best eye response

Spontaneously	4
To speech	3
To pain	2
No response	1

Best verbal response

Orientated	5
Confused	4
Inappropriate responses	3
Inappropriate sounds	2
No response	1

Best motor response

Obeys commands	6
Localises to pain	5
Withdraws from pain	4
Flexion (decorticate) to pain	3
Extension (decerebrate) to pain	2
No response	1

- Scoring system is used to monitor changes in the level of consciousness.
- The total score is the sum of eye, verbal and motor responses.
- The possible score ranges from 3 (worst) to 15 (normal).

Pupil size 1–8 mm and reaction

- +: reacts.
- −: no reaction.
- c: closed eyes.

Limb movement: arms and legs

Normal power
Mild weakness
Severe weakness
Spastic flexion
Extension
No response

Turn to the examiner and summarise your findings.

37 Examining visual fields

Introduction and consent

- Introduce yourself to the patient and ask permission to examine them.
- Ensure that you are in a darkened, quiet and private area.
- Position: the patient should sit in a chair and you should sit directly opposite, facing them.
- Testing the visual fields involves assessing the function of the peripheral and central retina, the optic pathways and the cortex.
- It is achieved by a method of confrontation and using accurate perimeters.
- Normal field extends 160° horizontally and 130° vertically, with a blind spot 15° from fixation in the temporal field.
- A crude test of visual fields can be done by moving your hand quickly towards the patient's face. The patient should blink.

Specific tests

- First, examine each eye separately.
- Ask the patient to cover one eye, and look straight at your opposing eye.
- Examine the outer aspects of the visual fields with a moving finger or with a red hat pin. Keep your finger mid-way between you and the patient, and extend your arm so that your finger is beyond your own peripheral vision. Then move your finger toward the midline until it is seen in your visual field. If you and the patient have normal fields, you will both see at the same time.

- Bring the finger into the field of vision in a curve. Approach from the periphery at several points in the circumference of the upper and lower, nasal and temporal quadrants of the fields.
- Ask the patient to respond as soon as the finger is seen moving.
- Map out the central field defects by moving the finger across the visual field.
- When using the red hat pin, ask the patient to tell you when the red colour is seen.
- Test for visual inattention by asking the patient to report when the finger is moved on one or both sides simultaneously. If inattention is present, the patient will detect single targets but will ignore objects when the two fields are stimulated.

Turn to the examiner and summarise your findings.

38 Examining the retina (ophthalmoscopy)

Introduction and consent

- Introduce yourself to the patient and ask permission to examine them.
- Ensure that you are in a quiet and private area.
- Position: ask the patient to sit in a chair.

Inspection

- Eyelids: look for ptosis, lid retraction, entropion (lids turned in), ectropion (lids turned out) and styes.
- Conjunctiva: look for conjunctivitis, chemosis and pallor.
- Sclera: look for yellow colour (jaundice), blue colour (iron-deficiency anaemia, osteogenesis imperfecta) or inflammation.
- Cornea: look for corneal arcus (hypercholesterolaemia) and Kayser–Fleischer ring (Wilson's disease).
- Iris: look for iritis.
- Pupils: may be miotic (constricted) or mydriatric (dilated). Test direct and consensual light reflex, and accommodation reflex.
- Ocular movements: test movements in all positions of gaze. Both eyes should move symmetrically.

Ophthalmoscopy (fundoscopy)

- It is much easier to examine through a dilated pupil (use tropicamide eye drops).
- Turn off the lights (the procedure is best performed in a darkened room).
- Elicit the red reflex.
- Use your right eye to look at the patient's right eye, and use your left eye to look at the patient's left eye.
- Initially focus on the anterior structures, before concentrating on the fundus systematically.
- Focus on the optic disc.
- Examine the surrounding structures.

Turn on the lights, face the examiner and summarise your findings.

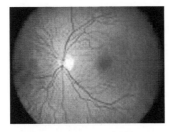

Figure 1   Fundus in normal eye.

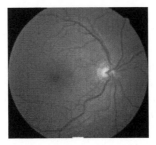

Figure 2   Fundus in diseased eye.

39 Assessing gait

Introduction and consent

- Introduce yourself to the patient and ask permission to examine them.
- Ensure that you are in a quiet and private area.
- Position: the patient should be standing.
- Expose the lower limbs, with socks and shoes removed.

Inspection

- Look at the soles of the patient's shoes and look for walking aids.
- Ask the patient to walk towards a specific point on the other side of the room and then turn to walk back to the starting point.
- Note whether the patient has difficulty in initiating movement (e.g. Parkinson's disease).
- Look for abnormalities of gait.

Type	Description
Antalgic	Decreased stance and increased swing phase
Cerebellar	Broad-based gait, often falling to one side
Hemiparesis	One leg is in extension, associated with foot drop; the leg swings out (circumducted to avoid falling)
High stepping	Foot lands flat or on the ball instead of the heel, with the foot slapping the ground
Parkinsonian	Unsteady, small steps, shuffling gait, difficult to start
Sensory ataxic	Foot-slapping gait due to loss of proprioception, associated with neuropathy
Short leg	Ipsilateral hip drops when weight is placed on the leg
Spastic	Hyperextended lower limbs using 'scissor'-like action
Waddling	Loss of control of the pelvis when one leg is lifted off the ground. Seen in muscular dystrophies and proximal weakness

Trendelenburg's test

Ask the patient to stand on their good leg and flex the other leg at the knee as you face them. The patient should rest the palms of their hands on your hands. This test is then repeated on the other leg. A positive test result is obtained if the pelvis on the unsupported side (the side where the leg is flexed) drops down. This is associated with hip abductor weakness.

Complete examination

- Examine the back and hips.
- Measure leg lengths.
- Examine lower limb neurology.

Thank the patient.

Turn to the examiner and summarise your findings.

40 Examining the breast

Introduction and consent

- Introduce yourself to the patient and ask permission to examine them.
- Ensure that you are in a quiet and private area.
- Position: the patient should be sitting in bed at an angle of 45°.
- There should be adequate exposure from the waist upward.

Inspection

This is best completed with the patient facing you with their hands pressed into their hips.

- General: for signs of weight loss, shortness of breath, jaundice or pallor.
- Breasts:
  - symmetry: size and shape
  - skin changes: surgical scars, redness, erythema, peau d'orange, ulceration, puckering, nodules
  - nipples and areolae: retraction, destruction or discharge.
- Axilla and arm: swelling or muscle wasting.
- Now inspect with the patient holding their arms over their head. Examine the breast and axilla for scars, puckering or tethering.

Palpation

Ask the patient to lie down on the bed, with their hands behind their head.

- Breast:
  - ask the patient whether they have any pain
  - palpate both breasts, starting with the normal breast
  - systematic review of all four quadrants
  - if a lump is found, assess the size, shape, surface, edges, consistency, mobility and site. Also assess the fixity of the lump (with the arms pressed in at the sides).
- Axilla:
  - assess the axillary lymph nodes (hold the patient's elbow and relax the arm)
  - identify the four walls and the apex.
- Neck:
  - palpate the supra- and infra-clavicular lymph nodes.
- Signs of metastasis can be detected by:
  - palpation of the liver and spine
  - auscultation of the chest (metastasis).

Complete examination

- Assess for nipple discharge.
- If a breast lump is found, refer the patient for triple assessment:
  - history and examination
  - imaging (ultrasound or mammography)
  - cytology (fine-needle aspiration or Trucut biopsy).

Cover and thank the patient.

Turn to the examiner and summarise your findings.

41 Examining a lump

Introduction and consent

- Introduce yourself to the patient and ask permission to examine them.
- Ensure that you are in a quiet and private area.
- Position: ensure that the patient is comfortable.

Inspection

- General:
  - note whether the patient is comfortable or in pain
  - note any surgical scars.
- Examine the lump systematically:
  - position
  - colour
  - texture of overlying skin
  - temperature
  - tenderness
  - shape
  - size
  - surface
  - edge
  - composition
  - consistency
  - compressibility
  - fluctuation
  - fluid thrill
  - fixity to surrounding structures
  - translucency
  - resonance
  - pulsatility
  - bruits
  - reducibility.
- Relation to surrounding structures (nerves and vessels):
  - test of neurological status: modalities, fine touch and vibration sense
  - test of vascular integrity: capillary refill time (CRT) and feel for regional pulses.
- State of the regional lymph nodes.

Complete examination

- Arrange follow-up to check that the lump remains unchanged.
- Based on clinical findings, biopsy or total excision of the lump can be performed.

Cover and thank the patient.

Turn to the examiner and summarise your findings.

42 Examining the neck and thyroid gland

Introduction and consent

- Introduce yourself to the patient and ask permission to examine them.
- Ensure that you are in a quiet and private area.
- Position: the patient should be sitting comfortably in a chair (away from the wall).
- Ensure that there is adequate exposure of the neck (ask the patient to unbutton blouse or take off shirt).

Inspection of the anterior triangle of the neck and thyroid

- Face: myxoedema, hyperthyroidism, plethoric faces.
- Neck: lump, swelling, goitre and surgical scars.
- Water test: ask the patient to swallow water, and note whether the lump moves on swallowing (if it does, it is a thyroid lump).
- Protrusion of the tongue: ascertain whether the lump moves on extending the tongue (if it does, it is a thyroglossal cyst).

Palpation of neck (from behind)

- Ask whether the patient experiences any pain.
- Describe any thyroid lumps or swelling that you find (*see* Topic 41):
  - position
  - colour
  - texture of overlying skin
  - temperature
  - tenderness
  - shape
  - size
  - surface
  - edge
  - composition
  - consistency
  - compressibility
  - fluctuation
  - fluid thrill
  - fixative to surrounding structures
  - translucency
  - resonance

- pulsatility
- bruits
- reducibility
- relationship to surrounding structures (nerves and vessels).
- Examine the lymph nodes.
- Ensure that the trachea is central.

Percussion

Assess retrosternal extension.

Auscultation

For a Graves' bruit.

Complete examination

Arrange follow-up to check that the lump remains unchanged.

Assess thyroid status

- Hands and pulse:
  - hyperthyroidism: tremor, increased sweating, thyroid acropachy, tachycardic irregular pulse
  - hypothyroidism: dry, cool and pale inelastic skin, paraesthesiae and bradycardia.
- Face and eyes:
  - Graves' disease: proptosis, exophthalmos, lid retraction, lid lag, chemosis and ophthalmoplegia
  - hypothyroidism: thin dry brittle hair, loss of outer third of eyebrows.
- Lower limb:
  - test ankle reflexes
  - look for pretibial myxodema.
- Ask how the lump affects the patient's life.
- Ultrasound with or without biopsy may be useful.

Thank the patient.

Turn to the examiner and summarise your findings.

43 Orthopaedic examination of the hip, knee, shoulder, spine and hand

Introduction and consent

- Introduce yourself to the patient and ask permission to examine them.
- Ensure that you are in a quiet and private area.
- Position: the patient should be sitting comfortably for upper limb examination, and lying down for lower limb examination.
- Adequate exposure of the joint is essential.
- Always ask the patient whether they are experiencing any pain.

For these orthopaedic examinations, four basic principles should be followed:

- Look.
- Feel.
- Move.
- Special tests.

Examining the hip

Look

- Front: pelvic tilting, muscle wasting, rotational deformity.
- Side: scars, lumbar lordosis.
- Behind: scoliosis, gluteal muscle wasting and scars.

Feel

- Temperature.
- Greater and lesser trochanter and head of femur.

Move

- **Thomas' test (testing for flexed flexion deformity).** Place your arm behind the lumbar spine, and fully flex the hip. The lumbar spine should flatten and the tested leg should remain in contact with the bed.
- **Active and passive movement:**
  - flexion, extension

- abduction, adduction (in extension)
- internal and external rotation (at 90°).
- **Special tests:**
  - assess shortening: true and apparent length
  - Trendelenburg's test (*see* Topic 38).

Complete examination

- Assessment of gait.
- Neurological examination.
- Radiographs (two views).

Cover and thank the patient.

Turn to the examiner and summarise your findings.

Examining the knee

Look

- Front: symmetry, swelling, scars, quadriceps wasting and deformity.
- Behind: swelling or sinus.

Feel

- Temperature.
- Effusion: stroke test, patella tap.
- Joint line.

Move

- Check that the extension apparatus is intact.
- Active and passive flexion and extension.

Special tests

- Collateral ligaments: varus and valgus stress test.
- Cruciate ligaments: anterior draw and Lachman's test, posterior draw.
- Menisci: McMurray's test.
- Patella: lateral apprehension test.

Complete examination

- Assessment of gait.
- Radiographs (two views).

Cover and thank the patient.

Turn to the examiner and summarise your findings.

Examining the shoulder

Look

- Front: asymmetry, wasting, deformity and scars.
- Above: scars, lumbar lordosis.
- Behind: winging of scapula.

Feel

- Temperature.
- Crepitus.
- Tenderness in sternoclavicular joint, clavicle, acromioclavicular joint, glenohumeral joint and axilla.

Move

Active and passive movement:

- abduction, (initiation, arc and holding arm up) (maxium degree of movement: 170°)
- adduction (hand on opposite shoulder)
- flexion (forwards)
- extension (backwards)
- internal rotation (hands behind back)
- external rotation (hands behind head).

Special tests

Deltoid power and sensation (regimental badge sensation).

Complete examination

- Cervical spine examination.

- Neurological examination of upper limb.
- Radiographs (two views).

Cover and thank the patient.

Turn to the examiner and summarise your findings.

Examining the spine

Position: the patient should be standing.

Look

- Side: kyphosis, scars and lumbar lordosis.
- Behind: scolisis, swellings and scars.

Feel

- Temperature.
- Tenderness in vertebrae, muscles and joints (also assessed by percussion).
- Feel for any steps.

Move

Active and passive movement:

- forward flexion
- extension
- lateral flexion
- rotation.

Special tests

Straight leg rise and then passive dorsiflexion.

Complete examination

- Neurological examination of upper and lower limb.
- Sphincter integrity.
- Abdominal examination.
- Radiographs (two views: AP and lateral films).

Cover and thank the patient.

Turn to the examiner and summarise your findings.

Examining the hand

Most frequently, you will be asked to examine a patient with rheumatoid hands.

- Position: ask the patient to rest their hands on a pillow, with their sleeves rolled up.

Look

- Symmetrical deformities (polyarthropathy of joints).
- Spindling of fingers.
- Sparing of distal interphalangeal (DIP) joints.
- Wasting of small muscles of hands.
- Thin and bruised skin.
- Ulnar deviation at metacarpophalangeal (MCP) joint.
- Radial deviation at wrist.
- Finger: swan-neck, Boutonnière's and Z-thumb deformity.
- Nail: pale beds, vasculitis lesions, pitting.
- Palms: pale palmar creases, palmar erythema.
- Elbow: nodules.

Feel

- Be careful – hands can be very tender.
- Temperature.
- Joints.
- Rheumatoid nodules.
- Heberden's node.

Move

- Active and passive movement at wrist and fingers.
- Flexion, extension, radial and ulnar deviation.

Functional assessment

Power grip, pincer grip (picking up a coin or keys), buttoning/un-buttoning shirt, holding a pen and writing name.

Sensation (fine touch)

Radial, median and ulnar nerves.

Special tests

Table top test: check whether hands can lie flat on a table.

Complete examination

- Neurological examination of upper limb.
- Assess for extra-articular manifestation of rheumatoid arthritis (eye, respiratory, cardiovascular, abdominal, dermatological and neuro-logical systems).
- Radiographs.

Cover and thank the patient.

Turn to the examiner and summarise your findings.

44 Gynaecological examination

Introduction and consent

- Introduce yourself to the patient and ask permission to examine them.
- Ensure that you are in a quiet and private area.
- Position: the patient should be lying on a bed.
- Ensure that there is adequate exposure.
- Ensure that a chaperone is present.

General examination

- Appearance and weight.
- Blood pressure, pulse and temperature.
- Colour: pale (anaemia) or yellow (jaundice).

Breast

(*see* Topic 40)

- Position: ask the patient to lie down on the bed, with their hands behind their head.
- Ask them whether they are experiencing any pain.
- Palpate both breasts, starting with the normal breast.
- Perform a systemic review of all four quadrants.
- If a lump is found, assess size, shape, surface, edges, consistency, mobility and site. Also assess the fixity of the lump (with the arms pressed in at the sides).

Axilla

- Assess the axillary lymph nodes (hold the patient's elbow and relax the arm).
- Identify the four walls and the apex.

Abdomen

(*see* Topic 29)
Position: lie the patient flat with their arms by their sides and ensure that there is exposure from the nipples to the knees.

Inspection

- Look for hernias: ask the patient to cough and to lift their head from the bed.
- Look for distension, swelling, scars, striae and distribution of body hair.

Palpation

- Kneel down at the side of the bed.
- Ask the patient whether they are experiencing any pain in their abdomen. Start with non-tender areas. Be systematic.
- Superficial and deep (nine quadrants) palpation.
- Assess for organomegaly and masses.
- If any masses are present, do they arise from the pelvis?

Percussion

Assess for shifting dullness (free fluid).

Auscultation

Bowel sounds.

Pelvic examination

Inspection

Note: During the examination this will be performed on a plastic model.

- Examine the vulva and vaginal orifices (assess colour, ulceration and/ or lumps).

Digital bimanual examination

- Put on gloves and apply lubricating jelly.
- Place your left hand on the abdomen, and insert two fingers of your right hand into the vagina.
- Assess the uterus, cervix, adnexa and pouch of Douglas.

Examination with Cusco's speculum

- In order to visualise the cervix, a speculum examination should be performed.
- Look for ulceration, bleeding or masses.
- A cervical smear can be taken.
- Withdraw the speculum slowly in order to visualise the vaginal vault.
- Close the speculum and withdraw it.

Examination with Sims' speculum

This allows better inspection of the vaginal walls and can be used to assess prolapse.
Position: left lateral position.

Digital rectal examination

This is used to assess prolapse or cervical disease.

Cover and thank the patient.

Turn to the examiner and summarise your findings.

45 Ear, nose and throat (ENT) examination

Introduction and consent

- Introduce yourself to the patient and ask permission to examine them.
- Ensure that you are in a quiet and private area.
- Position: sit the patient up.
- Equipment needed: otoscope, syringe for wax removal, light source and tongue depressor, direct endoscopy mirror and local anaesthetic spray.

Ears

- Examine the external auditory meatus and pinna: shape, symmetry and discharge.
- Use the otoscope to examine the meatus and the drum. To straighten the external auditory canal, pull the pinna up and backwards.
- Visualise the tympanic membrane and obtain the light reflex. Behind the posterior aspect of the drum is the posterior malleolar fold, the long process of the incus, and the facial nerve. Note the colour, translucency and any bulging of the membrane. Look for perforations and ensure that the margin extends to the periphery.
- Next ask the patient to perform the Valsalva manoeuvre. A patent Eustachian tube is demonstrated by movement of the drum.
- Test the cranial nerve (vestibulocochlear nerve – VIII) to assess auditory acuity (*see* Topic 34).

Nose and throat

- In the first instance, local anaesthetic spray can be applied.
- Apply a tongue depressor in order to visualise the oropharynx (dental hygiene, tonsils, pharynx and fauces).
- Examine the post-nasal space with direct flexible endoscopy. You should visualise the nasal septum, turbinates, nasopharnx, the opening of the Eustachian tubes, the pharyngeal recess and the adenoids.
- Using a mirror and with the tongue protruded, indirect laryngoscopy is possible (epiglottis, larynx and vocal cords may be seen).
- Flexible nasendoscopy allows more detailed examination if required.

- Test the following cranial nerves: glossopharyngeal (IX), vagus (X) and hypoglossal (XII) (*see* Topic 34).

Thank the patient.

Turn to the examiner and summarise your findings.

46 Examination of the newborn

APGAR scoring examination

The condition of the neonate should be determined at 1 and 5 minutes after birth.

Appearance
2: Entire body pink
1: Pink body and blue extremities
0: Entire body blue or pale

Pulse
2: > 100 beats/minute
1: < 100 beats/minute
0: Absent

Grimace
2: Cough, sneeze or vigorous cry
1: Grimace or slight cry
0: No response

Activity
2: Active movement
1: Some movement
0: Limp and motionless

Respirations
2: Strong crying
1: Slow, irregular crying
0: Crying absent

The total score is the sum of five assessments. It can range from 0 (worst) to 10 (best).

- Score of 7: good.
- Score of 4–6: assist, stimulate.
- Score of < 4: resuscitate.

Detailed examination of the neonate

- Introduce yourself to the parents and ask permission to examine the neonate in order to detect any abnormalities or problems.
- Wash your hands.
- Information required:
  - weight.
  - whether the pregnancy and birth were routine
  - Rhesus status of the mother.

Face

- Head: circumference, shape, fontelles (tense or sunken).
- Eyes: check red reflex, corneal opacities and conjunctivitis.
- Ears: symmetry, shape or position.
- Skin: complexion, colour and turgor.
- Mouth: look inside with a pen torch. Insert finger to assess sucking reflex.

Limb

- Position and shape.
- Hands/feet: assess palmar creases, and look for clinodactyly
- Ortolani and Barlow tests for congenital dislocation of the hip.

Thorax

- Respiratory movement and effort.
- Palpate the apex beat, and auscultate for heart and breath sounds.

Abdomen

- You should be able to palpate the liver and spleen. Feel for masses.
- Inspect the umbilicus.
- Examine the external genitalia (including the urinary meatus, and in males check whether the testicles are descended) and the anus.

Central nervous system

- Assess movement (power), tone and reflexes (e.g. Moro reflex).

Cover the neonate and thank the parents.

Turn to the examiner and summarise your findings.

47 Paediatric examination: assessment of developmental milestones

Age	Ability
Age	*Ability*
2 months	Smile, follow past midline, say 'ooh/aah', head to 45°
4 months	Regard hand, grasp rattle, squeal or laugh, bear weight on legs
6 months	Feed self, reach, imitate speech sounds, pull to sit, no head lag
9 months	Take two cubes, jabber, pull to stand, sit unsupported
12 months	Wave goodbye, play 'pat-a-cake', pincer grasp, say 'dada/mama', stand for 2 seconds
15 months	Play ball with examiner, scribble, speak two words, walk well
18 months	Use spoon and fork, drink from cup, build 2-cube tower, speak three words, able to run
24 months	Remove garment, build 4-cube tower, name six body parts, walk up steps
3 years	Wash and dry hands, build 8-cube tower, use two adjectives, broad jump
4 years	Dress without help, copy circle, speech all understandable, able to hop

Clinical skills

48 Basic life support

Basic life support (BLS) refers to the initial management of the airways and support of breathing and the circulation. Sudden cardiac death is a leading cause of death in the Western world, and in approximately 40% of patients the initial cardiac rhythm is ventricular fibrillation (VF). However, this rhythm rapidly deteriorates to asystole, which has an extremely poor prognosis for survival.

Early bystander recognition of the need for cardiac and cardio-pulmonary resuscitation, and their ability to perform this, can double or even triple survival from VF cardiac arrest, and it is therefore essential that all medical trainees are familiar with BLS and are aware of the recent changes to the BLS algorithm.

Scenario

You witness an elderly person collapse on the street. There is no one else around. Perform basic life support.

- Ensure that you, the patient and any bystanders are safe.
- Check whether the patient is responsive.
- 'Shake the patient's shoulders and ask in a loud voice 'Are you all right?'

If the patient responds:

- Leave him in the position in which you have found him, provided that he is safe.
- Ascertain what is wrong with him and get help if necessary.
- Reassess him regularly.

If the patient does not respond:

- Shout for help.

- Turn the patient on to his back.
- **Open the airway using head tilt** (place your hand on the patient's forehead and gently tilt his head back) and **chin lift** (place your fingertips under the patient's chin and lift his chin to open the airway).
- **Look** for chest movements, **Feel** for air on your cheek. **Listen** for breath sounds for up to **10 seconds.**
- If the patient is breathing, turn him into the recovery position.
- **If he is not breathing normally:**
  - send someone for help
  - if you are alone, leave the patient and call for an ambulance
  - then return to the patient and start chest compressions.

Chest compressions

- Kneel at the patient's side, positioned vertically above their chest.
- With your arms straight and fingers interlocked, perform compressions over the mid-lower portion of the sternum to a depth of 4–5 cm and at a rate of 100 compressions per minute.
- Combine compressions with rescue breaths at a ratio of 30 compressions to 2 rescue breaths.

Rescue breaths

- Open the airway using head tilt and chin lift.
- Pinch the soft part of the nose.
- Take a normal breath.
- Place your lips around the patient's mouth and maintain a tight seal.
- Blow steadily for about 1 second while watching for the chest to rise.
- Watch for the chest falling as air passes out, and perform another rescue breath before returning to perform 30 chest compressions.
- If the initial rescue breath does not cause the chest to rise:
  - check for airway obstruction and remove the obstacle
  - recheck that there is adequate chin lift and head tilt
  - do not attempt more than two rescue breaths before returning to chest compressions.
- Continue with chest compressions and rescue breaths at a ratio of 30:2 until help arrives, until the patient's breathing recovers or until you become exhausted.
- If there is more than one rescuer, change over every 1–2 minutes.

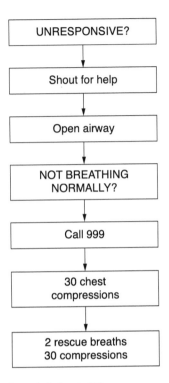

Figure 3   Algorithm for adult basic life support.

49 Airway adjuncts

In patients with a reduced Glasgow Coma Score, the tongue can fall backwards to obstruct the hypopharynx. Simple airway manoeuvres such as chin lift and jaw thrust can be employed to correct this, and the airway can then be temporarily maintained using airway adjuncts such as an oropharyngeal (Guedel) or nasopharyngeal airway.

Guedel airway

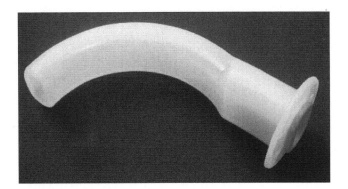

Figure 4   Guedel airway.

This should not be used in conscious patients, in whom the gag reflex is intact, due to the risk of vomiting and aspiration.

Procedure in adults

- Wash your hands and put on gloves and an apron.
- Select the appropriate size airway. When placed against the patient's face, the airway should extend from the tragus of the ear to the angle of the mouth.
- Open the mouth by using a chin lift manoeuvre and insert the airway into the patient's mouth in a reverse position.
- As the airway is advanced towards the back of the mouth, rotate the airway into its correct position.
- The airway should lie between the teeth.
- Note: in infants the airway should be inserted in the correct position.

Nasopharyngeal airway

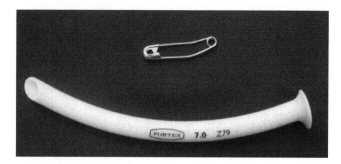

Figure 5   Nasopharyngeal airway.

- This is used when the patient has a gag reflex or in cases where there is lower facial trauma.
- It should be avoided in cases of nasal obstruction (e.g. by polyps or blood) or where a fracture of the base of the skull is suspected.

Procedure

- Wash your hands and put on gloves and an apron.
- Select the appropriate size airway (the lumen should have the same diameter as the patient's finger).
- Lubricate the tip of the airway with KY Jelly (note that the flange of the tube has a safety pin to prevent the airway being advanced too far).
- Insert the tip into the nostril, aiming towards the nasopharynx (downwards), and advancing until the flange rests on the patient's nostril.
- Stop if any resistance is encountered, and attempt to reinsert the airway in the other nostril.
- Ventilate the patient using a bag-and-mask device.

50 Intubation

A definitive airway is indicated if the airway needs to be protected or ventilation is inadequate. It can be achieved by endotracheal intubation, nasotracheal intubation or creation of a surgical airway (e.g. needle cricothyroidectomy or tracheostomy). Note that a laryngeal mask airway is not a definite airway, as there is still a risk of aspiration.

Indications

- Unconscious patient with GCS < 8 (i.e. unable to maintain airway)
- Risk of aspiration
- Risk of impending airway obstruction (e.g. laryngeal oedema (due to anaphylaxis or burns), neck haematoma, stridor)
- Inadequate respiratory effort
- Apnoea (e.g. due to neuromuscular paralysis)
- Requirement for general anaesthetic (e.g. for surgery)

Relative contraindications

- Maxillofacial trauma
- Suspected cervical spine injury

Absolute contraindications

- Fractured larynx

Scenario

You are part of the trauma team that is called to attend an emergency admission in Accident and Emergency. The patient has a GCS of 7 and you are required to intubate them.

Position patient

- The patient should be supine.
- In trauma, the head and neck should be immobilised and held in neutral by an assistant (e.g. in-line immobilisation).

Prepare equipment

- Wash your hands and put on a pair of gloves.
- Gather the following equipment:
  - endotracheal tube of internal diameter 7.0 mm for female patients and 8.0 mm for males. Inflate the tube cuff with a 10-ml syringe to check for leaks before use

- laryngoscope (size 3) handle and blade. Connect these, and check the light source by extending the blade
- suction
- stylet (may be useful in difficult intubations)
- bandage/tape to secure the tube
- stethoscope to check position.

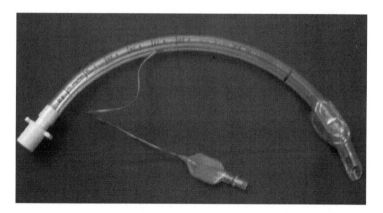

Figure 6 Endotracheal tube.

Procedure

- Pre-oxygenate the patient for 30 seconds using 100% oxygen, and ventilate for a minimum of 30 seconds via bag mask or mouth mask.
- Apply cricoid pressure to prevent aspiration.
- If the patient is conscious, perform rapid-sequence induction. Administer 3 mg/kg of succinylcholine (this produces paralysis lasting for 1–5 minutes).
- Hold the extended laryngoscope in your left hand.
- Remove loose dentures or any foreign bodies or fluid. Apply suction if necessary.
- Open the mouth with your right hand and, using the blade of the laryngoscope, displace the tongue to the patient's left.
- Advance the blade to visualise the vocal cords, and with your right hand insert the endotracheal tube to a distance of 21 cm in females and 23 cm in males (measured at the patient's incisors).
- Inflate the cuff with approximately 5 ml of air using a 10-ml syringe, to create a good seal.
- Release the cricoid pressure.

- Bag-valve-tube ventilate the patient and look for symmetrical movement of the chest wall. Auscultate the lungs for air entry.
- Avoid prolonged periods without ventilation. As a general rule of thumb, the patient needs to be ventilated within a single breath hold. If intubation within this time period is not successful, the patient should be bag-mask ventilated before any further attempt.

Closure

- Secure the tube in position.
- Check the position of the tube with a chest X-ray and/or attach a carbon dioxide calorimetric device to the tube (if no carbon dioxide is detected, this suggests oesophageal intubation).

51 Tracheostomy

Scenario

Can you tell me what this is and what it is used for?

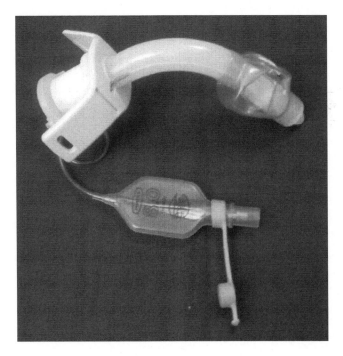

Figure 7   Tracheostomy tube.

This scenario requires you to correctly identify the instrument, and discussion may involve:

- indications for tracheostomy insertion
- the procedure
- complications.

Indications for tracheostomy

- In emergencies:
  - to maintain airway in congenital disorders (e.g. laryngeal atresia), acquired disorders (e.g. maxillofacial trauma), laryngeal oedema (e.g. due to burns, anaphylaxis) and obstruction of the upper airway by a foreign body.
- To facilitate ventilation:
  - to reduce work of breathing and deadspace (e.g. due to chronic obstructive pulmonary disease)
  - to enable respiratory toilet
  - in neurological disorders that lead to paralysis of the respiratory muscles (e.g. coma, bulbar palsy).
- Elective:
  - head and neck surgery.

Tracheostomy insertion

Consent

- Introduce yourself to the patient. Explain the procedure, its risks and benefits, and obtain written consent.
- Tracheostomy insertion is not an emergency procedure but should be performed in the operating theatre under a general anaesthetic with endotracheal intubation.

Position

- The patient is positioned supine with a sandbag placed between the shoulder blades and the neck hyperextended.

Procedure

- Scrub up, gown and glove.

- Prepare the skin of the neck with betadine, and create a sterile field around the incision site.
- Make a transverse incision at the midpoint between the cricoid cartilage and the sternal notch.
- Deepen to divide the platysma muscle. Retract the strap muscles to expose the trachea and the thyroid isthmus.
- Divide the thyroid isthmus.
- Incise the trachea from the second to the fourth tracheal cartilage to permit entry of the tracheostomy tube.
- Ask the anaesthetist to withdraw the endotracheal tube and insert the tracheostomy tube. Inflate the cuff and loosely suture the tissues around the tube.
- Secure the tracheostomy tube with ties.
- Change the tube after 24 hours.

Complications

- Immediate complications:
  - bleeding
  - oesophageal perforation
  - subcutaneous emphysema
  - aspiration.
- Early complications:
  - displacement
  - blockage
  - infection (e.g. with *Pseudomonas* spp., *E.coli*, *Staphylococcus aureus*.
- Late complications:
  - tracheo-innominate vein fistula
  - tracheal stenosis.

---

52 Oxygen delivery devices

Scenario

Mrs Jones is a post-operative patient who has had an open cholecystectomy. She has developed atelectasis and has reduced saturations. You have been called to the ward to assess her oxygen requirements.

Introduction

- Introduce yourself to the patient and check her identity.
- Discuss the requirement for supplemental oxygen with the patient and obtain verbal consent.

Position

- The patient should be seated upright.
- Ensure that they are comfortable.

Procedure

- Assess the patient's oxygen requirement. This may require interpretation of their arterial blood gases (ABG) and review of their chest X-ray.
- Decide on the amount of oxygen to be given, and prescribe this on the patient's drug chart if necessary.
- Select the appropriate oxygen delivery device (e.g. nasal cannulae, mask, mask and reservoir bag).
- Connect the mask/cannulae to the oxygen tubing, and then connect the tubing to the oxygen cylinder.
- Adjust the oxygen flow rate and apply the mask/cannulae, ensuring that they are comfortably placed.

Oxygen delivery device	Oxygen delivered (FiO_2)	Flow rate	Problems
Nasal cannulae	30–40%	4–6 litres/ minute	Variable oxygen delivery depending on patient's tidal volume, respiratory rate and whether nasal or oral breather
Face mask (e.g. Hudson)	40%	15 litres/ minute	Variable performance
Fixed-volume delivery masks (e.g. Venturi)	24%, 28%, 35%, 40% and 60% masks are available	Flow adjusted to mask	Maximum oxygen delivery 60% FiO_2
Reservoir bag attached to face mask	Approximately 95%	15 litres/ minute	–

Note: In patients with type II respiratory failure the oxygen delivered should be titrated up as tolerated due to hypercapnia. However, in an emergency maximum oxygen therapy should be used.

Closure

- Advise the patient on:
  - duration of oxygen therapy
  - monitoring (saturations monitor)
  - the need for repeat ABG (should be performed at least 20 minutes after initiating oxygen therapy to allow steady-state levels to be achieved).
- Ask the nursing staff to monitor the patient's saturations at regular intervals (i.e. hourly).
- Document your management plan.

53 Measuring peak expiratory flow rate (PEFR)

Scenario

Miss Molloy is a 33-year-old patient who presents to her GP with a persistent nocturnal cough that she has 'not been able to shake off' for the past month. You have been asked to take a PEFR recording.

Introduction

- Introduce yourself to the patient.
- Explain the procedure and obtain informed verbal consent.

PEFR

- Measures maximum flow rate in the first 2 ms of expiration.
- Cheap and simple test to perform.
- Is used to estimate airway calibre.
- Is useful for monitoring and assessing response to treatment in patients with respiratory disease.
- Is measured using a PEFR meter.
- The best of three PEFR readings is compared with the predicted PEFR value.

> - A ratio of actual to predicted PEFR of > 80% is considered normal, < 50% is seen in acute severe asthma and < 33% is seen in severe life-threatening asthma.

Preparation of equipment

- Wash your hands.
- Obtain peak flow meter and attach disposable mouthpiece.

Position

- Ask the patient to stand upright.

Procedure

- Demonstrate the technique to the patient by performing your own PEFR measurement as described below.
- Reset the pointer on the peak flow meter to zero before starting.
- Hold the peak flow meter in a horizontal position, ensuring that your fingers do not obstruct the scale.
- Take a deep breath, and create a tight seal around the mouthpiece.
- Blow as fast and as hard as you can and note the number reached on the scale.
- Check that the patient has understood the technique.
- Attach a fresh disposable mouthpiece.
- Reset the pointer to zero, ask the patient to perform the procedure and note the reading.
- Repeat the procedure two more times, and record the highest of the three readings (the patient's personal best) in the patient's notes or in their PEFR diary.

Closure

- Compare the patient's personal best PEFR reading with their normal predicted PEFR. This varies from person to person and depends on the patient's age, height and gender.
- *The patient's height is 1.6 m, and their best PEFR reading is found to be 350 litres/minute. According to the chart, the normal predicted PEFR is 365 litres/minute.* Advise the patient of the results.

- The patient's PEFR is 96% of the predicted value for their age and gender. This is essentially within the normal range.
- Offer to take a full history and examine the patient.
- Ask the patient to take their PEFR readings three times a day (in the morning, in the afternoon and at night) and to keep a PEFR diary for 2 weeks.
- Address any of the patient's concerns or questions.

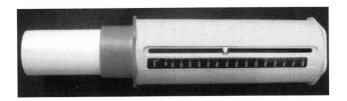

Figure 8   PEFR meter.

54 Arterial blood gas sampling

Scenario

Mr Jones is a 68-year-old post-operative patient with chronic obstructive pulmonary disease (COPD), who has just had an abdominal aortic aneurysm (AAA) repair. He becomes acutely short of breath and tachypnoeic, and you are asked to perform arterial blood gas sampling.

Introduction and consent

- Explain the procedure and its indication to the patient.
- Obtain informed verbal consent.

Risks of arterial puncture

- Pain
- Bleeding with or without haematoma
- Pseudoaneurysm
- Arterial dissection
- Distal limb ischaemia
- Failure of procedure

Positioning the patient

- Wash your hands or use alcohol gel.
- Ensure that the patient is seated or lying comfortably.
- Select the artery to be used, in the following order of preference: radial, femoral and brachial artery.
- If the radial artery is selected, an Allen's test (*see* p.83) should be performed prior to arterial sampling to ensure that the collateral blood supply to the hand from the ulnar artery is intact.
- Support the wrist on a pillow and ensure that any constricting clothing proximally is loosened.

Preparation

- Wash your hands and put on a pair of gloves.
- Gather the following equipment:
  - heparinised syringe
  - 23–25 gauge needle
  - alcohol swab.

Procedure

- Clean the arterial puncture site with an alcohol swab.
- Wait 30 seconds for the alcohol to evaporate.
- Hyperextend the wrist joint (helping to bring the artery to the surface) and palpate the radial artery proximally and distally, using the index and middle finger.
- Expel the heparin from the syringe completely and, holding the syringe like a pencil with the bevel pointed upwards, enter the skin at an angle of 60–90° between the two fingers.
- Advance the needle, maintaining a slight negative pressure until a bright red flashback is seen. Some syringes fill spontaneously due to the pressure in the artery, while others require gentle aspiration.
- When 1–2 ml of blood have been obtained, withdraw the needle and apply pressure to the puncture site for 5 minutes, or longer if the patient is on anticoagulation.
- Expel any air within the syringe. Remove the needle into a sharps container and cap the syringe.
- Analyse the blood sample obtained.

Closure

- Ensure that the patient is comfortable and advise them of the results of the test and of any action which needs to be taken.
- Document the results in the patient's notes, including the date, time and patient's inspired oxygen at the time of taking the sample.

Interpretation of arterial blood gas measurements

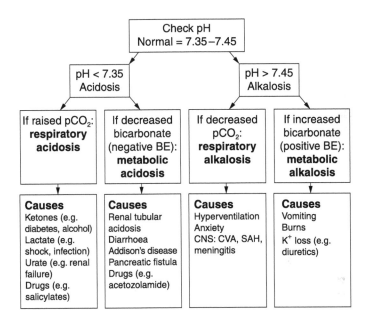

- Normal pCO_2 = 4.3–6.0 kPa; plasma bicarbonate = 22–26 mmol/l; base excess (BE) = ± 2.
- If the pH is normal but pCO_2 or bicarbonate is abnormal, this suggests compensation.

55 Pleural aspiration

Scenario

Mr Brown is a 56-year-old patient with a history of heart failure who has become acutely short of breath. On respiratory examination he is found to be tachypnoeic. His chest is dull to percussion on the left mid-lower zones with absent air entry. A chest X-ray reveals a pleural effusion which you are asked to tap.

Indications

- Therapeutic:
  - to relieve symptomatic effusion
  - to introduce an antibiotic (e.g. erythromycin)
  - to introduce a cytotoxic agent.
- Diagnostic:
  - to determine aetiology (e.g. transudate (protein < 30 g/l) versus exudate (protein > 30 g/l), malignancy, infection).

Introduction and consent

- Introduce yourself to the patient and confirm their identity.
- Discuss the procedure, explaining the reason for the investigation and what it entails, and the risks and benefits.
- Ascertain whether the patient has any allergies or contraindications (e.g. coagulopathy, pneumothorax, haemothorax) to the procedure, and obtain their informed consent.
- Check the patient's chest X-ray (AP and lateral views – blunting of the costophrenic angle suggests the presence of > 300 ml of fluid) and examine the patient to confirm the presence of a pleural effusion.

Preparation

- Wash your hands and put on a pair of gloves.
- Gather the following equipment:
  - dressing pack
  - 50-ml syringe, three-way tap and sterile tubing
  - wide-bore needle/cannula
  - kidney dish
  - specimen bottles
  - lignocaine (1%), 10-ml syringe and 25- and 22-gauge needle
  - Betadine.

Positioning

- The patient should be seated upright, leaning forward with their elbows resting on a table in front of them.
- Assist the patient into a comfortable position, ensuring that the back is exposed.
- Re-examine the patient, percuss the fluid level and mark the site of aspiration below this level, ideally in the eighth to ninth intercostal space in the posterior axillary line.

Procedure

- Scrub up, gown and glove.
- Prepare the aspiration site with Betadine and create a sterile field around the site using the sterile drapes within the dressing pack.
- Infiltrate the skin with 1% lignocaine using a 25-gauge needle. Change to a 22-gauge needle and infiltrate deeper down to the pleura, aspirating before injecting the local anaesthetic. Once a small volume of fluid has been aspirated, note the depth at which this occurs and remove the needle.
- Attach the wide-bore needle to the three-way tap, which at one port should be connected to a syringe and at the other port to sterile rubber tubing draining into a kidney dish.
- Insert the wide-bore needle through the anaesthetised area over the top of the rib (to avoid the neurovascular bundle). Gently aspirate while advancing the needle until fluid is encountered.
- Aspirate the fluid into the syringe, and then close the three-way tap and flush the contents through the tubing into the kidney dish. Repeat until no more fluid can be withdrawn.
- Fill the specimen bottles.
- *Do not remove more than 1000 ml of fluid at one sitting, due to the risk of mediastinal shift and hypovolaemia.*
- Withdraw the needle while asking the patient to exhale, and apply an occlusive dressing.
- Dispose of sharps and clinical waste appropriately.
- Wash your hands.

Closure

- Explain to the patient that the procedure is complete, and describe the next steps in their management. Address any questions or concerns.

- Organise and complete the appropriate form for a chest X-ray to confirm resolution of the effusion.
- Label the specimen bottles and appropriate investigation request forms for cytology, microbiology (MC&S) and biochemistry.
- Document the procedure in the patient's notes, including the colour, consistency and volume of fluid withdrawn, as well as any complications.

Complications

- Pneumothorax
- Haemothorax
- Infection
- Hypotension

---

56 Administering drugs via a nebuliser

Scenario

Miss Holmes is a 35-year-old asthmatic who presents to Accident and Emergency with increasing shortness of breath and a clearly audible wheeze. She has been prescribed a nebuliser, and you have been asked to administer this.

General information

- Nebulisers convert a drug in solution into a fine aerosol mist.
- Particles are typically 1–5 μm in diameter and are inhaled directly into the lungs.
- Larger particles are deposited in the nasopharynx.
- Nebulisers allow a large dose of drug to be administered effectively.
- *Note that only 10% of the prescribed dose will reach the lungs.*

Indications

- Emergency treatment of acute asthma and COPD.
- Long-term bronchodilator treatment in COPD.
- Antibiotic treatment for cystic fibrosis, bronchiectasis and HIV/ AIDS.
- Symptomatic relief in palliative care.

Introduction and consent

- Introduce yourself to the patient and confirm their identity.
- Consult the patient's prescription chart and establish the prescribed drug, the dose and the dilution, as well as the time and route of administration.
- Ascertain whether the patient has any allergies.
- Explain to the patient that you would like to administer a drug called salbutamol via a face mask, and obtain their informed, verbal consent.
- Wash your hands and put on gloves.

Positioning the patient

- Ensure that the patient is in the upright position and comfortable.

Preparing the equipment

Components of a nebuliser

- Face mask or mouthpiece.
- Nebuliser chamber, which converts the liquid drug into a mist.
- Compressor (power source) or a supply of compressed air or oxygen, which drives the nebuliser.

- Use a clean nebuliser.
- Connect the air tubing from the compressor to the nebuliser base.
- Attach the mask to the nebuliser.
- Check the name, strength and expiry date of the medication, either out loud or with a colleague.
- Measure the required dose of salbutamol (usually 2.5 or 5 mg) into the nebuliser chamber with a syringe.

Procedure

- Place the mask on the patient's face and ensure that the nebuliser chamber is in the upright position.
- Switch on the compressor to the recommended gas flow (nebulisers usually require flow rates of > 6 litres/minute).

- Check that the patient is comfortable.
- Tell the patient to breathe normally and inform them that the procedure should take approximately 10 minutes.
- Occasionally tap the side of the nebuliser to dislodge any deposits of the drug from the walls of the nebuliser chamber.
- Sign, date and time the patient's drug chart to indicate that the drug has been administered.
- Once the nebuliser has stopped misting, switch off the compressor and dismantle, clean and store the equipment.

Closure

- Ask the patient whether she feels that her condition has improved. Ascertain whether she is still short of breath, and confirm any improvement by taking a peak flow reading and comparing these results with the patient's results on admission.

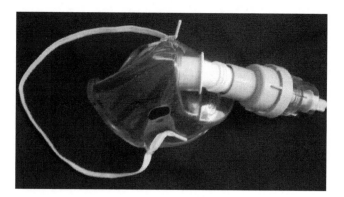

Figure 9 Nebuliser apparatus.

57 Setting up a blood transfusion

Scenario

Mrs Jennings is a 45-year-old inpatient who has just had a nephrectomy. Her haemoglobin level is 7.2 g/dl. You are asked to set up a two-unit blood transfusion. The blood has already been cross-matched, and the first unit is waiting on the ward for you. The patient already has an IV cannula in situ.

Introduction

- Introduce yourself to the patient and confirm her identity.
- Explain to the patient that she requires a blood transfusion because she lost a lot of blood during her operation.
- Address any of her concerns and obtain verbal consent for the procedure.
- Review the patient's prescription chart and confirm the date, time, number of units and rate of infusion requested for the transfusion.
- Establish whether the patient has any allergies or any history of any blood transfusion reactions, or whether she has been pregnant in the past 3 months.

Positioning the patient

- Ensure that the patient is either seated or lying in bed comfortably, with the arm in which the transfusion is to run supported by a pillow.
- Measure the patient's temperature, blood pressure and heart rate.

Preparing the equipment

Gather the following:

- normal saline flush
- unit of blood
- blood-giving set
- 250 ml of 0.9% normal saline.

Procedure

- Wash your hands and put on a pair of gloves.
- Flush the IV cannula which is currently *in situ* with 5–10 ml of saline to check its patency.
- Check the patient's surname, first name, gender, hospital number and date of birth against their identity band, drug chart and the blood compatibility report and blood unit label. These should all match.
- Check the patient's blood group on the compatibility report with that on the blood bag, and if possible against the current and previous laboratory reports.
- Finally, with a nurse or colleague double-check the serial number of the blood unit against that on the compatibility report.
- Inspect the blood bag for leaks, and ensure that the expiry date has not passed.

- Prime (flush through) the blood-giving set with 0.9% normal saline to remove any air (never use solutions containing dextrose). Attach the blood bag and start the transfusion.
- Using the roller clamp, alter the drip flow rate as necessary.
- Commence the blood transfusion within 30 minutes of receiving the blood.
- Advise the patient to notify either you or one of the nursing staff if she develops a fever, joint pain, breathing difficulties, itchiness or a rash.
- Run approximately 25–50 ml of blood in the first 15 minutes and re-check the patient's observations (temperature, blood pressure and heart rate). Then ask for observations to be made every 30 minutes until 1 hour after the transfusion (or as per hospital policy).
- Sign, date and time the drug chart and blood compatibility report.

Closure

- Check that the patient is comfortable.
- Address any concerns that may have arisen.
- Re-check the haemoglobin level after 24 hours.

Blood transfusion

- Blood is usually run at a rate of between 2- and 4-hourly.
- A 1-unit blood transfusion of packed cells will cause a 1 g/dl increase in haemoglobin concentration.
- In general, transfuse if the haemoglobin level is < 8 g/dl or if the patient is symptomatic.
- Frusemide 20–40 mg by mouth can be given with alternate bags of blood if there is concern about fluid overload.

---

58 Pulse oximetry

Pulse oximetry is a non-invasive, continuous method of measuring arterial oxygen saturation levels of haemoglobin. The pulse oximeter consists of a probe with two light-emitting diodes (LEDs), a photodetector and a microprocessor unit which displays a waveform, oxygen saturations and heart rate in beats per minute. The light absorption at the two different wavelengths (660 nm and 940 nm) depends on the degree of oxygen saturation of haemoglobin. The results are averaged over 5–20 seconds.

Introduction

- Introduce yourself to the patient. Explain that you wish to place a probe on their finger to measure the oxygen levels in their blood, and obtain verbal consent for this procedure.
- Wash your hands or apply alcohol gel.

Procedure

- Ensure that the pulse oximeter is plugged in or has sufficient battery power.
- Switch it on and wait for it to finish calibrating.
- Select the appropriate size probe and place it on the patient's digit (note that the ear lobe and nose can also be used). Ensure that the digit to be used is clean and free from nail varnish beforehand.
- Do not place the probe distal to a blood pressure cuff.
- Wait a few seconds for the pulse oximeter to detect the heart rate and calculate oxygen saturations. These will then be displayed as a digital readout.
- For the readings to be valid, a waveform should also be displayed.
- *Note:* The heart rate is usually accompanied by an audible signal which falls in pitch as levels of saturation decrease.

Closure

- Record both the heart rate and oxygen saturation in the patient's notes.
- Advise the patient of the results, their significance, and any further course of action that may be necessary.
- Address any questions or concerns that the patient may have. Thank the patient.

Factors that affect the accuracy of readings

- Ambient light (e.g. bright light)
- Peripheral vasoconstriction (e.g. hypovolaemia, hypotension, peripheral vascular disease, hypothermia)
- Venous congestion
- Shivering
- Nail varnish
- Methylene blue

- Saturations of < 70% are unreliable
- Diathermy can interrupt measurement

Note: Pulse oximetry:

- does not measure ventilation, so gives no information about CO_2
- does not measure PaO_2
- cannot distinguish between different forms of haemoglobin (e.g. carboxy- or methaemoglobin).

The results should always be interpreted in the context of the patient's clinical condition.

59 Blood pressure measurement

Scenario

Mrs Smith is a known hypertensive and has come in to have her blood pressure measured.

Introduction and consent

- Introduce yourself to the patient.
- Explain that you would like to take her blood pressure, and obtain verbal consent.
- Inform the patient that she may experience some temporary discomfort on inflation of the blood pressure cuff.

Positioning

- Ensure that the patient is seated comfortably and has been rested for at least 10 minutes prior to measurement of blood pressure.
- Adequately expose the right arm and remove any constricting clothing.

Procedure

- Ensure that the patient's arm is supported at the level of their heart and that the mercury manometer is upright and at your eye level.

- Select the appropriate size blood pressure cuff. (Note that small cuffs used in a large patient can give a falsely elevated result. Ideally the bladder of the cuff should encompass 80% of the patient's arm.)
- Place the sphygmomanometer cuff around the upper arm with the inflation bag overlying the brachial artery.
- Inflate the cuff above systolic blood pressure (i.e. so that the brachial artery is compressed and the radial pulse is impalpable). When this point is reached, inflate the cuff by a further 30 mmHg.
- Place the diaphragm of the stethoscope over the brachial artery, below the cuff.
- Release the cuff pressure slowly using the valve at a rate of 2–3 mmHg.
- The pressure at which the first Korotkoff sound (named after the Russian physician who first described it) is heard (phase 1) corresponds to the systolic blood pressure.
- The Korotkoff sound then gets louder before becoming muffled (phase 4) and then disappearing (phase 5). Phase 5 defines the diastolic blood pressure.
- After phase 5, deflate and release the cuff.
- Tell the patient and the examiner the blood pressure measurement (to the nearest 2 mmHg), and offer to document the result in the patient's notes.
- Offer to take the patient's blood pressure in the other (left) arm, and also with the patient standing.

Variations in blood pressure

- Hypertension is diagnosed when the systolic pressure is > 160 mmHg and the diastolic pressure is > 95 mmHg, when measured on at least three different occasions (WHO guidelines).
- The optimal target systolic pressure is < 140 mmHg, and the optimal diastolic pressure is < 85 mmHg. In patients with diabetes or renal disease the optimal target systolic pressure is < 130 mmHg and the optimal diastolic pressure is < 130 mmHg.
- A blood pressure difference of < 10 mmHg between the right and left brachial arteries is acceptable.
- On standing, a reduction in the systolic pressure (< 20 mmHg) and an increase in the diastolic pressure (< 10 mmHg) can also be expected.
- However, in postural (orthostatic) hypotension a fall in both the systolic and diastolic pressure of > 15 mmHg is seen. Causes include volume depletion, diabetes, peripheral vascular disease and surgical sympathectomy.

Closure

- Thank the patient.
- Elicit any concerns and address any questions.

60 Measuring ankle brachial pressure index

Scenario

Mr O'Neill is a 74-year-old man who has been complaining of right leg pain at rest. He is a known hypertensive and insulin-dependent diabetic. You are asked to measure his ankle brachial pressure index (ABPI).

Introduction and consent

- Introduce yourself to the patient and check his identity.
- Explain that you would like to measure his ABPI, outlining the reasons for the procedure and what it entails.
- Address any of the patient's concerns and obtain his informed consent.

Positioning the patient

- Assist the patient into a supine position with his arms exposed and shoes and socks removed.
- Ensure that the patient is comfortable, and allow him to rest for 20 minutes.

Procedure

- Wash your hands or use alcohol gel.
- Select the appropriately sized blood pressure cuff and place it around the patient's arm.
- Palpate for the brachial artery and apply ultrasound gel to the site.
- Using the Doppler probe (angled at approximately 45°), locate the brachial artery signal and inflate the cuff until the signal disappears.
- Deflate the cuff slowly (at a rate of 2–3 mmHg per second) until the signal reappears, and record this 'brachial pressure.'
- Clean the ultrasound gel from the patient's arm and repeat the same process for the other arm.
- Use the higher of the two readings to calculate the ABPI.

- Next select the appropriate sized cuff and place it around the patient's calf above the level of the malleoli, ensuring that any ulcers are covered beforehand.
- Palpate for the dorsalis pedis pulse (located between the first and second metatarsal bones) or anterior tibial pulse (located at the midpoint between the malleoli).
- Apply ultrasound gel at the site where the artery is palpable (if you are unable to palpate the artery, apply gel at the site where the artery should be palpated) and, using the Doppler probe, locate the optimal artery signal.
- Record the dorsalis pedis (DP) or anterior tibial (AT) pressure as for the brachial pressure reading.
- Palpate for the posterior tibial (PT) artery (located posterior to the medial malleolus) and apply ultrasound gel at the site where the artery is found.
- Using the Doppler probe, locate the optimal arterial signal and, as for the brachial and dorsal pedal pressures, measure and record the dorsal pedis pressure.
- Clean the ultrasound gel from the patient's leg and repeat the procedure for the other leg to obtain the DP/AT and PT pressures.
- Use the higher of the two pressure measurements to calculate the ABPI for each ankle.
- Wipe any ultrasound gel from the patient's skin, assist the patient with their clothing, and ensure that they are comfortable.
- Clean the gel from the probe.
- Wash your hands.

Closure

- Calculate the ABPI for each ankle. The ABPI is the highest pressure recorded at the ankle divided by the highest brachial pressure measured.
- Record the results in the patient's notes.
- Tell the patient the findings of the investigation, and address any questions or concerns they may have, as well as discussing further management (e.g. referral to a vascular specialist, Duplex arterial mapping, angiography, medical optimisation of risk factors for peripheral vascular disease).
- Thank the patient.
- Turn to the examiner and summarise your findings and your interpretation.

Interpreting ABPI measurements

- Normal ABPI value is > 1.0.
- ABPI values are falsely elevated in diabetics, in whom blood vessels are calcified and therefore incompressible.
- An ABPI value of < 0.9 suggests a degree of peripheral vascular disease.
- An ABPI value in the range 0.5–0.9 is seen in intermittent claudication.
- An ABPI value of < 0.5 suggests the presence of severe peripheral vascular disease, associated with rest pain, gangrene and ulcers.

---

61 Twelve-lead ECG

Scenario

Mr Young is a 74-year-old man who presents to Accident and Emergency with central chest pain. You are asked to perform an ECG.

Introduction and consent

- Introduce yourself to the patient and confirm their identity.
- Discuss the procedure, explaining the reason for the investigation and what it entails, and obtain informed consent.

Positioning the patient

- Wash your hands or use alcohol gel.
- Assist the patient into a supine position and ensure that they are comfortable.

Preparation

- Read the instructions on the ECG machine and familiarise yourself with the machine.
- Check that there is paper in the machine and that it functions.
- Gather the following equipment:
  - disposable adhesive electrode pads
  - alcohol swabs
  - razor.

- Ask the patient to remove any jewellery that may interfere with the ECG reading.
- Adequately expose the chest and limbs.
- Ensure that the lead attachment sites are clean, and shave any chest hair if necessary.

Procedure

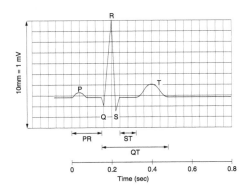

Figure 10   Twelve-lead ECG.

- Attach four limb electrodes proximal to the ankles and wrists over a bony prominence, and connect the limb leads from the ECG to each electrode. These are usually colour coded as follows:
  - AVR to the right arm (red)
  - AVL to the left arm (yellow)
  - AVF to the left leg (green)
  - neutral to the right leg (black)

  Note that this is the colour of traffic lights moving clockwise from right to left.
- Apply six electrodes to the chest at the following sites, and subsequently attach the corresponding (brown) chest lead from the ECG machine:
  - V1 – fourth intercostal space, right sternal edge
  - V2 – fourth intercostal space, left sternal edge
  - V3 – midway between V2 and V4
  - V4 – fifth intercostal space, mid-clavicular line
  - V5 – left anterior axillary line, between V4 and V6
  - V6 – fifth intercostal space, mid-axillary line
- Ensure that the ECG machine is set at a paper speed of 25 mm/second and calibrated to 10 mm/mV.

- Ask the patient to relax and keep still in order to reduce artefacts in the trace, and obtain a 12-lead recording with a longer rhythm strip (lead II).
- Check the quality of the recording and repeat if necessary.
- Detach the ECG printout and label it with the patient's full name, date of birth, hospital number and any other useful information (e.g. symptoms). Also record the date and time if this has not been done already.

Closure

- Indicate to the patient that the investigation is complete.
- Detach the leads and the electrode pads.
- Ensure that the patient is comfortable.
- Dispose of the clinical waste appropriately.
- Wash your hands or use alcohol gel.
- Interpret the ECG and discuss your findings and further management with the patient.

The ECG

P-wave

- First deflection preceding QRS complex.
- Represents atrial depolarisation.
- Normally inverted in AVR.
- Bifid P-wave (P-mitrale) suggests left atrial hypertrophy.
- Peaked P-wave (P-pulmonale) suggests right atrial hypertrophy.

QRS complex

- Represents ventricular depolarisation.
- Normal value is < 0.12 seconds.
- A value of > 0.12 seconds suggests bundle branch block.

Q-wave

- First negative deflection of the QRS complex.
- Normal if < 0.04 seconds wide; normal in leads AVR, II and V1.
- Pathological Q-waves seen in acute myocardial infarction.

R-wave

- First positive deflection.

S-wave

- Negative deflection following R-wave.

T-wave

- Represents ventricular repolarisation.
- Normally inverted in AVR; pathological if inverted in other leads.
- 'Tented' in hyperkalaemia and flattened in hypokalaemia.
- Inversion seen in subendocardial myocardial infarction, ischaemia, pulmonary embolism, left ventricular hypertrophy, left bundle branch block, right bundle branch block.

Interpretation of the ECG: the basics

- Before starting, confirm the following:
  - patient's name and date of birth
  - date and time of investigation
  - patient's symptoms at the time of the investigation (i.e. chest pain or pain free).
- Check the calibration. With the machine set at 25 mm/seconds
  - each small square equals 0.04 seconds
  - each large square equals 0.2 seconds.

The following information should then be extracted systematically.

Rate

- Rate equals 300 divided by the number of large squares per R-R interval.
- Normal rate = 60–100 beats/minute.
- A rate of < 60 beats/minute is a bradycardia.
- A rate of > 100 beats/minute is a tachycardia.

Rhythm

- P-waves preceding each QRS complex indicate sinus rhythm.
- An absence of P-waves suggests atrial fibrillation.

Axis

- The sum of vectors of electrical depolarisation of the ventricles.

- Normal axis is between −30 and 105 degrees.
- As a general rule of thumb, look at the lead AVF and the QRS in lead I:
  - normal axis: QRS is positive in I and positive in AVF
  - left axis deviation: QRS is positive in I and negative in AVF
  - right axis deviation: QRS is negative in I and positive in AVF.

QRS complex (see Figure 10)

Assess duration and look for pathological Q-waves.

Intervals

- PR:
  - period from start of P-wave to start of the QRS complex
  - normal range is 0.12–0.20 seconds
  - if prolonged, this suggests atrioventricular conduction defect
  - if shortened, this suggests fast atrioventricular conduction (e.g Wolff–Parkinson–White syndrome).
- ST:
  - period between the end of QRS and start of T-wave
  - normally isoelectric
  - in general, elevation by > 1 mm suggests myocardial infarction and depression by > 0.5 mm suggests ischaemia.
- QT:
  - period from start of QRS to end of T-wave
  - normal value is less than half the R-R interval
  - prolonged in ischaemia, myocarditis and bradycardia.

T-waves

Look for T-wave inversion.

Finally, summarise your findings.

62 Sizing a hard collar

Scenario

Mr Brock is a 40-year-old motorcyclist who was involved in a road traffic accident. You have found him at the scene and have been asked by the ambulance crew to immobilise his cervical spine.

Introduction and consent

- Introduce yourself to the patient (if he is conscious), and explain that you are going to fit a collar around his neck to protect his spine.
- In an emergency situation you are acting in the patient's best interest, and obtaining consent may not be possible or appropriate.
- Take universal precautions.
- Ask a colleague to maintain in-line immobilisation with the neck held in a neutral position.
- Measure the height from the angle of the patient's jaw to his shoulder using your hand.
- This distance should correspond to the distance between the lower border of the plastic portion of the hard collar and the plastic 'measuring post' in the appropriate size hard collar.
- The one-piece hard collar, which is flat-packed, is then applied by sliding it under the patient's neck and fastening it at the front.
- Three-point fixation to maintain the alignment of the spine should then be performed using sandbags/a head immobiliser on either side of the head, taped to the head and spinal board/trolley.
- The patient should be maintained in a hard collar until the cervical spine is cleared, and this should be explained to the patient if he is conscious.

Cervical spine immobilisation

Cervical spine immobilisation using a one-piece hard collar (stiff collar) and three-point fixation forms part of the initial management of patients in the trauma setting.

Indications

- The unconscious patient with a history of trauma.
- The conscious patient with:
  - a significant mechanism of spinal injury
  - polytrauma
  - significant injury above the clavicles
  - a history of neck trauma
  - neck tenderness
  - a decreased range of neck movements due to neck pain and neurological deficit.

In reality, all patients involved in trauma will have their cervical spine immobilised until it is cleared clinically and/or radiologically (with AP, lateral and odontoid views).

63 Urinary catheterisation

Scenario 1

Mr Bloggs is a 70-year-old man who underwent an inguinal hernia repair 1 day ago. He has not been able to pass urine for the past 10 hours, and is now complaining of abdominal pain. You have been asked to insert a catheter for him.

Introduction and establishment of rapport

Introduce yourself to the patient. For example, Hello, Mr Bloggs, my name is Karen Moss – I am a medical student. I understand that you had a hernia operation yesterday and you haven't been able to pass urine for the past 10 hours.

Confirmation of indication for catheterisation

- Establish whether the patient:
  - is in pain (and establish the site of pain)
  - experienced problems passing urine prior to surgery
  - has any history of prostate disease
  - has had a catheter inserted before.
- Offer to examine the patient's abdomen for a palpable bladder.

Indications for catheterisation

- Therapeutic:
  - to relieve urinary retention
  - for bladder irrigation (e.g. to remove clots or infection)
  - to monitor urine output (e.g. in cases of sepsis or dehydration)
  - to administer drugs (e.g. βHCG in bladder cancer).
- Diagnostic:
  - to perform investigations (e.g. cystogram).

Contraindication to catheterisation
Urethral disruption seen following pelvic trauma.

Explanation and consent

Explain to the patient that you wish to insert a urinary catheter, describe the procedure and obtain verbal consent.

For example, *Mr Bloggs, I would like to insert a catheter – a narrow tube – into your penis and into your bladder to drain the urine and so relieve the pain that you're experiencing. The procedure can be uncomfortable, and I will inject some local anaesthetic into the penis before I insert the tube, which should help. Do you have any questions?*

Positioning the patient

- For female patients, request the presence of a chaperone.
- Ensure that there is total privacy.
- The patient should be supine.
- In male patients, the legs should be extended. In females, the knees should be bent with the heels together and the thighs abducted.
- The patient's dignity should be maintained while you are preparing the equipment.

Preparation of equipment

- Wash your hands.
- Position yourself with your back to the patient and the procedure trolley in front of you.
- Open the non-sterile outer packaging of the catherisation pack and slide the sterile pack on to the procedure trolley.
- While maintaining asepsis, open the catherisation pack, thereby creating a sterile field. Pour sterile chlorhexidine solution into one of the galley pots in the pack, and open the following items on to the sterile field:
  - lignocaine gel
  - a 10-ml syringe to inflate the catheter balloon
  - a Foley catheter (the smallest practicable urinary catheter is used, typically 12-gauge in females and 14-gauge in males).

Procedure

- Put on sterile gloves.
- Place the sterile drapes (found in the pack) around the patient's perineum and thighs to create a sterile field around the penis in male patients, or the labia in female patients.

- For male patients, using your gloved hand closest to the patient (and/ or a swab), retract the foreskin and hold the penis until the procedure is complete. In the case of female patients, this hand should be used to hold the labia apart.
- The hand that is used to hold the penis or labia should not touch the catheter.
- For male patients, the 'clean' gloved hand should then be used to clean the glans penis with cotton swabs soaked in chlorhexidine solution. In female patients, the urethral meatus should be cleaned from the pubis towards the anus to avoid contamination from the perineum.
- Advise the patient of what you are about to do: *I am just about to clean the area. It will feel cold.*
- Holding the penis perpendicular to the body, the 'clean' hand should then introduce the nozzle of the lignocaine lubricating gel into the urethral meatus and discharge approximately 30–50 ml of gel into the urethra.
- Ideally, wait for 5 minutes for the local anaesthetic to take effect.
- Advise the patient: *I have injected the local anaesthetic gel. You may experience some burning sensation. It will take a few minutes to numb the area.*
- A sterile receiver containing the catheter should then be placed between the patient's legs, and the 'clean' hand should be used to insert the catheter.
- The catheter should be gently advanced to the hilt, and resistance may be felt at the level of the external sphincter/prostate.
- When urine is seen to flow, the balloon should be gently inflated with 5–10 ml of sterile water, after which the catheter should be slowly withdrawn so that the balloon rests at the bladder neck.
- Send a sample of urine for microscopy, culture and sensitivities (MC&S).
- The catheter should then be attached to a drainage system (e.g. leg bag, urometer or drainage bag) and secured.
- Replace the foreskin.
- Ensure that the patient is comfortable and that their modesty is restored.

Complications of urinary catheterisation

Immediate complications

- Failure to catheterise
- Bleeding
- Urethral and prostatic trauma (premature balloon inflation)

Early complications

- Infection
- Blockage
- Paraphimosis (failure to replace foreskin)

Late complications

- False passage
- Long-term catheter

Disposal of clinical waste

Dispose of all waste in the yellow clinical waste bags provided.

Documentation

Typical catheter procedure note

Date: 23 December 2006
Time: 17.00 hours
Indication: Urethral catheterisation for post-operative acute urinary retention
Procedure: Aseptic technique

- 14-gauge two-way catheter inserted
- Atraumatic; foreskin replaced.
- Residual volume 600 ml clear urine.

Signed: K Moss (medical student), Bleep 007

Closure

- Explain to the patient that you have successfully inserted a catheter, and describe the plan for the future. For example, *The catheter will remain for a further 48 hours to give you time to recover from the operation, and then we will take the catheter out.*
- Ask the patient whether they have any questions.

Classification of catheters

Catheters can be classified as two- or three-way, and can be made from latex, rubber or silastic (i.e. for long-term use).

Two-way catheter

- Two ports – one for balloon inflation and the other for drainage.
- Used to relieve obstruction and to monitor urine output.
- Typically 12- to 18-gauge.

Three-way catheter

- Three ports – the first for balloon inflation, the second for irrigation and the third for drainage.
- Used for bladder irrigation (e.g. in cases of clot retention).
- Typically 22- to 26-gauge.

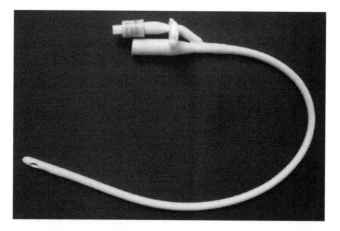

Figure 11   (a) Two-way catheter.

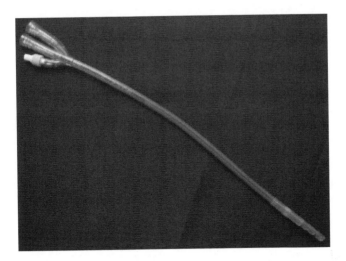

Figure 11   (b) Three-way catheter.

64 Suprapubic catheterisation (SPC)

Although it is unlikely that you will be asked to insert a suprapubic catheter, you may be asked to describe SPC insertion as part of a 'describing instruments' station.

Indications for SPC catheterisation

- Failed urethral catheterisation.
- Relative indication: urinary incontinence.

Contraindications to SPC catheterisation

- Bladder tumour.

Scenario

'Can you tell me what this is and what it is used for?'

This is a 16 French Ingram trocar suprapubic catheter. I've seen it used in suprapubic catheterisation where urethral catheterisation has failed.

Introduction and consent

- Introduce yourself to the patient.
- Explain the procedure and obtain verbal consent.
- Confirm the need for an SPC catheter.

Positioning the patient

- Ensure that the patient's dignity and privacy are maintained at all times.
- Assist the patient into a supine position.
- Examine the patient's abdomen and ensure that the bladder is distended and palpable between the pubis and the umbilicus.
- Check that the lighting is adequate.

Preparing the equipment

Gather the following:

- SPC catheter
- lumbar puncture needle (12–16 French)
- lignocaine (2%)
- 2 × 5 ml syringes
- 26-gauge needle
- dressing pack
- sterile water
- 1/0 silk suture
- urinary drain
- Betadine solution
- sterile gloves and gown.

Procedure

- Aseptic techniques should be used throughout.
- Scrub up and gown.
- Prepare the abdomen with Betadine and use the drapes provided in the dressing pack to create a sterile field.
- Starting with a 26-gauge needle, create a bleb with the local anaesthetic two finger breadths above the pubic symphysis. Switch to a larger, 18-gauge needle and infiltrate the deeper structures, remembering to withdraw gently before injecting any anaesthetic in order to avoid inadvertent injection into a blood vessel. Finally, aspirate a few millilitres of urine from the bladder.

- Wait 5 minutes for the local anaesthetic to take effect.
- Using a scalpel, make a small stab incision over the anaesthetised area at the point at which the needle was withdrawn.
- Using your right hand, insert the trocar catheter perpendicular to the skin, controlling the depth of penetration with your left hand.
- Once the bladder has been entered, urine will be seen to fill the catheter, and the latter should then be fully advanced into the bladder and the trocar withdrawn.
- Inflate the catheter balloon with 10 ml of water and connect the catheter to a drainage bag.
- Suture the catheter into position using the 1/0 silk stitch and the flange of the catheter.

Closure

- Thank the patient and ensure that they are comfortable.
- Explain that you have completed the procedure.
- Record the procedure and the residual volume in the patient's notes.
- Send a urine sample for microscopy and culture.

Complications of suprapubic catheterisation

- Failure of procedure
- Bleeding
- Infection
- Perforation of bowel
- Perforation of abdominal aorta

---

65 Urinalysis and interpretation

Scenario

Mr Bloggs has been complaining of a burning sensation when passing urine, and increased urinary frequency. He has been asked to produce a midstream urine sample, and you are asked to perform a urinalysis (urine dipstick) and discuss the results with the patient.

Introduction and consent

- Introduce yourself to the patient and indicate your intention to test his urine.
- Check the patient's name and date of birth against his notes and the sample bottle.
- Wash your hands and put on gloves.

Procedure

- Take the urine sample and assess its appearance: colour, turbidity and odour.

Appearance	Causes
Straw-coloured	Normal
Colourless	Diabetes insipidus Diuretics Excessive fluid intake
Dark	Acute intermittent porphyria Malignant melanoma
Cloudy	Pyuria (urinary tract infection) Blood Mucus Bilirubin
Pink/red	Blood/haemoglobin Myoglobin Beetroot
Orange	Rifampicin Bile pigments
Brown/black	Myoglobin Bile pigments Melanin Iron Nitrofurantoin
Green	Methylene blue Urobilinogen

- Open the specimen bottle and immerse the urine dipstick supplied (Labstix, Chemstix, etc.) into the urine for 1–2 seconds, ensuring that all of the pads are immersed, and then withdraw it.
- Start timing, keeping the dipstick horizontal throughout.
- Close the specimen bottle tightly and put it to one side.

- Read the results according to the colour chart and instructions on the urinalysis bottle. You may need to wait up to 60 seconds before reading some results (the times should be indicated on the chart).
- Do not touch the bottle with the reagent stick.
- Urinalysis dipsticks can test for pH, the specific gravity of the urine (an indicator of renal concentrating ability), and the presence of blood, glucose, ketones, nitrites, protein, bilirubin, urobilinogen and leucocytes.
- *The patient's urine is cloudy in appearance and offensive smelling, and contains nitrites and leucocytes.*
- Discard the urine dipstick appropriately in a clinical waste bag.
- Document your findings in the patient's notes.

Parameter	Value	Causes
pH	pH 5–8	Normal
	Acidic (< 5)	High-protein diet Acidosis (ketoacidosis) Renal tubular acidosis
	Alkaline (> 8)	UTI (urea-splitting organisms, e.g. *Proteus* spp.) Metabolic alkalosis (e.g. due to vomiting)
Specific gravity	Increased	Volume depletion Congestive heart failure Adrenal insufficiency SIADH Excretion of contrast media
	Decreased	Diabetes insipidus Pyelonephritis and/or glomerulonephritis Water overload
Bilirubin/urobilinogen	Positive	Obstructive jaundice Hepatitis/cirrhosis Blood

continued

Parameter	Value	Causes
	Positive	Urinary tract stones Trauma Tumours Coagulopathy Contamination (due to menses) Infection Instrumentation Haemolytic anaemia Transfusion reaction Polycystic kidneys/ interstitial nephritis
Glucose	Positive	Diabetes mellitus Pancreatitis Shock, burns, pain Endocrine disorders
Ketones	Positive	Starvation High-fat diet DKA Pregnancy Febrile states
Nitrites	Positive	Infection (bacteria convert nitrates to nitrites)
Protein	Positive	Renal tract disease (e.g. nephrotic syndrome) Myeloma Pre-eclampsia Malignant hypertension Fever, stress, heavy exercise Postural proteinuria
Leucocytes	Positive	UTI

UTI, urinary tract infection; SIADH, syndrome of inappropriate antidiuretic hormone secretion; DKA, diabetic ketoacidosis.

Closure

- Indicate your findings to the examiner and the patient.
- *Mr Bloggs, your urine has tested positive for both white blood cells and nitrites, which along with your history suggests that you have a urinary tract infection. I will send the rest of your urine sample for further testing (microscopy and culture) to see if any organisms can*

be grown, and I would like to start you on a 1-week course of antibiotics. It is also important that you drink plenty of water to help flush the infection through, and if you find that your symptoms are not getting better or are getting worse, or you develop a temperature, please come back and see me.

- Ask the patient whether they have any questions or concerns.
- Offer to label and complete the appropriate microbiology forms for the urine microscopy and culture.
- Tell the patient that the results of the urine test will be available in approximately 2 days, and that you will contact him with the findings.
- If a prescription pad is available, you may need to prescribe the antibiotics. It is important to check for any allergies before doing this.
- Finally, thank the patient.

Midstream urine (MSU) collection (guidance for patients)

In order to obtain an MSU specimen:

- The patient's bladder should be full.
- Your hands should be washed beforehand.
- In female patients, the labia are separated and the vulva cleaned from front to back with sterile swabs. The labia are then separated with the non-dominant hand.
- In male patients, the foreskin (if present) is retracted and the glans penis is cleaned using sterile swabs.
- The patient then voids into the toilet pan.
- When they are halfway through voiding, while the urine is freely flowing (i.e. without stopping), the sterile container should be placed directly in the stream using the dominant hand and a sample of urine collected.
- Voiding should then be completed into the toilet pan.
- Samples for urinalysis should be less than 1 hour old, or else refrigerated after collection.

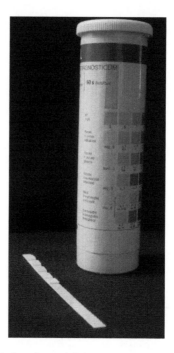

Figure 12   Urinalysis bottle and Stix.

66 Nasogastric (NG) tubes

Scenario

Mr Frith is a 78-year-old man who has recently suffered a stroke, since which he has had difficulty swallowing. You have been asked to insert a nasogastric tube for feeding.

Indications for insertion of a nasogastric tube

- Gastric lavage (e.g. following drug overdose).
- To reduce the risk of aspiration.
- Feeding.
- Gastrointestinal decompression (e.g. ileus, obstruction or post-operatively).

Introduction and consent

- Introduce yourself to the patient, confirm their identity and establish a rapport.
- Explain the procedure and obtain informed verbal consent.
- *Hello, my name is Tom Jones and I am a medical student. I have been asked to insert a nasogastric tube. This is a narrow tube which passes through your nasal passage, down the back of your mouth and into your stomach. This will enable us to feed you since you have been having problems swallowing. Would this be all right? Do you have any questions at all?*
- Allow the patient time to express any concerns.

Positioning the patient

- Assist the patient into an upright sitting position and ensure that he is comfortable.

Preparing the equipment

Gather the following:

- nasogastric tube of choice (in this case a feeding tube)
- lubricant KY Jelly
- catheter-tipped syringe
- glass of water
- stethoscope.

Types of nasogastric tube

Wide bore (e.g. Ryles tube)

- Can be single or double lumen.
- Size varies (10–18 French).
- Has perforations at tip and sides for aspiration.
- Can be attached to suction.
- Has radio-opaque markings.
- Designed for short-term use.

Fine bore (e.g. feeding tube)

- Smaller diameter (6–8 French).
- More pliable and comfortable.

- Can be used for up to 6 months.
- Has radio-opaque stylet.

Sengstaken–Blakemore tube

- Triple-lumen tube
- Used to tamponade bleeding oesophageal varices.
- One lumen is for gastric aspiration, and the other two are for the gastric and oesophageal balloons, respectively.

Procedure

- Wash your hands and put on gloves.
- Measure the anticipated length for which the tube will need to be inserted by measuring the cumulative distance from the patient's ear to their nose and then to two finger breadths above their umbilicus.
- Lubricate the distal few centimetres of the tube with KY Jelly.
- Stand on the same side of the patient as the nostril into which the tube will be inserted.
- Give the patient the glass of water and ask them to sip some water when they feel the tube is at the back of their mouth (oropharynx).
- Insert the tube gently into the nostril aiming towards the occiput (*not* upwards).
- Advance the tube a few centimetres at a time and continue as the patient swallows, but stop advancing and withdraw if the patient starts to cough.
- Stop once the tube is in the stomach (at approximately 30 cm).
- Check that the nasogastric tube is in the correct position before use. The position of fine-bore feeding tubes can only be confirmed using a chest X-ray, and they are packaged with a radio-opaque guidewire which needs to be removed prior to commencing feeding.
- Tape the nasogastric tube securely to the nose (avoiding the ala) and the side of the face.
- In the case of a nasogastric drainage tube, attach a drainage bag following insertion.
- Dispose of any clinical waste appropriately.

Closure

- Thank the patient. Explain that the nasogastric tube has been successfully inserted and that a chest X-ray will need to be taken prior to feeding.

Complications of nasogastric tube insertion

- Inadvertent passage into the trachea.
- Failure of insertion.
- Coiling of the tube in the oropharynx.
- Ischaemic necrosis of the nose.
- Bleeding.
- Intracranial passage through the cribriform plate (associated with basal skull fractures).

Methods of checking the position of the nasogastric tube

- Aspirate the nasogastric tube using a 50-ml syringe for stomach contents.
- Test the aspirate with litmus paper. If the pH is < 5, this is indicative of gastric contents (this method is inaccurate if the patient is on a proton pump inhibitor).
- Push 10 ml of air via syringe through the nasogastric tube while auscultating over the stomach.
- Take a chest X-ray, looking for the radio-opaque guidewire or tip in the stomach.

67 Digital rectal examination, proctoscopy and rigid sigmoidoscopy

Scenario

Mr Smith is a 67-year-old man with a history of bright red rectal bleeding. He has presented in clinic, and you are asked to perform a rectal examination, proctoscopy and rigid sigmoidoscopy.

Introduction and consent

- Introduce yourself to the patient and check their identity.
- Explain the need to perform the procedure, outlining the risks and benefits, and obtain the patient's verbal consent.
- Ascertain whether the patient is taking anticoagulants (a contraindication to biopsy), or has a heart valve or prostheses (in which case the patient will require antibiotic prophylaxis if a biopsy is taken).
- A chaperone will be required for female patients.

Positioning

- Assist the patient into a left lateral decubitus position, with their spine parallel to and at the edge of the bed and their knees drawn up to their chest.

Preparation

- Wash your hands and put on a pair of gloves.
- Gather the following equipment:
  - KY Jelly
  - tissues
  - occult blood stool test kit
  - proctoscope (consisting of an obturator, barrel and light source)
  - rigid sigmoidoscope (consisting of an obturator, barrel, light source and hand-held insufflation pump).

Procedure

- Talk to the patient throughout the procedure, and signpost your actions.
- Part the buttocks and examine the perianal region for:
  - skin tags
  - warts
  - fistulas
  - excoriation
  - prolapsed haemarrhoids
  - sentinel pile.
- Perform a digital rectal examination.
  - Apply KY Jelly to your index finger.
  - Introduce the pad of the index finger into the anus, assessing for pain (e.g. due to anal fissure).

- Palpate the posterior and then lateral rectal walls for masses and ulcers.
- Bend at the knees and rotate the index finger to palpate the anterior rectal wall for masses (cervix in females and prostate gland in males).
- Note any blood or faeces on withdrawal of the gloved finger.
- Perform a proctoscopy (this visualises the last 12 cm of the rectum).
  - Apply KY Jelly to the tip of the proctoscope.
  - Advance the proctoscope past the anal verge, and when the instrument is completely inserted remove the obturator.
  - Attach the light source and under direct vision slowly withdraw the instrument while checking the mucosa for ulcers, haemorrhoids (typically at the 3, 7 and 11 o'clock positions) and strictures.
  - If haemorrhoids are seen, they may be banded or injected with 2% phenol in almond oil using a Gabriel's needle.
- Perform a rigid sigmoidoscopy (this visualises the distal 40 cm).
  - Apply KY Jelly to the distal end of the sigmoidoscope.
  - Disposable sigmoidoscopes are lubricated by placing them under warm water.
  - Introduce the sigmoidoscope, aiming towards the umbilicus, and advance 2–3 cm beyond the internal anal sphincter.
  - Remove the obturator and attach the eyepiece, light source and insufflator.
  - Under direct vision with the aid of insufflation, advance the sigmoidoscope, following the curve of the sigmoid towards the sacrum past the rectosigmoid junction (identified by a change from smooth to concentric mucosa).
  - Advance as far as possible, and stop if the patient experiences pain.
  - Observe the mucosa for polyps, strictures, ulceration, bleeding and masses.
  - A biopsy can be taken for histology if a suspicious area is identified.
  - Release the air and withdraw the sigmoidoscope while continuing to observe.
- Assist the patient with any clothing, and ensure that they are comfortable.
- Dispose of the clinical waste appropriately.
- Wash your hands.

Closure

- Explain to the patient that the procedure is complete, and advise them of any findings and the next steps in their management (e.g. biopsy results, follow-up, further investigations). Address any questions or concerns that they may have.
- Tell the patient that they may experience mild cramps and bleeding per rectally, and advise them to avoid using laxatives for 1 week if a biopsy has been taken.
- Document the procedure in the patient's notes.

Complications

- Bleeding
- Perforation (rare)

---

68 Performing a Papanicolaou (PAP) smear test

Scenario

Mrs Jones is a 30-year-old woman who is attending her general practice for a routine cervical smear test.

Introduction and consent

- Introduce yourself to the patient and check their identity.
- Explain the need to perform the procedure and obtain their verbal consent.
- A female chaperone will be required.

Papanicolaou smear

- This is part of the national screening programme for pre-malignant disease (cervical intra-epithelial neoplasia, CIN).
- Cytology detects dyskaryosis.
- If dyskaryosis is moderate or severe, colposcopy is recommended. If it is mild, the smear should be repeated.
- Three-yearly screening is indicated between the ages of 20 and 60 years.
- If the patient is at high risk, annual screening is indicated.

Position

- The patient should be positioned supine with the knees bent and the heels together with the thighs abducted.
- Ensure that the patient is comfortable, with their underwear removed, and maintain their modesty until the actual procedure.
- Check that the lighting is adequate.

Preparation

- Wash your hands and put on a pair of gloves.
- Gather the following equipment:
  - vaginal speculum
  - slides, alcohol fixative
  - cervical spatula (Ayre's).

Procedure

- Talk to the patient throughout the procedure and warn them of each step beforehand.
- Observe the perineum for ulcers, warts and swellings.
- Separate the labia and inspect the clitoris, vestibule (for herpetic vesicles), urethral meatus (for Bartholin's cyst/abscess) and vaginal orifice (for discharge and prolapse).
- Warm the speculum with water and test the temperature against the patient's thigh.
- Insert the speculum at a 45° angle to the horizontal, part the labia and advance the speculum fully.
- Open the speculum to reveal the cervix.
- Inspect the cervix and vagina for masses, cysts and atrophy, and note the size, colour and shape of the cervical os.
- Rotate the Ayre's spatula 360° around the external os to obtain a sample of cells from the squamo-columnar junction.
- Smear the sample on to a frosted slide and fix the sample using alcohol.
- Using an endocervical brush, obtain another sample – this time from the endocervical canal.
- Smear the sample on to a slide and fix using alcohol as before.
- Remove the speculum and assess the mucosa of the vaginal wall on withdrawing.
- Assist the patient with any clothing and ensure that they are comfortable.

- Label the slides obtained with the patient's name, date of birth and hospital number.
- Dispose of the clinical waste appropriately.
- Wash your hands.

Closure

- Explain to the patient that the procedure is complete, tell them about any findings, and advise them of the next steps in their management (e.g. results, follow-up, further investigations).
- Tell the patient that they may experience some spotting of blood, and address any questions or concerns that they may have.
- Complete the appropriate investigation forms.
- Document the procedure in the patient's notes.

69 Measuring blood glucose

Scenario

Mrs Smith is a known insulin-dependent diabetic who has just had an incisional hernia repair. She has not started eating and drinking yet, and is on a subcutaneous insulin sliding scale. You are asked to measure her blood sugar level and manage her appropriately.

Introduction and consent

- Introduce yourself to the patient and establish a rapport.
- Indicate to the patient that you would like to measure her capillary blood glucose level, and obtain her verbal consent.
- *Hello, Mrs Smith. My name is Tom Jones and I'm a medical student. I've been asked to check your blood sugar. Would that be OK?*

Preparation of equipment

Prepare the following equipment:

- glucose meter – turn the meter on and insert a fresh enzyme-impregnated reagent strip
- attach a new lancet to the spring-loaded delivery device provided
- alcohol swab
- cotton wool.

Procedure

- Ask the patient to wash their hands.
- Make sure that the patient is seated comfortably.
- Wash your hands and put on gloves.
- Using an alcohol swab, clean the patient's fingertip and allow the alcohol to dry.
- Apply the spring-loaded lancet device firmly to the pulp/palmar aspect of the patient's finger. Warn the patient that they will feel a 'sharp scratch', and release the trigger.
- Dispose of the lancet in the sharps bin provided.
- Squeeze the patient's finger to express more blood. The resulting droplet should be transferred from the patient's finger on to the reagent strip. A cotton wool pad should then be applied to the finger and pressure applied.
- The glucose meter should count down to give a reading of capillary blood glucose levels.
- *The capillary blood glucose level (BM) is 16.7.*
- Dispose of the clinical waste appropriately.
- Advise the patient of their BM result.

Closure

- Document the BM in the notes.
- Thank the patient and ensure that they are comfortable. Inform them as to what will happen next, and elicit any concerns.
- *Thank you, Mrs Smith. Your blood sugar is on the high side – it is 16.7. I understand that you are taking insulin to control your blood sugar. I am just going to discuss your BM result with one of my senior colleagues, and then I will come back and talk to about what the plan is. Do you have any questions?*
- Offer to notify your senior colleagues of the result.

Your Registrar advises you that the patient is on a subcutaneous insulin sliding scale (see table below), and advises you to consult this and administer the appropriate amount of insulin (subcutaneous injection will be tackled separately). Calculate the amount of insulin which needs to be administered.

Blood sugar concentration	Rate (U/hour)
0.0–3.5	0
3.5–5.0	1
5.0–7.0	2
7.0–10.0	3
10.0–15.0	4
15.0–20.0	5
> 20	Call doctor

- Insulin is administered using a subcutaneous sliding scale every 4 hours. If the patient's blood sugar level is 16.7, they require 5 units in 1 hour, and therefore a dose of 20 units subcutaneously.

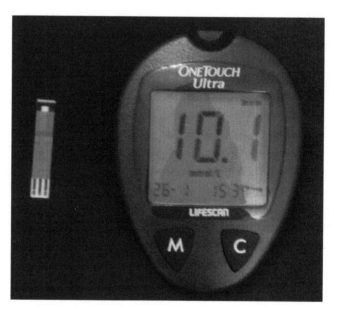

Figure 13   Blood glucose monitor.

70 Venepuncture

Scenario

Mr Thomas is being seen in a haematology clinic. He is on warfarin for a deep vein thrombosis, and you have been asked to take a blood sample from him to check his INR (international normalised ratio).

Introduction

- Introduce yourself to the patient and establish a rapport.
- Indicate to the patient that you would like to take a blood sample from him, and explain the reasons for the blood test.
- *Hello Mr Thomas, my name is Karen Moss and I'm a medical student. I understand that you are taking warfarin to treat a deep vein thrombosis (DVT), and I've been asked to take some blood from you so that we can check your INR, which tells us how thin your blood is.*

Consent

- Explain the procedure to the patient and obtain their verbal consent.
- *You've probably had this done before, but I will need to apply a tourniquet to your arm and insert a needle into one of your veins and withdraw some blood. Would that be OK? Do you have any questions?*
- Allow the patient time to ask questions and to express any concerns about the procedure.
- Confirm the patient's identity (name, date of birth and address).
- Talk to the patient throughout the procedure (even if a mannequin is used).

Preparation of equipment

Gather the following equipment and check that the packaging is intact:

- syringe and green/blue needle or a vacutainer and green/blue needle (or butterfly needle)
- the appropriate blood bottle (a blue-topped clotting bottle)
- alcohol swab
- cotton wool
- plaster

- tourniquet
- sharps container.

Positioning the patient

- Ensure that there is adequate lighting and privacy.
- Ask the patient to either sit in a chair or lie on a bed, and help them into a comfortable position.
- Select an arm (never draw blood proximal to an intravenous drip site, as the infusion invalidates the blood results), and place a pillow underneath the arm to support it.
- Make sure that the arm is adequately exposed and that any constricting clothing proximally is removed.

Procedure

- Wash your hands and put on a pair of gloves.
- Apply the tourniquet above the elbow (or at least 2–3 cm above the venepuncture site) and tighten it.
- Ask the patient to clench and unclench their hand to engorge and therefore accentuate the veins.
- Identify the target vein by palpation and/or visually.
- Clean the potential puncture site with an alcohol swab, using a circular motion, moving away from the centre to the periphery. Do not re-palpate this site once it has been cleaned.
- Allow the alcohol to evaporate.
- Select the appropriate size needle (blue/green or butterfly needle) and attach the needle to the syringe (or vacutainer).
- Unsheathe the needle and, holding the skin around the vein taut, advance the needle at an oblique 20–30° angle through the skin and subcutaneous fat into the vein.
- Gently draw back on the syringe while advancing it, and a flashback should be seen at the base of the syringe when the needle is successfully positioned in the vein. No flashback is seen with a vacutainer.
- Holding the needle and syringe (or vacutainer) still in the arm, withdraw the plunger of the syringe (or attach a blood bottle to the vacutainer) until enough blood is obtained.
- Release the tourniquet first, and then place a cotton wool ball above the venepuncture site and remove the needle.
- Apply digital pressure at the puncture site for approximately 1 minute using the cotton wool ball.

- As the patient is on warfarin, pressure may need to be applied for longer.
- Once the bleeding has stopped, apply a plaster to the venepuncture site, ensuring beforehand that the patient is not allergic to the plaster to be used.
- Decant the blood in the syringe into the blood bottle. Note that the clotting bottle needs to be filled to the top (approximately 4.5 ml).
- Transfer the sharps into the sharps container, and dispose of any other clinical waste appropriately.

Closure

- Label the blood bottle with the patient's details (name, date of birth, hospital number and date of sample), complete the accompanying request form (details of the patient's consultant and a brief clinical summary, e.g. patient on warfarin for DVT, required test and its urgency), and offer to send it to the laboratory.
- Advise the patient that the results will be available at the end of the day and that their next dose of warfarin will be determined by today's result.
- Finally, ask the patient whether they have any questions or concerns.

Potential sites for venepuncture

- Basilic vein
- Cephalic vein
- Median cubital vein (in the antecubital fossa)
- Dorsum of the hand
- Saphenous vein (anterior to the medial malleolus)
- External jugular vein

---

71 Intravenous cannulation

Scenario

Mr Smythe is a 40-year-old man who has been admitted with dehydration secondary to Crohn's related diarrhoea. You have been asked to insert a venflon and to start the patient on an intravenous fluid infusion as prescribed.

Introduction and consent

- Introduce yourself to the patient and establish a rapport.
- Explain that you would like to insert a venflon. Discuss the procedure and the reasons for it, and obtain the patient's verbal consent.
- *Hello, Mr Smythe, my name is Clare Jones and I am a medical student. I have been asked to insert a venflon – a plastic cannula/line that will sit in one of the veins in your arm. We will then be able to give you fluids via a drip, and this will help with the management of your diarrhoea. Would that be OK?*
- Ask the patient if they have any questions or concerns.
- Maintain conversation with the patient throughout the procedure (even if a mannequin is used).

Preparing the equipment

Prepare the following equipment and check that the packaging is intact prior to opening:

- venflon (a selection of sizes – blue, pink and green)
- tourniquet
- alcohol swab
- three-way tap
- 10-ml syringe
- 10 ml 0.9% sodium chloride flush
- cotton gauze
- venflon cover
- bandage
- tape.

Positioning the patient

- Ensure that there is adequate lighting and privacy.
- Ask the patient to either sit in a chair or lie on a bed, and help them into a comfortable position.
- Select an arm and place a pillow underneath the arm to support it.
- Make sure that the arm is adequately exposed and that any constricting clothing proximally is removed.

Procedure

- Wash your hands and put on a pair of gloves.

- Unpackage the three-way tap and flush the line through with a 0.9% normal saline flush to remove any air. Leave the syringe filled with the remainder of the 0.9% normal saline attached.
- Apply the tourniquet to the arm proximal to the elbow.
- Ask the patient to clench and unclench their hand to accentuate the veins.
- Select a vein.
- Clean the potential puncture site with an alcohol swab and allow the alcohol to evaporate (wait at least 30 seconds).
- Do not re-palpate the vein after cleaning.
- Select the appropriate cannula based on the size of the vein.
- Unsheathe the needle guard and inspect the venflon for any obvious defects.
- Stabilise/anchor the vein by applying traction to the skin a couple of centimetres distal to the proposed puncture site.
- Warn the patient that they will feel a 'sharp scratch' and advise them that it is important to keep their hand as still as possible.
- Ensure that the bevel of the cannula is facing upward, and firmly puncture the skin at an oblique angle along the line of the vein to enter the vein.
- Once the vein is punctured, a flashback will be seen in the flash chamber of the stylet.
- When the flashback is seen, reduce the angle of entry and advance the cannula a few more millimetres to ensure that the needle and the tip of the cannula have entered the vein.
- Carefully withdraw the needle/stylet while advancing the cannula of the stylet into the vein.
- Release the tourniquet.
- Compress the vein using your thumb proximal to the cannula to minimise blood loss, and connect the three-way tap.
- Flush the cannula with 5 ml of 0.9% normal saline using the syringe, and observe for any leakage or swelling. Ask the patient whether they are in any discomfort.
- Secure the cannula in place with the venflon plaster. It may be easier to remove your gloves in order to do this.
- Put on a fresh pair of gloves if the previous ones were removed, and bandage the venflon securely in place.
- Discard the waste and any sharps in the sharps bin.

Closure

Explain to the patient that you have inserted the venflon/cannula and that you are now going to start some fluids.

Optimal site for intravenous cannulation

- Non-dominant upper limb is the optimal site.
- Lower limb has increased risk of thrombophlebitis.
- Avoid veins which cross a joint line, as movement at the joint will be restricted by the cannula.
- Choose a distal site so that if vein 'tissues', the line can be sited more proximally.
- Avoid the arm if it is being considered for haemodialysis.
- If no extremity vein can be found, the external jugular vein can be used. Place the patient in reverse Trendelenburg position to help to distend the vein.

---

72 Intravenous infusions

Continuation from above: The cannula has already been inserted and consent obtained to start an intravenous infusion.

- Check the patient's prescription chart for the fluid instruction.
- *The patient is prescribed a 1-litre bag of 0.9% normal saline over 8 hours.*
- Check the patient's identity by comparing the details on the drug chart with the patient's identity bracelet.
- Check to see whether the patient has any allergies.

Preparing the equipment

Gather the following equipment and ensure that the packaging is intact:

- 1 litre of 0.9% normal saline
- fluid giving set
- alcohol swab
- kidney dish.

Positioning the patient

Ensure that the patient is positioned comfortably with a pillow support-ing the 'venflon arm', and that their dignity and privacy are maintained.

Procedure

- Wash your hands and put on a pair of gloves.
- Check the expiry date on the 0.9% normal saline bag (do not use if the expiry date has passed).
- Connect the giving set to the bag of fluids by breaking the seal on the fluid bag and puncturing the bag using the pointed end of the giving set.
- Run the fluid though the tubing into a kidney dish to remove any air bubbles. Then close the tap and apply the clamp to prevent any more fluid running through.
- Clean one port of the three-way tap using an alcohol swab.
- Wait 30 seconds for the alcohol to dry, and attach the connecting tubing to the port. Open the three-way tap and unclamp the connecting tubing to allow the normal saline to run through the cannula.
- Assess for any swelling or leakage, and check that the patient is not in any discomfort.
- Set the drip to run at the desired rate by adjusting the flow through the drip chamber.
- Dispose of any waste appropriately.

Adjusting the flow rate

In large drip chambers:

- 10 drops correspond to 1 ml
- therefore 10 drops/minute = 60 ml/hour
- therefore 16 drops/minute = 100 ml/hour.

Thus for 125 ml/hour (as in the above scenario):

- adjust the flow in the chamber to 20 drops per minute.

Closure

- Sign the drug chart against the fluid prescription. Also document the date and time when the infusion was started.
- Ensure that the patient is comfortable. Explain to them that you have started the fluid infusion, and that once the fluid bag has run out they will be reassessed to see whether further intravenous fluids are necessary.
- Ask the patient whether they have any questions.

73 Setting up a syringe driver

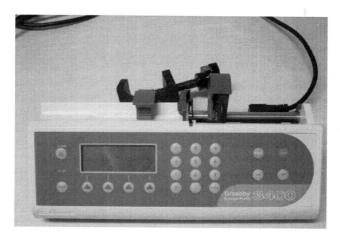

Figure 14   Syringe driver.

Scenario

Mr Grimes is a 64-year-old man with unstable angina. He has been admitted with continuous chest pain, and has been prescribed a glyceryl trinitrate (GTN) infusion (50 mg of GTN diluted in 50 ml of 0.9 % normal saline) run at a rate of 2 mg/hour (i.e. 2 ml/hour). You are asked to set up the infusion. Note: the patient has a peripheral line *in situ*.

Introduction and consent

- Introduce yourself to the patient and check their identity.

- Tell them that you are going to start an infusion of GTN. Explain that this is a medication which will help to relieve the chest pain they are experiencing.
- Advise the patient that they may experience headaches with the GTN, and that if this occurs they should inform the nursing staff, who will then alter the rate of the infusion.
- Obtain the patient's verbal consent to the procedure.
- Check the patient's drug chart and ascertain the following:
  - dose of drug, dilution and dilutant
  - rate of infusion
  - validity of prescription (signature of clinician)
  - date and time of drug administration.
- Also check whether the patient has any allergies or is being prescribed any medication which may be contraindicated with the GTN infusion (e.g. oral nitrates).

Positioning the patient

- Ensure that the patient is comfortable.
- Check that there is a cannula *in situ*.

Preparation and procedure

- Ask the nursing staff to take the patient's blood pressure (since GTN can lead to a fall in blood pressure).
- Select an infusion device and consult the manual if necessary.
- Check that the power source (mains or battery) is functioning.
- Wash your hands and put on a pair of gloves.
- Take a vial of the medication prescribed (GTN).
- Check the drug name, concentration and expiry date with a member of the nursing staff.
- Open the vial and draw up 50 mg of the drug into a 50-ml syringe which is compatible with the brand of device you have selected.
- Draw up 50 ml of 0.9% normal saline (the prescribed dilutant) into the same syringe.
- Using a sticky label, label the syringe with the drug and dilutant, the patient's name, the date and time the infusion was made up, and your signature.
- Ensure that the label does not obscure the scale or fluid level on the syringe and that it faces outwards.
- Attach the syringe to the infusion set and use the contents of the syringe to prime the tubing (expel the air in the tubing).

- Measure the length of fluid in the syringe, as this will give an indication of the time by which the infusion will run out.
- Secure the syringe on to the syringe driver, ensuring that the wings of the syringe fit snugly in the syringe slot.
- Slide the actuator until it rests against the plunger (there may be an actuator release button).
- Turn the syringe pump on.
- Set the syringe driver to the correct rate (i.e. 2 ml/hour) and turn the machine on.
- Press 'start' and check that the motor is audible, the 'on' light is flashing and the device is delivering correctly.
- Remove the bung/cap of the cannula which is *in situ*. Clean the injection port with an alcohol swab and allow the alcohol to evaporate. Flush the cannula with 5 ml of normal saline to confirm its patency.
- Attach the syringe tubing to the cannula and secure some of the tubing to the patient in order to relieve the tension and prevent the needle from being pulled out.
- Start the infusion.
- Ensure that the patient is comfortable.
- Dispose of any sharps and clinical waste appropriately.
- Wash your hands or use alcohol gel.

Closure

- Sign the drug chart and document the procedure where appropriate.
- Ask the nursing staff to monitor the infusion every 4 hours or as per hospital protocol.
- Start an infusion-monitoring chart if available.
- Explain to the patient that the infusion rate may be varied or stopped, depending on their symptoms.
- Address any concerns which may arise.

- Syringe pumps can be used for both intravenous and subcutaneous infusion sites.
- Intravenous infusions can run through either a peripheral or central line.
- In addition, certain drug infusions may be run concurrently with the use of multiple taps.

- Subcutaneous infusions can be set up at the following sites:
  - upper arm
  - anterior and posterior chest wall
  - anterior aspect of thigh
  - anterior abdominal wall.

74 Central venous line insertion

Scenario

Mr Everitt is a 55-year-old man who requires intravenous antibiotics and in whom peripheral venous cannulation has been unsuccessful. You are asked to insert a central line.

Central lines may be placed in the internal jugular, subclavian, brachial and femoral veins.

Uses of central venous line insertion

- Administration of fluids and medication.
- Administration of medication that is not tolerated peripherally (e.g. amiodarone, total parenteral nutrition).
- Measurement of central venous pressure (CVP).
- If a triple-lumen pulmonary artery (PA) catheter (Swan Ganz) is inserted, the following can be measured:
  - PA wedge pressure
  - cardiac output
  - CVP.

Introduction and consent

- Introduce yourself to the patient and check their identity.
- Explain the need to perform the procedure, outlining the risks and benefits, and obtain the patient's verbal consent.

Complications of central venous line insertion

- Pneumothorax
- Haemothorax
- Bleeding with or without haematoma
- Thrombosis of vein
- Inadvertent arterial cannulation
- Catheter tip embolus
- Air embolus
- Arrhythmias
- Infection

Position (for right internal jugular vein catheterisation)

- Assist the patient into a supine position in reverse Trendelenburg position to engorge the neck veins. Remove all pillows.
- Tilt the patient's head to the left side and explain to them the need to maintain this position and to keep still.

Preparation

- Wash your hands and put on a pair of gloves.
- Gather the following equipment on a procedure trolley:
    - sterile dressing pack
    - gown and sterile gloves
    - Betadine
    - lignocaine
    - central line
    - normal saline flush
    - guidewire
    - vessel dilator
    - introducer needle
    - 1/0 silk suture plus adhesive dressing.

Procedure

- Scrub up, gown and glove.
- Prepare the right side of the patient's neck with Betadine and create a sterile field around the puncture site using the sterile drapes within the dressing pack.

- Flush each central line lumen with normal saline.
- Palpate for the carotid artery with the left hand, and using the right hand infiltrate the skin lateral to the artery and between the heads of sternocleidomastoid with 1% lignocaine using a 23-gauge needle.
- Change to a larger 21-gauge needle. Angle the needle at 45° to the skin and, aiming towards the ipsilateral nipple, aspirate and infiltrate the subcutaneous tissues with local anaesthetic and locate the right internal jugular (RIJ) vein.
- When a flashback is seen, withdraw the needle and advance the larger-bore introducer needle (attached to a syringe) in the line of the previous needle and locate the RIJ vein.
- Once the vein has been punctured and dark non-pulsatile venous blood can be freely aspirated, detach the syringe from the needle and feed the guidewire through the lumen of the needle. There should be no resistance.
- Once approximately half the length of the guidewire has been inserted, remove the needle.
- Nick the skin at the puncture site with the scalpel provided, and thread the dilator over the guidewire to the hilt.
- Remove the dilator and feed the catheter over the guidewire. Once the central venous catheter is in place, remove the guidewire.
- Check that blood can be aspirated from each of the lumens, and flush each lumen with normal saline.
- Secure the central line in place using 1/0 silk and apply an adhesive dressing.
- Dispose of the clinical waste and sharps appropriately.
- Ensure that the patient is comfortable and wash your hands.

Closure

- Explain to the patient that the central line has been successfully inserted and that a chest X-ray will need to be performed (to exclude a pneumothorax) prior to its use.
- Document the procedure in the patient's notes.

75 Administering an intravenous injection

Scenario

Mr Jones has been admitted to hospital with heart failure. You have been asked to give him 40 mg of furosemide intravenously to 'offload' him. The patient has a peripheral cannula *in situ*.

Introduction and consent

- Introduce yourself to the patient and check their identity.
- Explain the need to perform the procedure, outlining the risks and benefits, and obtain the patient's verbal consent.

Positioning

- Ensure that the patient is lying or sitting comfortably.
- Check the position of the cannula *in situ*.

Preparation of equipment

- Check the patient's drug chart and determine the following:
  - drug name
  - dose
  - dilutant and volume of dilutant
  - route of administration (i.e. intravenous)
  - date and time of administration
  - validity of prescription (i.e. signature of clinician).
- In addition, ascertain whether the patient has any allergies specifically to the drug that you are going to administer.
- Check that the drug and dose are appropriate if you are unsure of the dose or if you have never administered the drug before (use the *British National Formulary*).
- Wash your hands and put on a pair of gloves.
- Check the name, strength and expiry date of the drug with a nurse/colleague.
- Check the name and expiry date of the fluid to be used for re-constitution with a nurse/colleague.
- Prepare the appropriate volume of drug, diluting according to the manufacturer's instructions, and draw it up into a syringe.
- Expel any excess air from the syringe and needle by inverting the syringe and tapping.

Procedure

- Draw up a 10-ml normal saline flush.
- Remove the bung/cap of the cannula which is *in situ*. Clean the injection port with an alcohol swab and allow the alcohol to evaporate. Flush the cannula with 5 ml of normal saline to confirm its patency.
- Inject the drug into the vein at the prescribed or recommended rate, and follow this with a 5-ml normal saline flush.
- Check that the patient is comfortable and feels well throughout the procedure.
- Replace the bung/cap on the injection port.
- Dispose of any sharps.
- Wash your hands or use alcohol gel.

Closure

- Explain that you have successfully administered the drug, and address any concerns that the patient may have.
- Advise the patient that they should feel their breathing improving, and that they are likely to pass large amounts of urine. Reassure them that this is normal.
- Sign the prescription chart, and note the date and time, to indicate that you have administered the drug.

Intravenous drug preparations

There are three main types.

Liquid that does not require reconstitution

- Open the seal.
- Draw up into a syringe.
- Usually administered slowly.

Liquid that requires reconstitution

- Open the seal.
- Draw the drug up into a syringe large enough to hold the final volume.
- Draw up the appropriate volume of sterile dilutant (usually normal saline or water).

Powder that requires reconstitution

- The drug vial will usually have a vacuum.

- Draw the required volume of sterile dilutant into a syringe.
- Pierce the rubber seal of the drug vial and withdraw air to create a vacuum (negative pressure) in the vial.
- Inject the dilutant into the vial with the help of the vacuum created.
- Repeat as necessary until all of the dilutant has been injected.
- Shake to dissolve the drug in the dilutant.
- To withdraw the reconstituted drug, inject air into the vial to create a positive pressure.
- Invert the vial and withdraw the reconstituted drug with the help of the positive pressure created.

76 Administering an intramuscular injection

Scenario

Mr Wilmer is a 35-year-old man with chronic osteomyelitis which is being treated with intramuscular injections of penicillin. You have been asked to administer his next dose.

Indications

- High-volume (up to 10 ml) medications.
- Parenteral medication that cannot be absorbed from the subcutaneous layer.

Contraindications

- Allergy to medication.
- Infection at the injection site.
- Coagulopathies.

Complications

- Bleeding.
- Arterial puncture with or without inadvertent injection.
- Nerve damage.
- Infection with or without abscess formation.

Introduction and consent

- Introduce yourself to the patient and check their identity.
- Explain the need to perform the procedure, outlining the risks and benefits, and obtain the patient's verbal consent.

Preparation of equipment

- Check the patient's drug chart and determine the following:
  - drug name
  - dose
  - dilutant and volume of dilutant
  - route of administration
  - date and time of administration
  - validity of prescription (i.e. signature of clinician).
- In addition, ascertain whether the patient has any allergies or is taking any anticoagulants.
- Wash your hands and put on a pair of gloves.
- Check the name, strength and expiry date of the drug with a nurse/colleague.
- Check the name and expiry date of the dilutant with a nurse/colleague.
- Prepare the appropriate volume of drug, diluting according to the manufacturer's instructions, and draw it up into a syringe.
- Gather a fresh sterile needle (a 22-gauge is appropriate) and attach it to the syringe, expelling any excess air from the syringe and needle.

Positioning the patient

- Select an appropriate injection site.
- Assist the patient into a comfortable position and expose the injection site, identifying any landmarks in order to avoid any blood vessels or nerves.

[Adapted from Sritharan K, Elwell VA. Tips on ... theatre etiquette. *BMJ Careers*. 2005; **13**: 177–220.]

Sites of intramuscular injection

- Body of deltoid muscle – lateral to and a few centimetres below the acromion process to avoid the radial nerve.
- Gluteus muscle – the upper outer quadrant to avoid the sciatic nerve and superior gluteal artery (i.e. posterior to and above an

> imaginary line drawn from the anterior superior iliac spine to the greater trochanter, bounded superiorly by the iliac crest),
> - Vastus lateralis muscle – safe, but can be more painful due to overlying fascia lata.

Procedure

- Clean the injection site using an alcohol swab, and allow the alcohol to evaporate (this takes approximately 30 seconds).
- Stretch the skin taut at the injection site, using one hand.
- With the other hand hold the syringe and needle at 90° and quickly plunge it into the patient's skin.
- Draw back on the plunger to ensure that a blood vessel has not been inadvertently entered (change the injection site if blood is aspirated) and inject the drug slowly at a rate of 1 ml every 10 seconds.
- Once the drug has been fully administered, wait 10 seconds and then rapidly withdraw the needle and apply pressure over the injection site.
- Document the details (signature, time, date and drug batch number) of drug administration on the patient's drug chart.
- Dispose of sharps and clinical waste appropriately.

Closure

- Ensure that the patient is comfortable and assist them with any clothing.
- Explain that you have successfully administered the drug, and address any concerns they may have.
- Wash your hands or use alcohol gel.

77 Administering a subcutaneous injection

Scenario

Mrs Wallace is a 42-year-old woman who has a deep vein thrombosis. She has been prescribed 12,000 units of dalteparin (Fragmin) subcutaneously once a day. She has come in to have her heparin injection, and you are asked to administer it.

Introduction and consent

- Introduce yourself to the patient and check their identity.
- Explain the need to perform the procedure, outlining the risks and benefits, and obtain the patient's verbal consent.

Positioning the patient

- Select an appropriate injection site. This should ideally contain a large amount of subcutaneous fatty tissue.
- Assist the patient into a comfortable position.
- Ensure that the patient has privacy, and then expose the injection site.

Preparation of equipment

- Check the patient's drug chart and confirm the following:
  - drug name
  - dose
  - dilutant and volume of dilutant if required
  - route of administration
  - date and time of administration
  - validity of prescription (i.e. signature of clinician).
- In addition, ascertain whether the patient has any allergies, in particular to the drug you are about to administer.
- Wash your hands and put on a pair of gloves.
- Check the name, strength and expiry date of the drug with a nurse/colleague.
- Check the name and expiry date of any dilutant with a nurse/colleague.
- Prepare the appropriate volume of drug, diluting according to the manufacturer's instructions, and draw it up into a syringe (note that heparin usually comes in pre-packaged syringes).
- Gather a 23- to 25-gauge sterile needle (a 22-gauge is also appropriate) and attach it to the syringe, expelling any excess air from the syringe and needle.

Procedure

- Clean the injection site using an alcohol swab, and allow the alcohol to evaporate (this takes approximately 30 seconds).
- The drug needs to be administered into the subcutaneous fat above the muscle layer.

- Pinch the skin up between your thumb and index finger, lifting it off the underlying muscle.
- Insert the needle rapidly at a 45° angle into the skin, giving the patient warning beforehand.
- Release the skin and draw back on the plunger to ensure that a blood vessel has not been inadvertently entered (change the injection site if blood is aspirated), and inject the drug slowly.
- Once the drug has been fully administered, wait 10 seconds and then rapidly withdraw the needle.
- Apply gentle pressure over the injection site.
- Document the details (signature, time, date and drug batch number) of drug administration on the patient's drug chart.
- Dispose of sharps and clinical waste appropriately.

Closure

- Ensure that the patient is comfortable and assist them with any clothing.
- Explain that you have successfully administered the drug, and address any concerns they may have.
- Wash your hands or use an alcohol gel.

Sites of subcutaneous drug administration

These include:

- outer surface of upper arm
- anterior surface of thigh
- lower abdominal wall – rotate injection sites (e.g. in diabetics to reduce the risk of fat necrosis).

Avoid:

- sites of infection
- scars
- irradiated skin
- bony prominences or joints
- the abdomen in patients with ascites.

78 Blood culture

Scenario

Mr Keats is a 45-year-old man who has recently returned from a 2-week holiday in Africa. He presents to Accident and Emergency with rigors and currently has a temperature of 38.5°C. You are asked to take a set of blood cultures.

Indications for blood culture

- Pyrexia of unknown origin (PUO).
- To identify subacute bacteraemia (e.g subacute bacterial endo-carditis).

Important points

- Blood cultures should be performed prior to commencing anti-biotics.
- Each set of blood cultures consists of an anaerobic and aerobic blood culture bottle.
- A fever occurs between 30 and 120 minutes after the introduction of bacteria into the circulation.
- Ideally, three sets of blood cultures should be performed from at least two different sites.
- If a central line is *in situ*, blood cultures should also be sent from blood taken from the line.

Introduction and consent

- Introduce yourself to the patient and check their identity.
- Explain the need to take blood cultures, and obtain the patient's verbal consent.

Positioning the patient

- Ensure that the patient is comfortable, in a lying or sitting position.
- Support the arm from which blood is to be taken with a pillow.

Preparation

- Gather the following equipment:
  - blood culture bottles (anaerobic and aerobic)
  - tourniquet
  - alcohol swab
  - two green/blue needles
  - cotton wool
  - 20-ml syringe.
- Wash your hands and put on a pair of gloves.

Procedure

- Apply a tourniquet proximal to the elbow crease, and palpate for and select a vein.
- Clean the venepuncture site with an alcohol swab and wait approximately 30 seconds for the alcohol to evaporate.
- Do not re-palpate the venepuncture site once it has been cleaned.
- Using a green/blue needle attached to a 20-ml syringe, enter the skin and vein to withdraw a minimum of 10 ml of blood.
- Remove the tourniquet, apply pressure over the venepuncture site and withdraw the needle.
- Apply pressure over the venepuncture site until the bleeding has stopped.
- Ensure that the patient is comfortable.
- Discard the needle used for venepuncture into a sharps container and replace it with a new sterile needle.
- Flip off the caps of the culture bottles and clean the rubber tops with an alcohol swab.
- Allow the alcohol to dry (this takes approximately 30 seconds), and inject 5–10 ml of blood into each culture bottle.
- *Note:* some authors advocate that the anaerobic culture bottle should be filled first.
- Dispose of the sharps and clinical waste appropriately.
- Label the blood cultures with the patient's details (name, date of birth and hospital number) and the date and time when the blood sample was taken.
- Complete the relevant microbiology investigation request form, stating the test required (MC&S – microscopy and culture), the indication for the test (PUO), the site from which the sample was taken and whether the patient is taking any antibiotics.
- Wash your hands or use alcohol gel.

Closure

- Offer to send the blood sample to the laboratory.
- Explain to the patient when the blood culture results will be available. A preliminary report can usually be obtained within 24 hours. However, full culture results including antibiotic sensitivities will take at least 48 hours.
- Address any concerns that the patient may have.

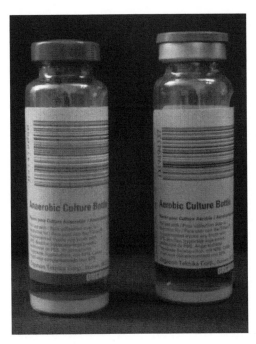

Figure 15 Blood culture bottles.

79 Taking a bacterial wound swab

Scenario

Mrs Walsh is a 77-year-old woman with chronic venous leg ulcers. She has noticed over the past week that the ulcers on her right leg have become more painful and hot, with an offensive discharge. You are asked to take a bacterial wound swab.

Introduction and consent

- Introduce yourself to the patient and confirm their identity.
- Explain the procedure to the patient, including the reasons why you wish to perform it, and obtain their verbal consent.
- It may be appropriate if the ulcers are painful to give the patient analgesia, especially if the dressing needs to be removed.

Positioning the patient

- Assist the patient into a comfortable position, preferably on a bed.
- Wash your hands and put on a pair of gloves.
- Remove any dressings and discard them into a clinical waste bag.

Preparing the equipment

- Wash your hands and put on a fresh pair of gloves.
- Gather a bacterial wound swab.

Procedure

- Open the outer packaging and remove the cotton swab from its plastic tube which contains culture medium at its base.
- Roll the swab in the area to be cultured and replace the swab back in its plastic case.
- Offer to redress the wound as appropriate.
- Discard any clinical waste.
- Assist the patient into a comfortable position.
- Wash your hands.

Closure

- Label the swab with the patient's name, hospital number, the site from which the swab was taken (right leg ulcer), the date and the ward number.
- Complete the accompanying investigation request form, stating the investigation (MC&S – microscopy and culture), indication for test (infected leg ulcer), site from which swab was taken, date, name of requesting clinician and details of any antibiotics the patient may be taking.
- Record the procedure in the patient's notes.

- Explain to the patient when the results of the investigation will be available (i.e. in 48 hours).

80 Performing a simple dressing change

Scenario

Mr Potts is a 54-year-old man who underwent a laparotomy 2 days ago. You are asked to change the wound dressing because it has 'soaked through.'

Introduction and consent

- Introduce yourself to the patient and check their identity.
- Explain that you would like to change their dressing and obtain verbal consent.
- Address any of the patient's concerns or questions.
- If the patient is experiencing pain from the wound, it may be appropriate to give analgesia beforehand.
- In addition, ascertain the patient's infection risk (e.g. MRSA, *Pseudomonas* spp.) beforehand and take the appropriate precautions.

Positioning

- Ensure that the patient is positioned in the supine position and is comfortable.
- Ensure that the patient has privacy, and adequately expose their abdominal wound.

Preparation

- On a procedure trolley open out a sterile dressing pack to create a sterile field.
- The dressing pack should contain a waste disposal bag. Attach this to the side of the procedure trolley for convenience.
- Pour sterile normal saline (available in bottles) into the gallipots in the dressing pack, maintaining the sterile field.

Procedure

- Remove the old dressing and discard it appropriately as clinical waste.
- Inspect the wound, assessing the following:
  - size of wound
  - presence of sutures/clips
  - healing – scar formation
  - inflammation
  - discharge and odour
  - dehiscence.
- In the case of ulcers or open wounds, assess:
  - size of defect
  - shape
  - edge – irregular, smooth
  - base – presence of granulation tissue, necrosis, or sloughing of tissue
  - discharge
  - surrounding tissue – healthiness or inflammation.
- Decide whether a dressing is required, and if so, on the appropriate dressing.
- Wash your hands or use alcohol gel.
- Open the new dressing on to the sterile field.
- Put on a pair of sterile gloves.
- If necessary take a wound swab.
- Clean the wound using cotton gauze and normal saline. Clean from the centre of the wound towards the periphery, and do not retrace old ground.
- Apply the new dressing.

Closure

- Tell the patient that the procedure is complete, and address any concerns they may have.
- Clear away and dispose of the waste appropriately.
- Disinfect the procedure trolley using an alcohol swab.
- Wash your hands or use alcohol gel.
- Document the procedure in the patient's notes.
- If a wound swab has been taken, label the specimen and complete the microbiology request form and offer to send the specimen to the laboratory.

81 Removing surgical skin clips and sutures

Scenario

Mr Lyle is a 45-year-old man who underwent repair of a perforated gastric ulcer 10 days ago. He has an upper midline incision and you have been asked to remove his surgical skin clips (or insoluble sutures).

Introduction and consent

- Introduce yourself to the patient and confirm their identity.
- Discuss the procedure with the patient and explain that it may be uncomfortable.
- Obtain their verbal consent.
- Assess whether the patient is currently in pain, and offer them analgesia before the procedure if appropriate.

Position

- Wash your hands or use alcohol gel.
- Put on a pair of gloves and an apron.
- Place the patient in a supine position and check that they are comfortable.
- Ensure that the patient has privacy, and adequately expose their abdominal wound.
- Remove the old dressing where appropriate, and discard in the clinical waste bin.
- Inspect the wound and ensure that there are clips (or insoluble sutures), and assess for any signs of infection (e.g. redness, discharge, hotness, tenderness).

Preparation

- Wash your hands and put on a new pair of gloves.
- Gather your equipment.
- On a procedure trolley open out a sterile dressing pack to create a sterile field.
- The dressing pack should contain a waste disposal bag. Attach this to the side of the procedure trolley for convenience.
- Pour sterile normal saline (available in bottles) into the gallipots in the dressing pack, maintaining the sterile field, and open a staple remover (or stitch cutter) on to the sterile field.
- Clean your hands with alcohol gel and put on a sterile pair of gloves.

Procedure

- Take a bacterial swab if necessary.
- Clean the wound using cotton gauze and normal saline. Clean from the centre of the wound towards the periphery, and do not retrace old ground.
- Use the sterile drapes in the dressing pack to create a sterile field around the abdominal wound.
- Place the teeth of the staple remover in the middle of each skin clip and squeeze the two handles to bunch and loosen the staple.
- A pair of forceps can then be used to free the staple from the skin. The staple should be collected into a gallipot.
- In the case of interrupted insoluble sutures, pick each knot up separately with a pair of forceps and cut only one end of the suture, flush to the skin. Gentle upward traction on the knot should free the suture.
- Where a continuous insoluble suture has been used, cut the suture at one end and apply gentle horizontal traction to the other end. The suture should pull smoothly through the wound.
- If the patient complains of pain, it may be necessary to stop the procedure and give analgesia or use a local anaesthetic.
- Once all the staples (or sutures) have been removed, reapply a fresh dressing.

Closure

- Tell the patient that the procedure is complete, and address any concerns they may have.
- Clear away and dispose of the waste, including sharps, appropriately.
- Disinfect the procedure trolley using an alcohol swab.
- Wash your hands or use alcohol gel.
- Document the procedure in the patient's notes.
- If a wound swab has been taken, label the specimen and complete the microbiology request form and offer to send the specimen to the laboratory.

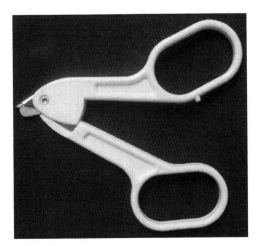

Figure 16   Clip remover.

82 Joint aspiration

Scenario

Mr Jones is a 65-year-old man who has been admitted with fever and a swollen tender left knee with no history of trauma. You have been asked to aspirate the knee joint because septic arthritis is suspected.

Indications

- Diagnostic (e.g. septic arthritis, to exclude acute or chronic infection, joint effusion).
- Therapeutic (e.g. administration of steroid, drainage of infection).

Contraindications

- Coagulopathy or anticoagulation.

Risks

- Pain.
- Bleeding.
- Infection.

Introduction and consent

- Introduce yourself to the patient and confirm their identity.
- Explain the procedure, including the indication, risks and benefits, and obtain the patient's verbal consent.

Positioning the patient

- Wash your hands and put on a pair of gloves.
- Ensure that the patient is comfortable in a supine position with the knee fully extended and exposed.
- Identify the optimal site of aspiration – the medial aspect of the patella in the patellar-femoral groove of the left knee – and mark it.

Preparation

- Gather the following equipment:
  - lignocaine 2%
  - Betadine
  - dressing pack
  - specimen pot
  - syringe
  - 25-gauge and 21-gauge needles
  - glucose tube.
- On a procedure trolley open out a sterile dressing pack to create a sterile field.
- The dressing pack should contain a waste disposal bag. Attach this to the side of the procedure trolley for convenience and, while maintaining the sterile field, open all the equipment.

Procedure

- Scrub up, gown and glove.
- Clean the left knee with Betadine and, using the drapes within the dressing pack, create a sterile field around the marked puncture site.
- Allow the Betadine to dry, and clean the puncture site with an alcohol swab (as Betadine can invalidate culture results).
- Anaesthetise the skin at the puncture site with lignocaine (2%), raising a bleb with a 25-gauge needle (note that lignocaine is bactericidal). Wait for the anaesthetic to take effect.
- Insert the needle through the skin and into the knee joint, aspirating as you advance the needle. Stop when fluid is encountered.

- Withdraw as much of the fluid as possible and fill the two specimen pots and the glucose tube.
- Never inject an infected joint with steroids. However, you may need to inject a joint in which you have aspirated a reactionary effusion. If the latter is the case, following aspiration leave the needle *in situ* in the knee joint, detach the syringe and replace it with a syringe containing the steroid (20–40 mg of methylprednisolone). Inject the steroid.
- Withdraw the needle and apply pressure.
- Tell the patient that the procedure is complete, and address any concerns they may have.
- Clear away and dispose of the waste appropriately.
- Disinfect the procedure trolley using an alcohol swab.

Closure

- Wash your hands or use alcohol gel.
- Document the procedure in the patient's notes, including the amount and colour of the effusion aspirated (clear, viscous, bloodstained, etc.).
- Label the specimens collected and complete the relevant microscopy and culture, cytology and glucose (biochemistry) request forms.

83 Surgical scrubbing, gowning and gloving

Scenario

You are asked to assist with an operation, and are required to scrub, gown and glove.

Preparation

- Remove wrist watch and hand jewellery, including rings.
- Staff must report open wounds or infections (e.g. boils) of the forearms, hands and nails, and should not scrub.
- Nails should be short and clean, ideally with no nail varnish.
- Surgical scrubs (greens), shoes/clogs and disposable cap must be worn in the operating room.
- Apply a face mask before scrubbing. This should fit snugly around the nose and mouth, and must be changed after each procedure.

- Open out a sterile gown pack. Open the outer pack consisting of a sterile pair of gloves, dropping the sterile inner gloves into the sterile field created by opening out the gown pack.

Procedure

- The first scrub of the day should last 5 minutes, and subsequent scrubs should last 3 minutes.
- Turn on the tap and adjust the water temperature.
- Open a sterile sponge/brush pack. Note that the sponge may or may not be impregnated with surgical scrub (e.g. Betadine), and leave to one side.
- Keep your hands above your elbows and do not touch any non-sterile objects/surfaces. In addition, hold your body away from your arms.
- Wet your forearms and hands, allowing the water to drain downwards from your hands to your elbows. Do not shake your hands or arms, but allow the water to drip away.
- Using your elbow, dispense Betadine or chlorhexidine scrub. Lather the detergent and perform a pre-scrub, washing from the hands to 2 cm above the elbow and then rinsing.
- Scrub one arm completely as described below before proceeding to the other arm.
- Using the brush and nail file, brush and file under the fingernails for 30 seconds per hand.
- Scrub each of the four surfaces of each finger, the palm, the back as well as the heel of the hand for a further minute per hand.
- Discard the sponge.
- Wash from the hands to the elbows for 1 minute without retracing your steps and then rinse, allowing the water to run away from your hands to your elbow.
- Pick up the towel, ensuring that it does not make contact with either your body or any non-sterile surface, and step away from the gowning table.
- Continue to hold your hands above your elbows, and dry your hands and forearms from distal to proximal using opposite sides of the same towel for each hand and forearm. Discard the towel on completion.
- Pick up your gown with one hand. Hold the gown away from you at the neck and at chest level and allow it to unfold.
- Slip your arms into the sleeves of the gown and advance your fingertips as far as but not beyond the proximal border of the gown cuffs.
- Ask a colleague to fasten the ties at the back of the gown.

- Open out the inner glove package.
- Pick up the left glove with your sleeve-covered left hand and place it on the opposite sleeve gown with the palm of the glove facing down and the fingers pointing towards you.
- Taking the folded edge of the glove with the thumb and index finger of your sleeve-covered left hand (palm facing upwards), use your sleeve-covered right hand to stretch the glove over the sleeve-covered left hand by grasping on the outer edge of the glove fold.
- Pull any excess sleeve from inside the glove using your sleeve-covered right hand.
- Pick up the right glove under its fold with your gloved left hand and pull the glove over your right hand.
- As before, draw any excess sleeve from the gown cuffs using your left hand.
- This is the closed technique for gloving and gowning.
- Finally, take the paper belt tab found at the front of the gown and pass it to the scrub nurse/assistant. The assistant will take the paper tab and move behind you to pass the belt (but not the paper tab) back to you.
- Tie the belt at the front to complete gowning.

- The purpose of scrubbing is to remove/kill surface organisms, and it is thought to be effective for up to 2 hours.
- The scrubbing brush should not be applied to skin, as this disturbs the normal skin flora.

---

84 Suture material and suturing

Suture material

- The *site*, *type of tissue* and *physician preference* determine the suture material and needle to be used.
- Suture material can be classified as absorbable or non-absorbable, and as synthetic or non-synthetic.
- The higher the number the smaller the size of the suture (e.g. 5.0 is a smaller suture than a 2.0 suture).
- Sutures are usually mounted on needles and pre-packaged.

- Needles can be classified as cutting (used in tough tissues such as skin or tendons) or round-bodied/blunt (used in delicate tissues such as bowel or muscle).

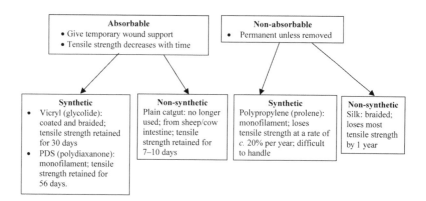

Suturing

Scenario

You are on call in Accident and Emergency. Mr Ingram has been admitted with a clean 5-cm laceration to his arm which you have been asked to suture.

Introduction

- Introduce yourself to the patient and confirm their identity.
- Explain the procedure and obtain verbal consent.
- Ascertain whether the patient has any allergies, in particular to the anaesthetic.
- Check their tetanus status.
- Do *not* suture contaminated wounds, wounds that are more than 24 hours old, or bites.

Positioning the patient

Ensure that the patient is comfortable and that the area to be sutured is exposed.

Preparation of equipment

- Wash your hands and put on a pair of gloves.
- Prepare the following on a procedure trolley:
    - appropriate local anaesthetic
    - 10-ml syringe and 25-gauge needle
    - dressing pack
    - Betadine
    - appropriate suture material and needle.

Local anaesthetics and suturing

- Maximum safe dose varies with anaesthetic used and patient's weight:
    - lignocaine (Xylocaine) safe dose: 5 mg/kg
    - lignocaine plus adrenaline: 7 mg/kg
    - bupivacaine (Marcain): 3 mg/kg.
- Concentration in mg can be calculated by multiplying percentage concentration by 10 (e.g. 1% lignocaine contains 10 mg/ml).

Procedure

- Scrub up, gown and glove.
- Clean the wound with Betadine, starting at the centre and working outwards without retracing old ground.
- Infitrate the wound with local anaesthetic using a 25-gauge needle, not exceeding the maximum safe amount.
- Aspirate before injecting to avoid inadvertent intra-arterial injection. (*Do not use adrenaline in digits*, as its peripheral vasoconstriction effect can cause ischaemia).
- Select the appropriate suture and needle.
- Hold the forceps between thumb and index finger and use it to manipulate (*not to crush*) the skin edges. Forceps may be toothed (used for skin and tough tissue) or non-toothed (used for bowel and blood vessels).
- Hold the needle holder with the thumb and index fingers inserted in the bows advanced no further than the distal phalanx. Extend the index finger to steady the scissors over its joint.
- Mount the needle two-thirds of the way from its tip.
- Insert the needle at right angles to the skin, advance the needle through one skin edge, pick the needle up using forceps (*not* hands),

remount and advance the needle through the opposite skin edge. (The distance from the skin edge should be roughly equal to the thickness of the wound for each stitch.)

- Pull the suture through, leaving the non-needle end short.
- Either instrument or hand-tie the suture, forming a reef knot, ensuring that the skin edges are *approximated not strangulated.*
- Hold the scissors in a similar manner to the needle holder and cut using the tips of the scissors. Use the index finger of the opposite hand to support the scissors underneath while cutting.
- Successive sutures should be equidistant at a distance of twice the wound depth.
- The resulting closure should be 'tension free.'
- Apply the dressing.
- Dispose of sharps and clinical waste appropriately.

Closure

- Ensure that the patient is comfortable.
- Advise the patient about:
  - what has been done
  - the type of suture used (i.e. 6/0 or 5/0 for face and dorsum hands; 3/0 or 4/0 for limbs)
  - whether the sutures need to be removed and when (i.e. skin and face on days 3–5; chest and abdomen on day 10; scalp on days 5–7)
  - dressing care
  - follow-up.

85 Preparing baby formula milk

Scenario

You are requested to make up powder formula milk for a 2-month-old baby who weighs 10 pounds.

Breastfeeding is always preferable. However, formula milk may be used:

- if the mother decides not to breastfeed
- if the mother stops breastfeeding when the child is less than 1 year old
- to supplement breastfeeding.

Background

- Baby formulas are designed to give the baby all its essential nutrients in the necessary quantities.
- Essentially there are three types of formula – powder, concentrated and ready-to-use formulas.
- Powder and concentrated formulas are cheaper, but need to be mixed with water before use.
- Whole cow's milk should not be given to babies under 1 year old, due to the increased risk of allergies.

Preparation

- Wash your hands.
- Ensure that the bottles, artificial nipples, rings and bottle caps are clean.
- Calculate the amount of formula required per feed by dividing the baby's weight (in pounds) by 2.
- The number of feeds per day depends on the baby's age. However, no baby should drink more than 32 ounces of formula per day.
- Using this knowledge, the amount of formula required for the day can be calculated (e.g. a 2-month-old baby that weighs 10 pounds will require 25–30 ounces of formula per day).

Number of feeds required per day

First month:	6–8 feeds
1–3 months:	5–6 feeds
3–7 months:	4–5 feeds
7–12 months:	3–4 feeds

Procedure

- Water used for mixing formula should be boiled beforehand and allowed to cool.
- Mix the powder formula according to the manufacturer's instructions.
- In general, each level scoop of powdered formula is mixed with 2 ounces of water. (Concentrated formula is usually mixed with water in a 1:1 ratio.)

- Measure the required amount of water into a clean container.
- Using the scoop accompanying the can, measure the required amount of formula, levelling each scoop with a clean knife, and add to the water.
- Mix well and pour the formula into the clean bottles and cap.
- Never over-concentrate or dilute the formula.

Closure

- Store the prepared formula according to the manufacturer's guidelines.
- In general, formula can be stored in the fridge (below 4°C) until ready to use, but should be discarded if not used within 48 hours.
- In addition, if the formula is left at room temperature for more than 2 hours or warmed and not used it should be discarded.
- Formula can be warmed by holding the bottle under a warm tap or standing it in a container of warm water.

86 Stomas and stoma care

Stomas may be encountered either in the context of a short case or in the surgical equipment station.

- Stomas are classified as either *temporary* (e.g. defunctioning loop ileostomy) or *permanent* (e.g. end colostomy/ileostomy or ileal conduit), and by their contents (e.g. ileostomy, colostomy, jejunostomy, urostomy, gastrostomy or caecostomy).

Indications for a stoma

- Feeding (e.g. percutaneous endoscopic gastrostomy, PEG).
- Decompression (e.g. caecostomy, transverse colostomy).
- Diversion (e.g. post-cystectomy ileal conduit, loop ileostomy to protect a distal bowel anastomosis).
- Exteriorisation – for example, where primary anastomosis is not possible due to ischaemia, perforation or distal obstruction, or a permanent stoma is formed (e.g. following abdomino-perineal resection for a low rectal tumour or panproctocolectomy for ulcerative colitis).
- Lavage (e.g. appendicostomy).

Scenario 1

Inspect this man's abdomen.

Introduction and consent

- Introduce yourself to the patient and obtain their consent to examination.
  Hello sir, my name is John Smith and I am a medical student. Would you mind if I examine your abdomen?
- Tell the examiner your findings throughout the examination.
- Ensure that the patient is positioned flat and ideally exposed from nipple to knee.

Inspection

- Inspect the patient in general and the abdomen initially from the end of the bed.
- Comment on the patient's general condition first and then on the abdomen.
  The patient looks well/cachectic/jaundiced, etc., at rest. The most obvious abnormality on inspection of the abdomen is a stoma.
- Comment on any scars, old drain sites or healed stoma scars.
- Assess the following.

Site of the stoma

- Right-sided: usually ileostomy or ileal conduit.
- Left-sided: usually colostomy or mucous fistula.
- Midline: transverse loop colostomy.
- Epigastric: percutaneous endoscopic gastrostomy (PEG).

Appearance

Assess the healthiness of the mucosa (if a stoma bag is present, ask to remove it).

Presence of spout

- An ileostomy has a spout to minimise the corrosive effect of the effluent on the skin.
- A colostomy is flush to the skin (unless prolapsing).

Number of lumen

- One: indicates an end stoma.
- Two (i.e. an afferent and efferent loop): indicates a loop or double-barrel stoma.

Bag contents

- Urine (ileostomy).
- Formed stool (colostomy).
- Semi-formed or liquid stool (ilesostomy).

Assess for any complications of stoma formation

Ask the patient to cough and/or raise their legs, so that you can look for a parastomal hernia.

Complications

These are classified as either *specific* or *general*.

Specific complications

- Ischaemia
- Parastomal hernia
- Haemorrhage
- Stenosis
- Prolapse
- Obstruction
- Retraction
- Skin excoriation
- Local recurrence of disease

General complications

- Stoma diarrhoea – resulting in electrolyte imbalance (especially lowered K^+ levels).
- Malnutrition – vitamin B_{12} and iron deficiencies (absorbed in terminal ileum and jejunum, respectively).
- Renal complications plus gallstones – due to increased water loss and loss of bile salts (usually reabsorbed in terminal ileum).
- Psychosexual complications.
- Recurrence or residual disease (e.g. Crohn's parastomal fistula).
- Problems with stoma management (e.g. odour, flatus, leakage).

- Tell the examiner that you would also like to:
    - perform a full abdominal examination (i.e. palpate, percuss and auscultate the abdomen)
    - examine the perineum (in abdomino-perineal resection the anus is oversewn)
    - perform a digital per stoma examination (looking for blood, stenosis and polyps).
- Finally, thank the patient.

Scenario 2

Can you tell me what this is?

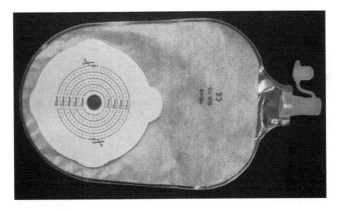

Figure 17   Stoma bag.

This scenario requires you to:

- identify the appliance
- describe the features of the appliance.

- A stoma bag can be either a one-piece or a two-piece device.
- A one-piece stoma bag is attached to the skin with adhesive, and needs to be changed in its entirety.
- A two-piece stoma bag has a base-plate with a flange which attaches to the skin, and only the pouch needs to be changed regularly.
- Some pouches may have a tap which facilitates measurement of output (if large) or drainage of the contents (useful for ileal conduits).

- Classify the stoma as above (temporary/permanent or type).
- Give the indications for its formation.
- Describe the complications.
- You may also be asked to discuss the pre- and post-operative management of a stoma.

Stomas should be created where possible in conjunction with a specialist stoma nurse specialist.

Pre-operatively:

- obtain informed consent
- give the patient psychosexual counselling
- mark the site of the stoma, which ideally should be:
  - away from any bony prominences, scars, skin creases and the waistline of clothes
  - 5 cm from the umbilicus
  - within easy reach by the patient to enable bag changes
  - within the rectus sheath.

Post-operatively:

- ensure that the patient receives counselling and support
- give stoma care advice: number of bag changes per day (colostomy requires 1–2 changes per day; ileal conduit requires more frequent changes); monitor output
- give dietary advice.

---

87 DVT prophylaxis

Scenario

Can you tell me what this is and what it is used for?

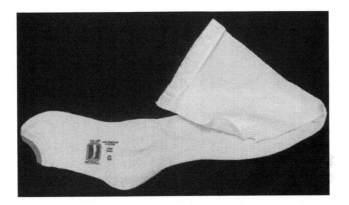

Figure 18   Thromboembolic deterrent stockings (TEDS).

This scenario requires you to correctly identify the surgical appliance, and the discussion may cover the following areas:

- indications for the use of thromboembolic deterrent stockings (TEDS)
- application of TEDS
- risk factors for deep vein thrombosis (DVT)
- preventive strategies for DVT
- diagnosis, treatment and management of DVT.

Indications for the use of TEDS

- A DVT is a thrombosis that occurs within the deep venous system of the lower limb.
- The incidence of DVT following major abdominal, pelvic or ortho-paedic surgery without prophylaxis is 40–50%, and its most life-threatening complication is a pulmonary embolism (PE).
- Around 0.1–0.2% of patients with a DVT die from a pulmonary embolism.
- Thigh-length TEDS are used peri-operatively and reduce the risk of DVT.

- Contraindications to the use of TEDS include patients with peripheral vascular disease with an ankle brachial pressure index (ABPI) of < 0.8.

Application of TEDS

- TEDS are sized according to measurements of a patient's thigh and calf circumference and leg length.
- TEDS apply graduated compression (12–14 mmHg at the ankle).

Risk factors for DVT

- Virchow's triad describes the factors involved in the pathogenesis of DVT, namely factors that affect:
  - blood flow (e.g. stasis)
  - the vessel wall (e.g. compression, trauma)
  - the blood constituents (e.g. hyperviscosity, hypercoagulability).
- The risk factors for DVT can be divided into patient factors and operative factors. Patients can be risk stratified into high-, medium- or low-risk groups.

Risk factors for DVT

Patient factors

- Age > 40 years
- Female gender
- Pregnancy
- Obesity
- Oral contraceptive pill
- Previous DVT/pulmonary embolism
- Thrombophilia (protein C, protein S or factor V deficiencies)

Operative/pathological factors

- Surgery duration > 150 minutes
- Laparoscopic procedure
- Post-operative immobility > 4 days
- Major abdominal or pelvic surgery
- Sepsis
- Pelvic or long bone fracture
- Malignancy

Preventive strategies for DVT

- DVT prophylaxis can be classified as either mechanical or pharmacological, and measures may be taken in the pre-, intra- and post-operative period to reduce the risk of DVT.

DVT prophylaxis

Pre-operative measures

- Weight loss
- Smoking cessation
- Hydration
- TEDS
- Subcutaneous heparin injections (continued until the patient is mobile post-operatively)

Intra-operative measures

- Foot pedals
- Ankle rests (to elevate calves)
- Intermittent pneumatic compression
- Electrical calf muscle stimulation
- TEDS

Post-operative measures

- Early mobilisation
- Hydration
- Avoiding crossing legs
- TEDS plus heparin

Diagnosis, treatment and management of DVT

- Diagnosis involves taking a full history and examining the patient, but this is often unreliable, and the patient should be treated as having suspected DVT until this has been confirmed by tests.
- History: the patient may complain of a swollen, painful calf or symptoms of a pulmonary embolism (haemoptysis, shortness of breath and pleuritic chest pain).
- Examination: pyrexia (typically days 6–8 post-operatively), calf swelling and a positive Homan's test (pain on passive ankle dorsiflexion) may be present.

- Investigations include D-dimer and Duplex scanning of the deep venous system of the lower limb as first line. Venography (the gold standard), plethysmography and radioisotope-labelled fibrinogen uptake scanning may also be employed.
- <u>Treatment</u> should include anticoagulation, initially with heparin, followed by warfarin for 3–6 months.
- Thrombolysis, venous thrombectomy and inferior vena caval filter insertion may also form part of the management of DVT in a few cases.

88 Surgical drains

Scenario

Can you tell me what this is and what it is used for?

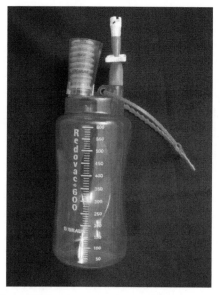

Figure 19 Redivac drain.

This station requires you to correctly identify the instrument, and discussion may involve:

- indications for insertion of a drain
- classification of drains
- complications.

This is a Redivac drain, which is an example of a closed active drainage system. I've seen it used following mastectomy, to abolish dead space.

Indications for insertion of a drain

- Drainage of a collection (e.g. pus, blood, fluid, air).
- Abolition of dead space.
- Removal of a potential collection (e.g. post-mastectomy seroma).

Classification of drains

- Drains can be classified as active or passive systems.
- Both systems can be further subdivided into closed and open systems.
- Drains may be made of latex, PVC, silastic or polyurethane.

Active systems

- Closed system drains (e.g. Redivac drain):
  - create a vacuum which draws fluid into the reservoir chamber
  - have a reservoir capacity of approximately 300 ml
  - are disposable
  - non-return valves prevent reflux
  - low pressure suction of 100 mmHg is typically generated
  - reduce risk of infection.
- Open system (sump) drains:
  - an inner tube under suction is protected from blockage by an outer vented/irrigated tube
  - are more efficient than closed suction systems
  - require a non-portable suction system
  - allow irrigation and aspiration.

Passive systems

- Closed system drains (e.g. Robinson drain):
  - drainage relies entirely on the siphoning of fluid down the pressure gradient into a collecting bag.
- Open system drains (e.g. stoma bag):
  - rely on capillary action or gravity
  - therefore position and site of drain are important.

Complicatons of surgical drains

Immediate

- Bleeding at drain insertion site.
- Perforaton of adjacent structures.

Early

- Occlusion.
- Displacement.
- Infection.

Late

- Pressure/suction necrosis of bowel or blood vessels.

Note: Drains should be removed within 5 days to reduce the risk of infection. Typically they are removed when output is < 50 ml/ 24 hours.

89 Chest drains

Scenario

Can you tell me what this is and what it is used for?

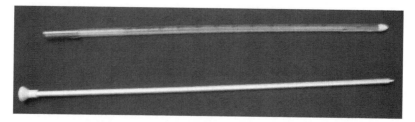

Figure 20 24 French chest drain tube and trocar.

This is a scenario which may be encountered in an OSCE instruments station. It requires you to correctly identify the instrument and its use.

This is a 24 French chest drain tube and trocar. I have seen it used in Accident and Emergency for the draining of a traumatic haemothorax.

The following areas may then be discussed:

- open and tension pneumothorax

- needle thoracentesis
- chest drain insertion, including indications and complications.

Classification of pneumothorax

Simple pneumothorax

- Air within the pleural cavity.

Open pneumothorax

- Air within the pleural cavity.
- Caused by large defect of chest wall.
- If defect is more than two-thirds of the tracheal diameter, air passes preferentially through chest defect.
- Management involves closing defect with dressing taped on three sides.

Tension pneumothorax

- This is a surgical emergency.
- A one-way valve is created.
- Air enters the pleural cavity on inspiration but cannot escape.
- The affected lung is collapsed and mediastinum displaced to the opposite side with subsequent reduced venous return and cardiac arrest.
- The patient presents with respiratory distress.
- Tracheal deviation is a late sign.
- Diagnosis is clinical.
- Chest X-ray should not be performed.

Needle thoracentesis

- Used in the management of life-threatening pneumothorax.
- On suspicion of tension pneumothorax, follow the procedure described below.
  - Ensure that the patient is receiving high-flow oxygen.
  - Place the patient in the upright position if a cervical spine injury has been excluded.
  - Identify the second intercostal space in the mid-clavicular line on the affected side.
  - Prepare the area with Betadine.

- Infiltrate the skin and deeper tissue with local anaesthetic if time permits.
- Insert a 16-gauge (large-bore) cannula over the rib into the pleural space and listen for a sudden escape of air when the needle enters the parietal pleura, as this indicates relief of the tension pneumothorax.
- Remove the needle, leaving the cannula *in situ*, and attach a three-way tap and aspirate using a 50-ml syringe.
- Stop if resistance is met or the patient coughs excessively.
- Request a chest X-ray to assess for residual pneumothorax.
- Prepare for chest drain insertion.

Indications for chest drain insertion

- Pneumothorax
- Haemothorax
- Chylothorax
- Drainage empyema

Preparation for insertion of chest drain

- Introduce yourself to the patient.
- Explain the procedure (including the reasons for it and the possible complications), and obtain informed verbal consent.
- Review a chest X-ray unless it is an emergency situation and time does not permit.
- Place the patient in either a sitting or supine position, if the cervical spine has not been cleared, with their arm, on the side that the chest drain will be placed, behind the head.
- Identify the fifth intercostal space in the mid-axillary line and mark it.
- Gather the following equipment:
    - trocar-mounted chest drain (20–36 French)
    - 1% lignocaine plus syringe and 26-gauge needle
    - minor procedures tray
    - Betadine
    - 0 silk suture
    - underwater seal drainage system.

Procedure

- Aseptic technique should be observed.
- Scrub up and gown.
- Prepare the chest drain insertion site with Betadine and drape the patient to create a sterile field.
- Infiltrate the skin and tissues down to the pleura with local anaesthetic (always drawing back on the syringe before injecting, to avoid injecting into blood vessels).
- Wait a few minutes for the anaesthetic to take effect.
- Make a 2-cm transverse incision over the upper border of the sixth rib to avoid the neurovascular bundle.
- Bluntly dissect the subcutaneous tissue and puncture the parietal pleura using either the tip of a clamp or a gloved finger.
- Remove the chest drain trocar.
- Clamp the proximal end of the thoracostomy to help to guide the drain into position, and introduce the drain, aiming for the apex (pneumothorax) or base (haemothorax) of the lungs.
- Attach the end of the chest drain to an underwater seal system and observe for bubbling.
- Using the 0 silk suture, tie the chest tube in place using a purse-string suture.
- Apply an airtight dressing and secure the tube to the patient's chest with tape (Sleek).
- Take a chest X-ray to confirm the position of the drain.

Complications of chest drain insertion

- Pain.
- Bleeding (with or without haemothorax).
- Inadvertent puncture of lungs, heart, great vessels or abdominal organs.
- Damage to the intercostal vein, artery and nerve.
- Infection.
- Subcutaneous emphysema.
- Blockage of tube.
- Recurrence of pneumothorax.
- Persistent pneumothorax (air leak).
- Failure of lung to expand (may require bronchoscopy).

90 Diagnostic peritoneal lavage (DPL)

Scenario

You are part of the trauma team and have been asked to perform a diagnostic peritoneal lavage in an unconscious 55-year-old man who was admitted following a road traffic accident with unexplained hypotension.

Diagnostic peritoneal lavage

- This is a rapidly performed, invasive procedure.
- It is 98% sensitive for intraperitoneal bleeding

Indications for DPL in trauma

- Intra-abdominal trauma where examination is unequivocal or unreliable.

Contraindications

- Clear indication for laparotomy.

Relative contraindications

- Previous abdominal surgery.
- Morbid obesity.
- Liver cirrhosis.
- Coagulopathy.
- Pregancy.

Explanation and consent

The patient is unconscious and therefore the procedure is performed in the patient's best interests.

Positioning

- Ensure that the patient is supine.
- Make sure that a urinary catheter and a nasogastric tube are already in place to decompress the bladder and stomach, respectively.

Preparation of equipment

Gather the following:

- 1% lignocaine
- Betadine
- peritoneal dialysis catheter
- procedure pack
- bag containing 1 litre of warmed, normal saline solution
- IV connecting tubing
- 2/0 vicryl suture
- 26-gauge needle.

Procedure

- Scrub, glove and gown.
- Prepare the abdomen using Betadine, and create a sterile field extending from above the umbilicus to the pubic symphysis.
- Infiltrate the skin and subcutaneous tissue in the midline, one-third of the distance from the umbilicus to the pubic symphysis, with 1% lignocaine using a 26-gauge needle and syringe.
- Make a vertical incision through the skin extending into the subcutaneous tissue.
- Grasp the linea alba between forceps, and then elevate and carefully divide the peritoneum, avoiding damage to the bowel.
- Advance the dialysis catheter towards the pelvis.
- Attach a syringe to its free end and aspirate.
- If no blood is aspirated, instil up to 1 litre of warmed, normal saline into the peritoneum via a connecting tube attached to the dialysis catheter.
- Allow the fluid to remain within the abdomen for 5 minutes while gently agitating the abdomen. Then allow the fluid to drain into a vented container.
- After the fluid has been collected, send a sample for analysis for white and red blood cells.
- Note: *In pregnancy or in patients with pelvic fractures, a supra-umbilical approach is advised.*

Positive result of DPL

- Initial aspiration of 5 ml of frank blood, bile or faeces.
- Red blood cell count > 100,000/mm^3.
- White blood cell count > 500/mm^3.
- *Note: a negative lavage does not exclude retroperitoneal injury.*

---

91 Ascitic tap

Scenario

Mr Laphroaig, an unemployed 52-year-old man with a history of alcoholism, presents to Accident and Emergency with gross ascites. You are asked by your registrar to perform an ascitic tap.

Indications

- Therapeutic: relief of tense ascites or distension that is causing respiratory distress.
- Diagnostic: to determine the cause of ascites (e.g. bacterial, malignancy).

Contraindications

- Coagulopathy.

Introduction and consent

- Introduce yourself to the patient.
- Explain the procedure and obtain the patient's informed verbal consent.
- Check the patient's clotting results and if they are abnormal, correct them before proceeding.

Position

- Ask the patient to empty their bladder.
- Place the patient in the supine position.

- Percuss the abdomen for the ascitic level and mark the point of drainage, avoiding old surgical scars where the bowel may be adherent to the abdominal wall.

Preparation of equipment

Gather the following:

- 21-gauge needle
- 20-ml syringe
- 1% lignocaine
- Betadine
- procedure pack
- specimen bottles.

Procedure

- Scrub up.
- Prepare the skin with Betadine and drape the abdomen.
- Infiltrate the skin with lignocaine at the marked site.
- Using a 21-gauge needle attached to a 20-ml syringe, advance through the skin while gently aspirating until fluid is withdrawn.
- Remove the needle and apply a sterile dressing.
- Send fluid specimens for biochemistry, protein, glucose, lactate dehyrogenase (LDH), amylase, bacteriology and cytology.
- For therapeutic taps do not remove more than 500 ml in the first 10 minutes or 1 litre at one sitting, due to the risk of hypotension.
- Tell the patient that the procedure is completed and that you will inform them of the results when they are available.

Complications

- Intra-abdominal haemorrhage.
- Perforated viscus (e.g. bladder or bowel).
- Peritonitis.
- Hypotension.
- Precipitation of hepatic coma if the patient has severe liver disease.

---

92 Lumbar puncture

Scenario

Can you tell me what this is and what it is used for? (Spinal needle)
This is a scenario which may be encountered in an OSCE instruments station. It requires you to correctly identify the instrument and its use.
This is a spinal needle. I have seen it used to perform a lumbar puncture.
The following areas may then be discussed:

- indications and contraindications for lumbar puncture
- performing a lumbar puncture
- complications
- differential diagnosis of CSF.

Indications

- Diagnostic:
  - to obtain a sample of CSF for assessment of infection (e.g. meningitis), blood (e.g. subarachnoid haemorrhage), malignant cells, abnormal proteins (e.g. myeloma)
  - injection of contrast (e.g. myelogram).
- Therapeutic:
  - administration of intrathecal drugs (e.g. chemotherapy drugs).

Contraindications

- Raised intracranial pressure (if suspected, perform a CT scan of the head before proceeding).
- Local infection near lumbar puncture site.
- Coagulopathy (platelets < 40).
- Suspicion of a spinal cord or posterior fossa mass.

Performing a lumbar puncture

Introduction and consent

- Introduce yourself to the patient.
- Explain the procedure to the patient, as well as the indication and risks, and obtain their verbal consent.

- Advise the patient that the procedure takes approximately 30 minutes, is not painful but is uncomfortable, and that you will be using a local anaesthetic. Elicit any allergies or contraindications to the procedure (e.g. anticoagulants, papilloedema), and review CT head scan if performed.
- Allow time to address any concerns that the patient may have.

Preparation of equipment

Gather the following on to a procedure trolley:

- spinal needles (21-gauge and 23-gauge)
- procedure pack (containing gallipot, gauze, sterile drapes)
- antiseptic Betadine/chlorhexidine solution
- sterile gloves and gown
- 2% lignocaine (local anaesthetic)
- syringe
- manometer.

Positioning the patient

Help to place the patient in the lateral decubitus position with the spine parallel to and at the edge of the bed. Ask the patient to draw their knees up to their stomach and flex their head to their chest, thereby flexing the vertebral column and widening the intervertebral spaces.

Procedure

- Locate the L3–4 interspace which is found along the supracristal line (an imaginary line between the iliac crests) and mark the puncture site.

- The spinal cord terminates at L1–2 in adults and at L2–3 in children.
- Lumbar puncture should be performed in the L3–4 or L4–5 interspace.
- L4–5 is found along the supracristal line.

- The procedure should be performed using aseptic techniques.
- Open the procedure pack and prepare and check the equipment.

- Scrub and gown.
- Prepare (prep) the skin over the puncture site and overlying several intervertebral spaces with Betadine/chlorhexidine solution applied in a circular fashion from the centre to the periphery.
- Drape the patient.
- Using 2% lignocaine with a 25-gauge needle, raise a wheal over the puncture site to anaesthetise the skin, and then use a 21-gauge needle to infiltrate into the interspinous ligament.
- Wait a few minutes for the local anaesthetic to take effect.
- Holding the spinal needle in the index and middle finger, with the thumb holding the stylet in place, direct the needle between the spinous processes, aiming towards the umbilicus.
- Advance the needle through the skin, supraspinous ligament, interspinous ligament and ligamentum flavum, epidural space, dura and subarachnoid membrane into the subarachnoid space.
- A 'give' is felt on puncturing the ligamentum flavum, and a loss of resistance is felt as the dura is penetrated.
- Withdraw the stylet periodically to check for CSF return. If no CSF is seen, continue to advance the needle a few millimetres.
- Once a CSF flashback is seen, remove the stylet, attach the manometer and measure the pressure. Normal opening pressure is in the range 80–180 mmHg.
- Finally, collect up to 2 ml of CSF into three specimen bottles (one for biochemistry, the second for bacteriology and the third for cytology).
- Withdraw the needle, and apply a dry sterile dressing.
- Dispose of the waste and sharps appropriately.

Closure

- Ask the patient to lie flat and drink plenty of fluid to reduce the risk of post-lumbar-puncture headache.
- Fill out the appropriate forms, label the specimens and dispatch them.
- Write a procedure note.

Complications of lumbar puncture

- Headache (common):
  - relieved by lying down, and worse on standing
  - occurs during the first 24 hours
  - can last up to 1 week.

- Nerve root or conus medullaris damage:
  - rare below L3
  - stop the procedure if the patient complains of paraesthesia.
- Herniation of the medulla or cerebellum through the foramen magnum:
  - seen with raised intracranial pressure.
- Meningitis.
- Bleeding into the subarachnoid or subdural space (can rarely lead to paralysis).

Differential diagnosis of CSF

Pathology	Appearance	Opening pressure	Protein (g/l)	Glucose (mg/ml)	Lymphocytes (mm^{-3})	PMNs (mm^{-3})
Normal	Clear	70–180	0.2–0.4	> 50% (serum)	< 5	Nil
Viral	Clear/ turbid	Normal /↑	Normal /↑	> 50% (serum)	10^{100}	Nil
Bacterial	Turbid/ purulent	↑	0.5–2	< 50% (serum)	< 50	200–3,000
Myco-plasma	Turbid/ viscous	↑	< 500	< 1/3 (serum)	100–300	0–200

PMNs, polymorphonuclear neutrophils.

Radiology

93 Interpreting chest X-rays

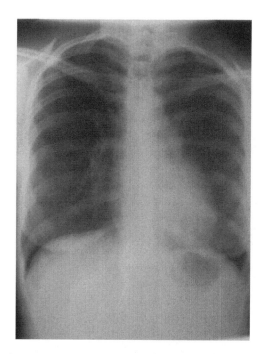

Figure 21   Chest X-ray.

General approach

Name, age and date of radiograph.

Quality of the radiograph

- Rotation: Identify the medial ends of the clavicles and select one of the vertebral spinous processes that fall between them. The medial ends should be equidistant from the spinous process.

- Penetration: Look at the lower part of the cardiac shadow. The vertebral bodies should be just visible through the cardiac shadow.
- Degree of inspiration: Count the number of ribs above the diaphragm. The midpoint of the right hemidiaphragm should be between the fifth and seventh ribs anteriorly.

Orientation (PA, AP or lateral)

Look for the radiographer's marking (left or right).

Trachea

Ensure that the trachea is central. A shift may represent mediastinal or lung pathology.

Mediastinum

- Check for a clear edge.
- If the mediastinal diameter is more than 30% of the intrathoracic diameter, the mediastinum is enlarged.
- Causes include:
  - aortic dissection
  - lymph nodes
  - thymus
  - thyroid
  - tumour.

Heart

- The cardiothoracic ratio is the ratio of the heart width to the chest width. It should be less than 50%.
- The heart should be normal shape.

Lung hilum

- Composed of pulmonary arteries and veins, lymph nodes and airways.
- Compare shape and density.
- The left hilum is higher than the right (by 1 cm).
- Describe hilar abnormalities.

Lung fields

- These should be of equal transradiancy.
- Identify the horizontal fissure and check its position.
- Identify the costophrenic angles and ensure that they are well defined.
- Identify discrete or generalised shadows.
- Increased translucency may indicate:
  - pneumothorax
  - bullous change
  - hyperinflation in chronic obstructive pulmonary disease
  - pulmonary hypertension
  - pulmonary embolism.
- Abnormal opacities may indicate:
  - consolidation
  - collapse
  - coin lesion, ring, shadows, linear opacities or diffuse shadows.

Diaphragm

- Expansion: 6 ± 1 anterior ribs or 9 ± 1 posterior ribs.
- The right hemidiaphragm should be higher than the left by 3 cm.

Soft tissues

- These include:
  - breast shadow
  - subcutaneous fat distribution.
- Look for enlargement.

Bones

- Look at the ribs, scapula and vertebrae.
- Look for fractures.

Summary and diagnosis

Ensure radiograph is reviewed by a radiologist

94 Interpreting abdominal X-rays

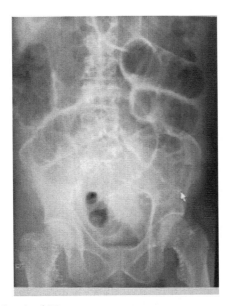

Figure 22 Abdominal X-ray.

General approach

Name, age, date of radiograph and orientation.

Quality of the radiograph

Orientation

Erect or supine.

Contrast present

Bones of spine and pelvis

Look for moderate degenerative change in lumbar spine or in hips, metastases, or collapse.

Calcification in abdomen and pelvis

Arteries (look for a calcified abdominal aortic aneurysm or iliac arteries), lymph nodes, phleboliths and stones.

Soft tissue

Look for psoas line and kidney size and shape.

Bowel and gas pattern

Look for small bowel (central position, valvulae conniventes) or large bowel (more peripheral, haustra) obstruction and gas distribution (air in liver, biliary, GU, peritoneum and colonic wall).

Summary and diagnosis

Ensure radiograph is reviewed by a radiologist

95 Interpreting orthopaedic X-rays

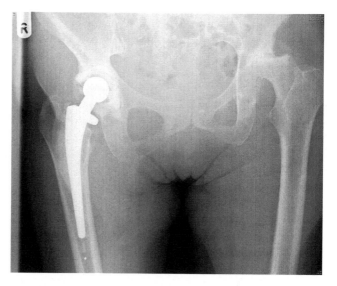

Figure 23 AP X-ray of the pelvis demonstrating avascular necrosis of the left hip and a right THR.

General approach

Name, age, date of radiograph and orientation.

Quality of the radiograph

Orientation

Be systematic

Distant and then close up.

Bone quality

Density and thickness.

Bone alignment

Dislocations, subluxations or fractures, or deformity.

Examination

- Look specifically for fracture lines.
- Fractures appear as a lucent line.
- Trace outline of cortical bone for breaks in integrity.
- Look for bulging or puckering of the cortex.
- Examine joint space and cartilage.
- Examine the soft tissue for swelling or free air.
- Use a Hotlamp if available.
- Always ask to see the two views/orientations (i.e. AP and lateral).

Summary and diagnosis

- Present films at the Trauma Meeting.

Ensure radiographs are reviewed by a radiologist

96 Interpreting computerised tomography (CT) scans of the head

CT scans of the head can be obtained for a number of different reasons – for example, in cases of trauma, stroke, subarachnoid haemorrhage, degenerative disease, infection or tumour.

General approach

Name, age and date of radiograph.

Quality

Orientation (i.e. coronal, sagittal or transverse sections)

Contrast present

Brain parenchyma

Look for symmetry. Is there a suspicious lesion in one half of the brain but not in the other half? Is there a shift of the midline, indicating a mass effect?

- The junction of grey matter and white matter adjacent to the cortex and the basal ganglia should be well defined. Poor delineation should raise the possibility of cerebral oedema.
- Hyperdensity within the parchenchyma is due to either haemorrhage or calcification. A haematoma will produce a mass effect upon adjacent structures. Calcification will usually be punctuate and have no mass effect.

Ventricles and subarachnoid spaces

Look for enlargement of the ventricles and the subarachnoid spaces. Children usually have narrow spaces, and the elderly usually have large ventricles and subarachnoid spaces, due to brain atrophy.

- Hyperdensity within the subarachnoid spaces and the ventricles usually indicates haemorrhage.

Dura and subdural space

Always check the subdural windows for subdural haemorrhage.

Bone and air spaces

Check for fractures, bone destruction and other bone lesions.

Skin and subcutaneous tissues

Check for swelling or free air in the soft tissues.

Note: Hounsfield units: bone, +1000; water, 0; fat, −1000.

Summary and diagnosis

Ensure radiographs are reviewed by a radiologist

Example 1

Skull fractures are categorised as linear or depressed, depending on whether the fracture fragments are depressed below the surface of the skull. Linear fractures are more common. The bone windows must be examined carefully.

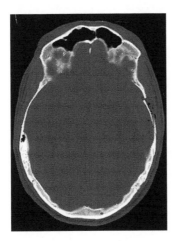

Example 2

Extradural haemorrhages arise between the skull and the dura. They usually develop from injury to the middle meningeal artery or one of its branches. A temporal bone may be fractured.

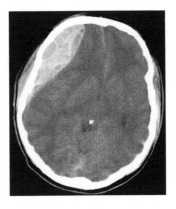

Example 3

Subdural haematomas arise between the dura and the arachnoid, often from ruptured veins crossing this potential space. The space enlarges as the brain atrophies, and thus subdural haematomas are more common in the elderly.

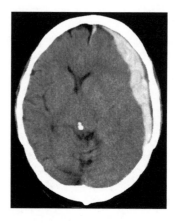

Written skills

97 Requesting a blood transfusion: crossmatching and complications

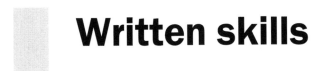

BLOOD TRANSFUSION

Hospital No. 123456 B D.O.B. 23/3/46	Consultant/GP: MR JONES
Surname SMITH	
First Name JOHN	
Affix Addressograph label here	Tests Required
28. FLOWER POT LANE	Group and Screen ☐ Crossmatch ☑
NORTHUMBRIA NW8 7JX	Other tests No. Units Required 8
Patient Location (Ward) A&E	Please note that this hospital operates a maximum surgical blood order schedule MSBOS Requests for crossmatch exceeding this schedule must be clarified with the laboratory staff
NHS ☑ Private ☐	
In pt. ☐ Out pt. ☐	
Theatre ☐	Date Required 23/1/07 Time Required ASAP
Specimen taken by (sign and date) 23/1/07	
Clinical Details/Relevant drugs, etc.	Blood retained for 48 hours only
- Ruptured AAA	Requesting Physician E. SPRATT
- URGENT	Bleep 009 Ext - Date 23/1/07
Ethnic Origin: Caucasian	
Previous Transfusion: Y (N)	
Date of most recent transfusion N/A	
Antibodies (if known) Not known.	
Special Requirements	

Figure 24   Crossmatch blood form.

Complications of blood transfusion are related to the mechanisms of transfusion (cannula site sepsis, haematoma or air embolism) or to transfusion itself.

Early complications

- Non-haemolytic transfusion (HLA mediated).
- Circulatory overload.

Delayed complications

- Delayed haemolytic reaction.
- Infection and septicaemia: hepatitis B and C, HIV, cytomegalovirus, syphilis, malaria.
- Iron overload.
- Immunosuppression (therapy in renal transplant).

Massive transfusion (replacement of the entire circulating blood volume within 1 day)

- Hypothermia.
- Citrate toxicity.
- Hypocalcaemia – citrate binding.
- Hyperkalaemia.
- Dilutional coagulopathy.
- Acute respiratory distress syndrome (ARDS).

98 Completing blood forms

- Fill out blood forms with a black indelible pen.
- Clearly print the patient's details (surname, first name, date of birth and hospital number).
- Complete the requested investigations.
  - Haematology: group and antibody screen (G+S), crossmatch and the number of units required, full blood count (FBC), clotting screen, INR, D-dimers, activated partial thromboplastin time (APTT), fibrinogen.
  - Biochemistry: urea and electrolytes (U&E), liver function tests (LFTs), thyroid function, troponin T, tumour markers, glucose, lactate, C-reactive protein (CRP).
  - Microbiology (blood culture): microscopy, sensitivity and culture (MC+S).
- Clearly print your name, contact bleep number and position.
- Print the consultant's name and team.
- State whether the patient is an inpatient or outpatient.
- Give the indication for performing the test.
- State the speed of processing (routine or urgent).
- Ring the laboratory if it is an urgent or out-of-hours request.
- Sign the completed form.

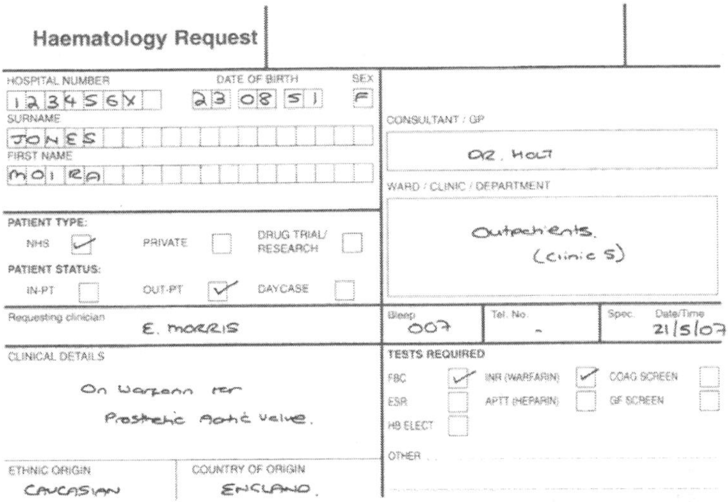

Haematology Request

HOSPITAL NUMBER 123456X | DATE OF BIRTH 23 08 51 | SEX F

SURNAME JONES

FIRST NAME MOIRA

CONSULTANT / GP: DR. HOLT

WARD / CLINIC / DEPARTMENT: Outpatients. (clinic 5)

PATIENT TYPE: NHS ✓ | PRIVATE | DRUG TRIAL/ RESEARCH

PATIENT STATUS: IN-PT | OUT-PT ✓ | DAYCASE

Requesting clinician: E. MORRIS

Bleep: 007 | Tel. No. - | Spec. | Date/Time: 21/5/07

CLINICAL DETAILS: On Warfarin for Prosthetic Aortic Valve.

TESTS REQUIRED: FBC ✓ | INR (WARFARIN) ✓ | COAG SCREEN | ESR | APTT (HEPARIN) | GF SCREEN | HB ELECT | OTHER

ETHNIC ORIGIN: CAUCASIAN | COUNTRY OF ORIGIN: ENGLAND.

Figure 25 (a) Haematology form.

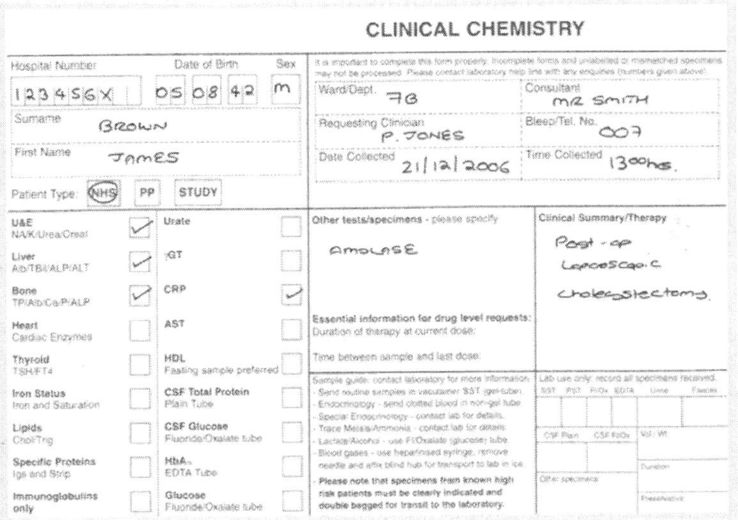

CLINICAL CHEMISTRY

Hospital Number 123456X | Date of Birth 05 08 42 | Sex M

Surname BROWN

First Name JAMES

Patient Type: (NHS) | PP | STUDY

It is important to complete this form properly. Incomplete forms and unlabelled or mismatched specimens may not be processed. Please contact laboratory help line with any enquiries (numbers given above)

Ward/Dept. 7B | Consultant MR SMITH

Requesting Clinician P. JONES | Bleep/Tel. No. 007

Date Collected 21/12/2006 | Time Collected 1300hrs.

U&E NA/K/Urea/Creat ✓ | Urate

Liver Alb/TBil/ALP/ALT ✓ | γGT

Bone TP/Alb/Ca/P/ALP ✓ | CRP ✓

Heart Cardiac Enzymes | AST

Thyroid TSH/FT4 | HDL Fasting sample preferred

Iron Status Iron and Saturation | CSF Total Protein Plain Tube

Lipids Chol/Trig | CSF Glucose Fluoride/Oxalate tube

Specific Proteins Igs and Strip | HbA1c EDTA Tube

Immunoglobulins only | Glucose Fluoride/Oxalate tube

Other tests/specimens - please specify: AMYLASE

Clinical Summary/Therapy: Post-op Laparoscopic Cholecystectomy.

Essential information for drug level requests: Duration of therapy at current dose: Time between sample and last dose:

Sample guide: contact laboratory for more information
- Send routine samples in vacutainer SST (gel-tube)
- Endocrinology - send clotted blood in non-gel tube
- Special Endocrinology - contact lab for details
- Trace Metals/Ammonia - contact lab for details
- Lactate/Alcohol - use F/Oxalate (glucose) tube
- Blood gases - use heparinised syringe, remove needle and affix blind hub for transport to lab in ice

Please note that specimens from known high risk patients must be clearly indicated and double bagged for transit to the laboratory.

Lab use only: record all specimens received. SST | PST | F/Ox | EDTA | Urine | Faeces | CSF Plain | CSF F/Ox | Vol / Wt | Duration | Other specimens | Preservative

Figure 25 (b) Biochemistry form.

99 Writing prescription charts on the ward

- There are a number of general scenarios for which you will be required to write up a prescription chart.
- Each hospital has a different chart, but all charts have general similarities.
- Before writing the chart you must gather an accurate history from the patient and perform an examination to try to determine which drugs are needed.

General scheme

- Introduce yourself to the patient.
- Establish a rapport.
- Take a full history and perform an examination.
- Explain the diagnosis to the patient.
- Agree on a mutual management plan.
- Tell the patient what the management plan entails.
- Describe any precautions that the patient should take while being treated with the drugs.
- Discuss the patient's current medications.
- Ask them about any allergies.
- Discuss the risks and benefits of each drug.
- Ask the patient to contact you or any other medical staff if they have any further questions.
- Ask the patient to look out for symptoms like vomiting, diarrhoea or rashes.
- Give them information leaflets as appropriate.
- Give them your contact details.
- Tell them that if they develop any side-effects they must stop the medication and get medical help.
- Ask them if they have any questions.
- Thank the patient.

General details on prescription chart

- Name of patient.
- Identity number.
- Date of birth.
- Consultant's name.
- Junior doctor's name.
- Junior doctor's bleep.
- Date of admission.
- Allergies.

- Each chart has the following sections:
  - stat or once only drugs
  - regular drugs
  - as required drugs (PRN)
  - fluid chart (may be included).

Prescribing exercise

- A sample of a filled out drug chart will be included to help you.
- You will be required to fill out a drug chart for the following conditions:
  - chronic obstructive pulmonary disease (COPD)
  - myocardial infarction
  - atrial fibrillation
  - acute left ventricular failure
  - peptic ulcer disease
  - acute gout
  - lobar pneumonia.

Scenario 1

Mr Francis is a 60-year-old man who has been admitted with breathlessness. He has been coughing up a greenish-brown coloured sputum. He is known to have chronic obstructive pulmonary disease (COPD). He is currently using inhalers (salbutamol 2 puffs PRN and Seretide 2 puffs PRN). In addition, he suffers from insomnia and has been taking diazepam. He has widespread crackles on his chest and is finding it difficult to breathe. His date of birth is 23/09/1947. His consultant is Dr Philips and his identity number is 56786.

Please write this patient's prescription chart.

Points to note

- This patient is suffering from acute exacerbation of COPD.
- You need to write out his current medication on the chart.
- Diazepam needs to be stopped, as it is a respiratory depressant.
- You will need to give him oxygen at a low percentage (i.e. 24% or 28%, depending on blood gases). COPD relies on carbon dioxide drive.
- You need to give him nebulised salbutamol for the wheezing.
- Give regular nebulised saline to aid expectoration of secretions.
- You need to prescribe him antibiotics for 5 days to cover community acquired infections.
- The antibiotics may be changed depending on the sputum culture.
- The patient needs a short course of steroids (e.g. prednisolone) that needs to be tapered off.

HAMMERSMITH HOSPITALS NHS TRUST
MEDICINE PRESCRIPTION CHART

DRUGS SENSITIVITIES AND FOOD ALLERGIES

NK DA

Weight (kg)		AFFIX ADDRESSOGRAPH LABEL HERE	
Height (m)		SURNAME FRANCIS	
Surface Area (m²)		FIRST NAME(S) JOHN	
		HOSPITAL NUMBER 5678C	
		DATE OF BIRTH 23/9/1947	

Date of Admission	Ward	Consultant
23/8/07	ARE	DR PHILIPS

Pharmacy Cost Centre	Tick box if Private Patient

ONCE ONLY PRESCRIPTIONS

Date	Time	Drug	Dose	Route	Additional Instructions	Signature / Print Name / Bleep	Time Given	Given by	Pharm.
23/8/07	06ʰˢ	SALBUTAMOL	5 mg	neb		S Byp 123 SK SRITARAN			
23/8/07	06ʰˢ	IPRATROPIUM BROMIDE	0.5 mg	neb		S Byp R3 SK SRITARAN			
23/8/07	06ʰˢ	PREDNISOLONE	30 mg	Po		S Byp 123 SK SRITARAN			
23/8/07	06ʰˢ	CEFUROXIME	750 mg	iv		S Byp 123 SK SRITARAN			
23/8/07	06ʰˢ	ERYTHROMYCIN	500 mg	Po		S Byp 123 SK SRITARAN			

VARIABLE PRESCRIPTIONS
(e.g. Steriods, Insulin)

	Month ⟶			
	Date ⟶			

Pharm.	DATE ⟶	Start	Change	Change	Change
	TIME ⟶	Dose	Dose	Dose	Dose
Drug					
Route					
Additional Instructions					
Signature					
Print Name Bleep No.					

Pharm.	DATE ⟶	Start	Change	Change	Change
	TIME ⟶	Dose	Dose	Dose	Dose
Drug					
Route					
Additional Instructions					
Signature					
Print Name Bleep No.					

ORAL ANTICOAGULANTS

TARGET INR RANGE

Drug	INR
Time	DOSE
Signature	SIGNATURE
Print Name Bleep No.	
Pharmacy	GIVEN BY

DISCHARGE MEDICATION (TO BE PRESCRIBED ON SEPARATE DISCHARGE & TTO FORM)	Seen by Pharmacist		Given to Patient on Ward (Nurse to sign here)
	Initials	Date	

WMD001

REGULAR PRESCRIPTIONS

PATIENT'S NAME:		HOSPITAL No:

MONTH	YEAR	DATE →
		TIMES →

DRUG (Approved Name) OXYGEN

Dose	Route	Frequency	Start Date
28%	Face mask	—	23/8/07

Signature	Pharmacy	Stop Date
S		

Print Name / Bleep No. K. SRINIVASAN Bip 123

Additional Instructions	Stopped by

DRUG (Approved Name) SALBUTAMOL

Dose	Route	Frequency	Start Date
5 ms	neb	qds	23/8/07

Signature	Pharmacy	Stop Date
S		

Print Name / Bleep No. K. SRINIVASAN Bip 123

Additional Instructions	Stopped by

DRUG (Approved Name) IPRATROPIUM BROMIDE

Dose	Route	Frequency	Start Date
0.5mg	neb	qds	23/8/07

Signature	Pharmacy	Stop Date
S		

Print Name / Bleep No. K. SRINIVASAN Bip 123

Additional Instructions	Stopped by

DRUG (Approved Name) NORMAL SALINE NEBS

Dose	Route	Frequency	Start Date
5ml	neb	qds	23/8/07

Signature	Pharmacy	Stop Date
S		

Print Name / Bleep No. K. SRINIVASAN Bip 123

Additional Instructions	Stopped by

DRUG (Approved Name) PARACETAMOL

Dose	Route	Frequency	Start Date
1g	po/iv/pr	qds	23/8/07

Signature	Pharmacy	Stop Date
S		

Print Name / Bleep No. K. SRINIVASAN Bip 123

Additional Instructions	Stopped by

DRUG (Approved Name) SERETIDE

Dose	Route	Frequency	Start Date
Tt	inh	bd	23/8/07

Signature	Pharmacy	Stop Date
S		

Print Name / Bleep No. K. SRINIVASAN Bip 123

Additional Instructions	Stopped by

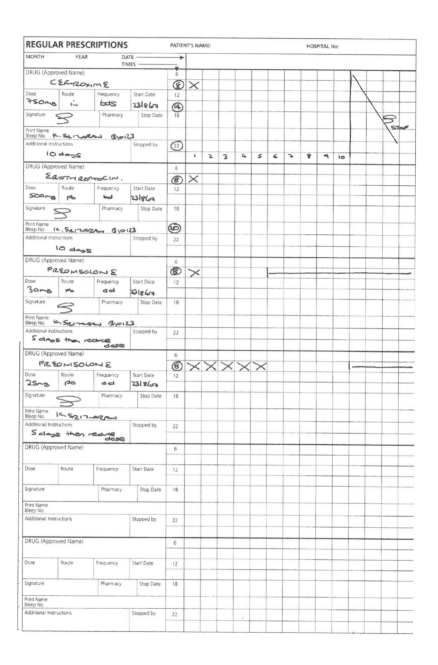

NOTES ON THE USE OF THE PRESCRIPTION SHEET

A. Print legibly in black ink using approved drug names.

B. The prescription sheet is valid for 2 weeks only. After this time, the chart must be re-written to allow further drug administration to be recorded.

C. Any changes in drug therapy must be ordered by a new prescription. DO NOT alter existing instructions.

D. 'Regular prescriptions' should be prescribed indicating the frequency and time of administration.

E. When a drug is not administered record the appropriate number in the administration record box and initial:
1. – Patient away from ward.
2. – Patient could not receive drug (e.g. nil by mouth, vomiting, no venous access).
3. – Patient refusing drug.
4. – Drug not available.
5. – On instructions of doctor.
6. – Patient did not require drug.
7. – Patient self-administering.
8. – Illegible.

F. Enter dietary regimens in the 'Regular Prescriptions' section. Do not use the intravenous chart.

G. Discharge drugs. These should be prescribed on the separate Discharge & TTO Prescription Sheet. The pharmacist should indicate on the front of this chart that the Discharge Prescription has been seen by the pharmacy and the nurse should indicate that the patient has been given the discharge drugs.

H. Sliding scale insulin should be prescribed on the separate insulin prescription chart. Additionally, on the Regular section of this chart a cross-reference to that chart should be added, e.g. "insulin – see sliding scale insulin chart".

PREPARATIONS ADMINISTERED BY REGISTERED NURSE OR MIDWIFE UNDER PATIENT GROUP DIRECTIONS

DRUG (Approved Name)	Dose	Date	Time	Given by	Dose	Date	Time	Given by	Pharm

MONTH   YEAR   DATE ➤

WHEN REQUIRED PRESCRIPTIONS

DRUG (Approved Name) SALBUTAMOL

Dose	Route	Max Frequency	Start Date
5mg	neb	PRN	23186?

Signature	Pharmacy	Stop Date

Print Name Bleep No. KSETHARAN	BIP.23

Additional Instructions	Stopped by

DRUG (Approved Name) TEMAZEPAM

Dose	Route	Max Frequency	Start Date
10mg	po	nocte	23186?

Signature	Pharmacy	Stop Date

Print Name Bleep No. SZITHARAN	BIP.123

Additional Instructions	Stopped by

DRUG (Approved Name)

Dose	Route	Max Frequency	Start Date

Signature	Pharmacy	Stop Date

Print Name Bleep No.	

Additional Instructions	Stopped by

DRUG (Approved Name)

Dose	Route	Max Frequency	Start Date

Signature	Pharmacy	Stop Date

Print Name Bleep No.	

Additional Instructions	Stopped by

DRUG (Approved Name)

Dose	Route	Max Frequency	Start Date

Signature	Pharmacy	Stop Date

Print Name Bleep No.	

Additional Instructions	Stopped by

DRUG (Approved Name)

Dose	Route	Max Frequency	Start Date

Signature	Pharmacy	Stop Date

Print Name Bleep No.	

Additional Instructions	Stopped by

continued overleaf

)se	Sig.	Time	Dose	Sig.	Time	Dose	Sig.	Time	Dose	Sig	Time	Dose	Sig.	Time	Dose	Sig.	Time	Dose	Sig	Time	Dose	Sig.	Time	Dose	Sig
		STOPPED																							
		EXACERBATION																							
		COPD																							

INTRAVENOUS INFUSION THERAPY
Record time of changing syringe pump. Administration of blood products and some medicines require two signatures. See the Trust's Medicines Policy.
Do not use more than 2 continuation sheets.

PATIENT'S NAME

HOSPITAL NUMBER

Date	Time	Intravenous Fluid	Volume	Additives and Special Instructions	Dose	Running Time or Flow Rate	Signature/ Print Name/ Bleep	Unit/Batch Number (Blood Products only)	Time Begun	Administration Signature	Witness Signature	Time Ended	Pharm. Initials
23/8/17	0600hrs	0.9% normal Saline	1 L	20mmol KCL		80	S.K.Sachardena Bleep 123						
23/8/17		5% DEXTROSE	1 L	20mmol KCL		80	S.K.Sachardena Bleep 123						

Scenario 2

Mr Stewart is a 40-year-old man who is admitted to Accident and Emergency with crushing central chest pain. ECG shows widespread ST elevation. A blood test for troponin T is positive. He has a history of hypertension and was taking verapamil. His identity number is 256748. His consultant is Dr Bloggs and his date of birth is 24/07/1967.

Please write this patient's prescription chart.

Points to note

- This patient has suffered an ST-elevation myocardial infarction.
- You need to stop the verapamil, as calcium-channel blockers are contraindicated in myocardial infarction.
- You need to give adequate oxygen, painkillers and anti-sickness medication, and treat the hypertension.
- Lifestyle modification such as cholesterol treatment needs to be added.
- In addition, an ACE inhibitor and beta-blocker should be commenced within 24 hours.
- The use of anti-platelet and anti-thrombotic medication needs to be considered.
- The issue of thrombolysis needs to be considered, but only a senior doctor can sign for it.

HAMMERSMITH HOSPITALS NHS TRUST
MEDICINE PRESCRIPTION CHART

DRUGS SENSITIVITIES AND FOOD ALLERGIES

NKDA

Weight (kg)	70ks
Height (m)	
Surface Area (m²)	

AFFIX ADDRESSOGRAPH LABEL HERE

SURNAME   STEWART

FIRST NAME(S)   EDWARD

HOSPITAL NUMBER   256748

DATE OF BIRTH   24/7/1967

Date of Admission	Ward	Consultant
23/8/67	A&E	DR BLOGGS

Pharmacy Cost Centre

Tick box if Private Patient

ONCE ONLY PRESCRIPTIONS

Date	Time	Drug	Dose	Route	Additional Instructions	Signature / Print Name / Bleep	Time Given	Given by	Pharm.
23/8/67	1400	GTN	÷	SL		S K. Srinivasan 3623			
23/8/67	1400	ASPIRIN	300 mg	PO		S K. Srinivasan 8123			
23/8/67	1400	CLOPIDOGREL	300 mg	PO		S K. Srinivasan 8123			
23/8/67	1400	MORPHINE	10 mg	iv		S K. Srinivasan 8123			
23/8/67	1400	METOCLOPRAMIDE	10 mg	im/iv		S K. Srinivasan 8123			

VARIABLE PRESCRIPTIONS
(e.g. Steriods, Insulin)

Month ➔
Date ➔

	Start	Change	Change	Change
Pharm. DATE ➔ TIME ➔	Dose	Dose	Dose	Dose
Drug				
Route				
Additional Instructions				
Signature				
Print Name Bleep No.				

	Start	Change	Change	Change
Pharm. DATE ➔ TIME ➔	Dose	Dose	Dose	Dose
Drug				
Route				
Additional instructions				
Signature				
Print Name Bleep No.				

ORAL ANTICOAGULANTS

TARGET INR RANGE

Drug	INR
Time	DOSE
Signature	SIGNATURE
Print Name Bleep No. Pharmacy	GIVEN BY

DISCHARGE MEDICATION (TO BE PRESCRIBED ON SEPARATE DISCHARGE & TTO FORM)

Seen by Pharmacist		Given to Patient on Ward (Nurse to sign here)
Initials	Date	

WMD001

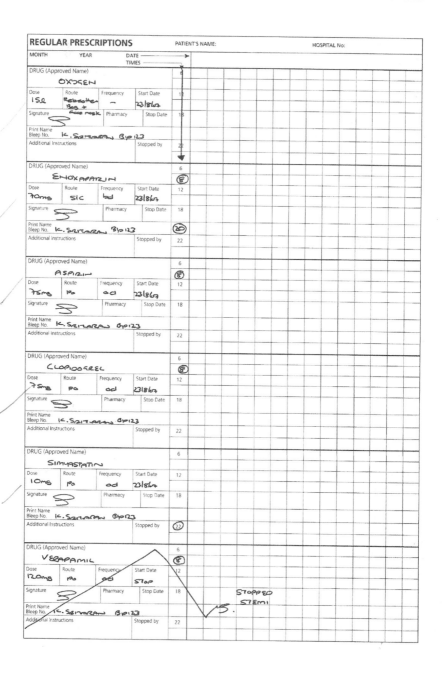

REGULAR PRESCRIPTIONS

PATIENT'S NAME:

HOSPITAL No:

MONTH   YEAR   DATE ———→
                         TIMES ———→

DRUG (Approved Name)
OXYGEN

Dose	Route	Frequency	Start Date
15L	Rebreather Bag + face mask	—	23/8/67

Signature

Print Name / Bleep No. K. Sritaran Bip 123

Additional Instructions   Stopped by

DRUG (Approved Name)
ENOXAPARIN

Dose	Route	Frequency	Start Date
70mg	SC	bd	23/8/67

Signature   Pharmacy   Stop Date

Print Name / Bleep No. K. Sritaran Bip 123

Additional Instructions   Stopped by

DRUG (Approved Name)
ASPIRIN

Dose	Route	Frequency	Start Date
75mg	PO	od	23/8/67

Signature   Pharmacy   Stop Date

Print Name / Bleep No. K. Sritaran Bip 123

Additional Instructions   Stopped by

DRUG (Approved Name)
CLOPIDOGREL

Dose	Route	Frequency	Start Date
75mg	PO	od	23/8/67

Signature   Pharmacy   Stop Date

Print Name / Bleep No. K. Sritaran Bip 123

Additional Instructions   Stopped by

DRUG (Approved Name)
SIMVASTATIN

Dose	Route	Frequency	Start Date
10mg	PO	od	23/8/67

Signature   Pharmacy   Stop Date

Print Name / Bleep No. K. Sritaran Bip 123

Additional Instructions   Stopped by

DRUG (Approved Name)
VERAPAMIL

Dose	Route	Frequency	Start Date
120mg	PO	od	Stop

Signature   Pharmacy   Stop Date

STOPPED
STEMI
S.

Print Name / Bleep No. K. Sritaran Bip 123

Additional Instructions   Stopped by

REGULAR PRESCRIPTIONS

PATIENT'S NAME: HOSPITAL No:

MONTH	YEAR	DATE ➤		
		TIMES		

DRUG (Approved Name)				6	
ATENOLOL				⑧	
Dose	Route	Frequency	Start Date	12	
50mg	po	od	23/8/67		
Signature S		Pharmacy	Stop Date	18	
Print Name Bleep No. K.SRITARAN B/p123					
Additional Instructions			Stopped by	22	

DRUG (Approved Name)				6	
RAMIPRIL					
Dose	Route	Frequency	Start Date	12	
5mg	po	od	24/8/67		
Signature S		Pharmacy	Stop Date	18	
Print Name Bleep No. K.SRITARAN B/p123					
Additional Instructions monitor renal function.			Stopped by	㉒	

DRUG (Approved Name)				6	
Dose	Route	Frequency	Start Date	12	
Signature		Pharmacy	Stop Date	18	
Print Name Bleep No					
Additional Instructions			Stopped by	22	

DRUG (Approved Name)				6	
Dose	Route	Frequency	Start Date	12	
Signature		Pharmacy	Stop Date	18	
Print Name Bleep No.					
Additional Instructions			Stopped by	22	

DRUG (Approved Name)				6	
Dose	Route	Frequency	Start Date	12	
Signature		Pharmacy	Stop Date	18	
Print Name Bleep No.					
Additional Instructions			Stopped by	22	

DRUG (Approved Name)				6	
Dose	Route	Frequency	Start Date	12	
Signature		Pharmacy	Stop Date	18	
Print Name Bleep No					
Additional Instructions			Stopped by	22	

NOTES ON THE USE OF THE PRESCRIPTION SHEET

A. Print legibly in black ink using approved drug names.

B. The prescription sheet is valid for 2 weeks only. After this time, the chart must be re-written to allow further drug administration to be recorded.

C. Any changes in drug therapy must be ordered by a new prescription. DO NOT alter existing instructions.

D. 'Regular prescriptions' should be prescribed indicating the frequency and time of administration.

E. When a drug is not administered record the appropriate number in the administration record box and initial:
1. – Patient away from ward.
2. – Patient could not receive drug (e.g. nil by mouth, vomiting, no venous access).
3. – Patient refusing drug.
4. – Drug not available.
5. – On instructions of doctor.
6. – Patient did not require drug.
7. – Patient self-administering.
8. – Illegible.

F. Enter dietary regimens in the 'Regular Prescriptions' section. Do not use the intravenous chart.

G. Discharge drugs. These should be prescribed on the separate Discharge & TTO Prescription Sheet. The pharmacist should indicate on the front of this chart that the Discharge Prescription has been seen by the pharmacy and the nurse should indicate that the patient has been given the discharge drugs.

H. Sliding scale insulin should be prescribed on the separate insulin prescription chart. Additionally, on the Regular section of this chart a cross-reference to that chart should be added, e.g. "insulin – see sliding scale insulin chart".

PREPARATIONS ADMINISTERED BY REGISTERED NURSE OR MIDWIFE UNDER PATIENT GROUP DIRECTIONS

DRUG (Approved Name)	Dose	Date	Time	Given by	Dose	Date	Time	Given by	Pharm

---

MONTH   YEAR   DATE ────▶

WHEN REQUIRED PRESCRIPTIONS

DRUG (Approved Name) MORPHINE

Dose 5– 10mg	Route im iv	Max Frequency 4o	Start Date 23|8|o9
Signature		Pharmacy	Stop Date
Print Name Bleep No. K. SRITARAN Bp123			
Additional Instructions See Stat section			Stopped by

DRUG (Approved Name) METOCLOPRAMIDE

Dose 10mg	Route iv im po	Max Frequency 6dS	Start Date 23|8|o9
Signature		Pharmacy	Stop Date
Print Name Bleep No. K. Sritaran B1p123			
Additional Instructions See Stat section			Stopped by

DRUG (Approved Name) GTN

Dose -7-	Route S1l	Max Frequency PRN.	Start Date 23|8|o9
Signature		Pharmacy	Stop Date
Print Name Bleep No. K. Sritaran Bp123			
Additional Instructions with chest pain			Stopped by

DRUG (Approved Name)

Dose	Route	Max Frequency	Start Date
Signature		Pharmacy	Stop Date
Print Name Bleep No.			
Additional Instructions			Stopped by

DRUG (Approved Name)

Dose	Route	Max Frequency	Start Date
Signature		Pharmacy	Stop Date
Print Name Bleep No.			
Additional Instructions			Stopped by

DRUG (Approved Name)

Dose	Route	Max Frequency	Start Date
Signature		Pharmacy	Stop Date
Print Name Bleep No.			
Additional Instructions			Stopped by

continued opposite

se	Sig.	Time	Dose	Sig.	Time	Dose	Sig.	Time	Dose	Sig.	Time	Dose	Sig.	Time	Dose	Sig.	Time	Dose	Sig.	Time	Dose	Sig.	Time	Dose	Sig.

INTRAVENOUS INFUSION THERAPY
Record time of changing syringe pump. Administration of blood products and some medicines require two signatures. See the Trust's Medicines Policy.
Do not use more than 2 continuation sheets.

PATIENT'S NAME

HOSPITAL NUMBER

Date	Time	Intravenous Fluid	Volume	Additives and Special Instructions	Dose	Running Time or Flow Rate	Signature/ Print Name/ Bleep	Unit/Batch Number (Blood Products only)	Time Begun	Administration Signature	Witness Signature	Time Ended	Pharm. Initials

Scenario 3

Mrs Edwards is a 77-year-old woman. Her date of birth is 5/12/1930. She is admitted with palpitations. An ECG shows absent P-waves. She has heart failure and is taking ramipril 5 mg. Her identity number is 356789 and her consultant is Dr Brooks.

Please write this patient's prescription chart.

Points to note

- This patient is suffering from atrial fibrillation.
- As the patient is elderly and has heart failure, digoxin is the treatment of choice.
- Consider giving an anti-thrombotic such as heparin, whilst simultaneously loading with warfarin.
- The heparin will be stopped once the desired INR is reached.
- Digoxin levels need to be measured regularly to avoid toxicity.
- A loading dose of digoxin is needed, and a reduced dose of digoxin thereafter due to the patient's age.

HAMMERSMITH HOSPITALS NHS TRUST **MEDICINE PRESCRIPTION CHART**	Weight (kg)	AFFIX ADDRESSOGRAPH LABEL HERE
DRUGS SENSITIVITIES AND FOOD ALLERGIES	Height (m)	SURNAME _EDWARDS_
		FIRST NAME(S) _AMANDA_
NKDA	Surface Area (m²)	HOSPITAL NUMBER _356789_
		DATE OF BIRTH _5/12/1930_

Date of Admission 30/5/07	Ward A&E	Consultant DR BROOKS

ONCE ONLY PRESCRIPTIONS

Pharmacy Cost Centre	Tick box if Private Patient

Date	Time	Drug	Dose	Route	Additional Instructions	Signature / Print Name / Bleep	Time Given	Given by	Pharm.
30/5/07	1200	DIGOXIN	500 mcg	PO		S K. SRITHARAN B4623			
31/5/07	0800	DIGOXIN	500 mcg	PO		S K. SRITHARAN B4623			
31/5/07	1200	DIGOXIN	500 mcg	PO		S K. SRITHARAN B4623			

VARIABLE PRESCRIPTIONS
(e.g. Steroids, Insulin)

	Month ➤				
	Date ➤				

Pharm.	DATE ➤		Start	Change	Change	Change
	TIME ➤		Dose	Dose	Dose	Dose
Drug						
Route						
Additional Instructions						
Signature						
Print Name Bleep No.						

Pharm.	DATE ➤		Start	Change	Change	Change
	TIME ➤		Dose	Dose	Dose	Dose
Drug						
Route						
Additional Instructions						
Signature						
Print Name Bleep No.						

ORAL ANTICOAGULANTS

TARGET INR RANGE 2.5 - 3.5

Drug WARFARIN	INR	
Time 1800hrs	DOSE	10 mg
Signature S	SIGNATURE	S
Print Name K. SRITHARAN Bleep No. B4623	GIVEN BY	
Pharmacy		

DISCHARGE MEDICATION (TO BE PRESCRIBED ON SEPARATE DISCHARGE & TTO FORM)	Seen by Pharmacist	Given to Patient on Ward (Nurse to sign here)
	Initials	Date

WMD001

REGULAR PRESCRIPTIONS

PATIENT'S NAME: HOSPITAL No:

MONTH	YEAR	DATE	
		TIMES	

DRUG (Approved Name)				6	ⓔ
DIGOXIN					

Dose	Route	Frequency	Start Date	12
125mcg	Po	od	1/6/07	

Signature	Pharmacy	Stop Date	18

Print Name Bleep No.	K.Sriniraran		
Additional Instructions		Stopped by	22

DRUG (Approved Name)				6
RAMIPRIL				

Dose	Route	Frequency	Start Date	12
5mg	Po	od	30/5/07	

Signature	Pharmacy	Stop Date	18

Print Name Bleep No.	K.Sriniraran Bp12		
Additional Instructions		Stopped by	(22)

REGULAR PRESCRIPTIONS   PATIENT'S NAME: HOSPITAL No:

MONTH		YEAR		DATE ➤ TIMES												

DRUG (Approved Name)				6											
Dose	Route	Frequency	Start Date	12											
Signature		Pharmacy	Stop Date	18											
Print Name Bleep No.															
Additional Instructions			Stopped by	22											

DRUG (Approved Name)				6											
Dose	Route	Frequency	Start Date	12											
Signature		Pharmacy	Stop Date	18											
Print Name Bleep No.															
Additional Instructions			Stopped by	22											

DRUG (Approved Name)				6											
Dose	Route	Frequency	Start Date	12											
Signature		Pharmacy	Stop Date	18											
Print Name Bleep No.															
Additional Instructions			Stopped by	22											

DRUG (Approved Name)				6											
Dose	Route	Frequency	Start Date	12											
Signature		Pharmacy	Stop Date	18											
Print Name Bleep No.															
Additional Instructions			Stopped by	22											

DRUG (Approved Name)				6											
Dose	Route	Frequency	Start Date	12											
Signature		Pharmacy	Stop Date	18											
Print Name Bleep No.															
Additional Instructions			Stopped by	22											

DRUG (Approved Name)				6											
Dose	Route	Frequency	Start Date	12											
Signature		Pharmacy	Stop Date	18											
Print Name Bleep No.															
Additional Instructions			Stopped by	22											

NOTES ON THE USE OF THE PRESCRIPTION SHEET

A. Print legibly in black ink using approved drug names.

B. The prescription sheet is valid for 2 weeks only. After this time, the chart must be re-written to allow further drug administration to be recorded.

C. Any changes in drug therapy must be ordered by a new prescription. DO NOT alter existing instructions.

D. 'Regular prescriptions' should be prescribed indicating the frequency and time of administration.

E. When a drug is not administered record the appropriate number in the administration record box and initial:
1. – Patient away from ward.
2. – Patient could not receive drug (e.g. nil by mouth, vomiting, no venous access).
3. – Patient refusing drug.
4. – Drug not available.
5. – On instructions of doctor.
6. – Patient did not require drug.
7. – Patient self-administering.
8. – Illegible.

F. Enter dietary regimens in the 'Regular Prescriptions' section. Do not use the intravenous chart.

G. Discharge drugs. These should be prescribed on the separate Discharge & TTO Prescription Sheet. The pharmacist should indicate on the front of this chart that the Discharge Prescription has been seen by the pharmacy and the nurse should indicate that the patient has been given the discharge drugs.

H. Sliding scale insulin should be prescribed on the separate insulin prescription chart. Additionally, on the Regular section of this chart a cross-reference to that chart should be added, e.g. "insulin – see sliding scale insulin chart".

PREPARATIONS ADMINISTERED BY REGISTERED NURSE OR MIDWIFE UNDER PATIENT GROUP DIRECTIONS

DRUG (Approved Name)	Dose	Date	Time	Given by	Dose	Date	Time	Given by	Pharm

---

MONTH	YEAR	DATE ──────▶	

WHEN REQUIRED PRESCRIPTIONS

DRUG (Approved Name)			
Dose	Route	Max Frequency	Start Date
Signature		Pharmacy	Stop Date
Print Name Bleep No.			
Additional Instructions			Stopped by

DRUG (Approved Name)			
Dose	Route	Max Frequency	Start Date
Signature		Pharmacy	Stop Date
Print Name Bleep No.			
Additional Instructions			Stopped by

DRUG (Approved Name)			
Dose	Route	Max Frequency	Start Date
Signature		Pharmacy	Stop Date
Print Name Bleep No.			
Additional Instructions			Stopped by

DRUG (Approved Name)			
Dose	Route	Max Frequency	Start Date
Signature		Pharmacy	Stop Date
Print Name Bleep No.			
Additional Instructions			Stopped by

DRUG (Approved Name)			
Dose	Route	Max Frequency	Start Date
Signature		Pharmacy	Stop Date
Print Name Bleep No.			
Additional Instructions			Stopped by

DRUG (Approved Name)			
Dose	Route	Max Frequency	Start Date
Signature		Pharmacy	Stop Date
Print Name Bleep No.			
Additional Instructions			Stopped by

continued overleaf

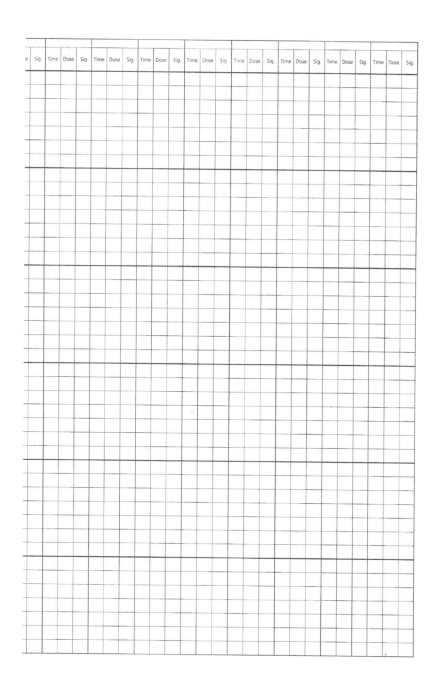

e	Sig.	Time	Dose	Sig.	Time	Dose	Sig.	Time	Dose	Sig.	Time	Dose	Sig.	Time	Dose	Sig.	Time	Dose	Sig.	Time	Dose	Sig.

INTRAVENOUS INFUSION THERAPY
Record time of changing syringe pump. Administration of blood products and some medicines require two signatures. See the Trust's Medicines Policy.
Do not use more than 2 continuation sheets.

PATIENT'S NAME

HOSPITAL NUMBER

Date	Time	Intravenous Fluid	Volume	Additives and Special Instructions	Dose	Running Time or Flow Rate	Signature/ Print Name/ Bleep	Unit/Batch Number (Blood Products only)	Time Begun	Administration Signature	Witness Signature	Time Ended	Pharm. Initials

Scenario 4

Mr Abrahams is an 80-year-old man who is admitted with acute shortness of breath. He is coughing up frothy sputum which is white in colour with a hint of pink. On auscultation there is widespread wheeze and crackles on his chest. He is known to have heart failure, and was recently started on atenolol 100 mg for his heart failure and hypertension. In addition he has angina (he uses a glyceryl trinitrate spray, 2 puffs) and takes 20 mg atorvastatin for cholesterol. His consultant is Dr Adams and his identity number is 87678. His date of birth is 28/04/1927.

Please write this patient's prescription chart.

Points to note

- This patient is suffering from acute left ventricular failure.
- This patient requires high-flow oxygen.
- Nitrate infusion may help to stop the chest pain.
- Adequate pain relief (i.e. morphine) is needed, with an anti-sickness medication.
- Frusemide or another diuretic is needed to relieve the pulmonary oedema.
- Nebulised salbutamol may help with wheezing.

HAMMERSMITH HOSPITALS NHS TRUST
MEDICINE PRESCRIPTION CHART

DRUG SENSITIVITIES AND FOOD ALLERGIES

NKDA

Weight (kg)		AFFIX ADDRESSOGRAPH LABEL HERE
		SURNAME ..... ABRAHAMS
Height (m)		FIRST NAME(S) ..... JOHN
Surface Area (m²)		HOSPITAL NUMBER 87678
		DATE OF BIRTH 28/4/27
Date of Admission 30/5/07	Ward MAU	Consultant DR ADAMS

ONCE ONLY PRESCRIPTIONS

Date	Time	Drug	Dose	Route	Additional Instructions	Signature / Print Name / Bleep	Time Given	Given by	Pharm.
30/5/07	10⁰⁰	FRUSEMIDE	40 mg	iv		S (B/p 5854) K. SRITHARAN			
30/5/07	10⁰⁰ hrs	GTN	2 puffs	s/l	monitor BP	S (B/p 5854) K. SRITHARAN			
30/5/07	10⁰⁰ hrs	MORPHINE	5 mg	iv	—	S (B/p 5854) K. SRITHARAN			
30/5/07	10⁰⁰ hrs	METOCLOPRAMIDE	10 mg	iv/im		S (B/p 5854) K. SRITHARAN			
30/5/07	10⁰⁰ hrs	SALBUTAMOL	5 mg	neb		S (B/p 5854) K. SRITHARAN			

VARIABLE PRESCRIPTIONS
(e.g. Steroids, Insulin)

Month ———▶
Date ———▶

Pharm.	DATE ———▶		Start	Change	Change	Change								
	TIME ———▶		Dose	Dose	Dose	Dose							
Drug													
Route													
Additional Instructions													
Signature													
Print Name Bleep No.													

Pharm.	DATE ———▶		Start	Change	Change	Change								
	TIME ———▶		Dose	Dose	Dose	Dose							
Drug													
Route													
Additional Instructions													
Signature													
Print Name Bleep No.													

ORAL ANTICOAGULANTS

TARGET INR RANGE

Drug	INR
Time	DOSE
Signature	SIGNATURE
Print Name Bleep No.	GIVEN BY
Pharmacy	

DISCHARGE MEDICATION (TO BE PRESCRIBED ON SEPARATE DISCHARGE & TTO FORM)	Seen by Pharmacist		Given to Patient on Ward (Nurse to sign here)
	Initials	Date	

REGULAR PRESCRIPTIONS		PATIENT'S NAME:			HOSPITAL No:												
MONTH	YEAR	DATE → TIMES →															

[handwritten left margin:] ucu, *subractive*, eucropeyin

DRUG (Approved Name) OXYGEN				6													
Dose 15 l	Route inh	Frequency —	Start Date 30/5/07	12													
Signature S		Pharmacy	Stop Date	18													
Print Name Bleep No. K. SRITHARAN (Bp S854)																	
Additional Instructions			Stopped by	22													

DRUG (Approved Name) ATENOLOL				6													
Dose 100 mg	Route PO	Frequency od	Start Date 30/5/07	12													
Signature S		Pharmacy	Stop Date	18													
Print Name Bleep No. (S854 Bp) K-SRITHARAN																	
Additional Instructions			Stopped by	22													

DRUG (Approved Name) ATORVASTATIN				6													
Dose 20mg	Route PO	Frequency od.	Start Date 30/5/07	12													
Signature S		Pharmacy	Stop Date	18													
Print Name Bleep No. K. SRITHARAN (Bp S854)																	
Additional Instructions			Stopped by	22													

DRUG (Approved Name)				6													
Dose	Route	Frequency	Start Date	12													
Signature		Pharmacy	Stop Date	18													
Print Name Bleep No.																	
Additional Instructions			Stopped by	22													

DRUG (Approved Name)				6													
Dose	Route	Frequency	Start Date	12													
Signature		Pharmacy	Stop Date	18													
Print Name Bleep No.																	
Additional Instructions			Stopped by	22													

DRUG (Approved Name)				6													
Dose	Route	Frequency	Start Date	12													
Signature		Pharmacy	Stop Date	18													
Print Name Bleep No.																	
Additional Instructions			Stopped by	22													

REGULAR PRESCRIPTIONS			PATIENT'S NAME:							HOSPITAL No:						
MONTH		YEAR	DATE → TIMES →													
DRUG (Approved Name)				6												
Dose	Route	Frequency	Start Date	12												
Signature		Pharmacy	Stop Date	18												
Print Name Bleep No. Additional Instructions			Stopped by	22												
DRUG (Approved Name)				6												
Dose	Route	Frequency	Start Date	12												
Signature		Pharmacy	Stop Date	18												
Print Name Bleep No. Additional Instructions			Stopped by	22												
DRUG (Approved Name)				6												
Dose	Route	Frequency	Start Date	12												
Signature		Pharmacy	Stop Date	18												
Print Name Bleep No. Additional Instructions			Stopped by	22												
DRUG (Approved Name)				6												
Dose	Route	Frequency	Start Date	12												
Signature		Pharmacy	Stop Date	18												
Print Name Bleep No. Additional Instructions			Stopped by	22												
DRUG (Approved Name)				6												
Dose	Route	Frequency	Start Date	12												
Signature		Pharmacy	Stop Date	18												
Print Name Bleep No. Additional Instructions			Stopped by	22												
DRUG (Approved Name)				6												
Dose	Route	Frequency	Start Date	12												
Signature		Pharmacy	Stop Date	18												
Print Name Bleep No. Additional Instructions			Stopped by	22												

NOTES ON THE USE OF THE PRESCRIPTION SHEET

A. Print legibly in black ink using approved drug names.

B. The prescription sheet is valid for 2 weeks only. After this time, the chart must be re-written to allow further drug administration to be recorded.

C. Any changes in drug therapy must be ordered by a new prescription. DO NOT alter existing instructions.

D. 'Regular prescriptions' should be prescribed indicating the frequency and time of administration.

E. When a drug is not administered record the appropriate number in the administration record box and initial:
1. – Patient away from ward.
2. – Patient could not receive drug (e.g. nil by mouth, vomiting, no venous access).
3. – Patient refusing drug.
4. – Drug not available.
5. – On instructions of doctor.
6. – Patient did not require drug.
7. – Patient self-administering.
8. – Illegible.

F. Enter dietary regimens in the 'Regular Prescriptions' section. Do not use the intravenous chart.

G. Discharge drugs. These should be prescribed on the separate Discharge & TTO Prescription Sheet. The pharmacist should indicate on the front of this chart that the Discharge Prescription has been seen by the pharmacy and the nurse should indicate that the patient has been given the discharge drugs.

H. Sliding scale insulin should be prescribed on the separate insulin prescription chart. Additionally, on the Regular section of this chart a cross-reference to that chart should be added, e.g. "insulin – see sliding scale insulin chart".

PREPARATIONS ADMINISTERED BY REGISTERED NURSE OR MIDWIFE UNDER PATIENT GROUP DIRECTIONS

DRUG (Approved Name)	Dose	Date	Time	Given by	Dose	Date	Time	Given by	Pharm

MONTH	YEAR	DATE ➤	

WHEN REQUIRED PRESCRIPTIONS

DRUG (Approved Name) MORPHINE

Dose	Route	Max Frequency	Start Date
5–10mg	IV/IM	4°	30/5/07

Signature	Pharmacy	Stop Date

Print Name / Bleep No. K. SRITHARAN (Bp 5854)

Additional Instructions	Stopped by
See stat section before	

DRUG (Approved Name) METOCLOPRAMIDE

Dose	Route	Max Frequency	Start Date
10mg	IV/IM/PO	tds	30/5/07

Signature	Pharmacy	Stop Date

Print Name / Bleep No. K. SRITHARAN (Bp 5854)

Additional Instructions	Stopped by
See stat section before giving	

DRUG (Approved Name) GTN

Dose	Route	Max Frequency	Start Date
↑↑	SL	PRN	30/5/07

Signature	Pharmacy	Stop Date

Print Name / Bleep No. K. SRITHARAN.

Additional Instructions	Stopped by
Check BP before giving. NOT ē GTN infusion	

DRUG (Approved Name)

Dose	Route	Max Frequency	Start Date

Signature	Pharmacy	Stop Date

Print Name / Bleep No.

Additional Instructions	Stopped by

DRUG (Approved Name)

Dose	Route	Max Frequency	Start Date

Signature	Pharmacy	Stop Date

Print Name / Bleep No.

Additional Instructions	Stopped by

DRUG (Approved Name)

Dose	Route	Max Frequency	Start Date

Signature	Pharmacy	Stop Date

Print Name / Bleep No.

Additional Instructions	Stopped by

continued opposite

se	Sig.	Time	Dose	Sig.	Time	Dose	Sig.	Time	Dose	Sig.	Time	Dose	Sig.	Time	Dose	Sig.	Time	Dose	Sig.	Time	Dose	Sig.	Time	Dose	Sig.

INTRAVENOUS INFUSION THERAPY

Record time of changing syringe pump. Administration of blood products and some medicines require two signatures. See the Trust's Medicines Policy.
Do not use more than 2 continuation sheets.

PATIENT'S NAME

HOSPITAL NUMBER

Date	Time	Intravenous Fluid	Volume	Additives and Special Instructions	Dose	Running Time or Flow Rate	Signature/ Print name/ Bleep	Unit/Batch Number (Blood Products only)	Time Begun	Administration Signature	Witness Signature	Time Ended	Pharm. Initials
3/5/12	10:30	GTN	50 mg	in 50mL 0.9% N/Saline		0-10mL/h Titrate to keep systolic BP >...	Dr WSMITH 5617760						

Scenario 5

Mr Brown is a 35-year-old man who has vomited up what look like coffee grounds.

Two days previously he passed black motions. He is now tachycardic, his blood pressure has dropped and he is unresponsive. He had been taking aspirin for joint pain.

Please write up the necessary drugs on the prescription chart.

Points to note

- This patient has had an upper gastrointestinal bleed.
- Aspirin needs to be stopped.
- He needs adequate oxygen (high flow).
- He needs to be given adequate fluids and blood.
- He needs proton pump inhibitor (PPI) infusion at the start and then regular PPIs.
- He needs painkillers.
- You may want to prescribe antibiotics – cefuroxime and metronidazole.
- You want to give him Heliclear or a combination of PPI and antibiotics to treat *H. pylori*.

HAMMERSMITH HOSPITALS NHS TRUST	Weight (kg)	AFFIX ADDRESSOGRAPH LABEL HERE
MEDICINE PRESCRIPTION CHART		SURNAME _BROWN_
DRUGS SENSITIVITIES AND FOOD ALLERGIES	Height (m)	FIRST NAME(S) _BEN_
NKDA.	Surface Area (m²)	HOSPITAL NUMBER _65413_
AVOID NSAIDS - GI Bleed		DATE OF BIRTH _2/7/1972_

Date of Admission	Ward	Consultant
3d5/07	ARE	DR DAVIES

ONCE ONLY PRESCRIPTIONS

Pharmacy Cost Centre		Tick box if Private Patient

Date	Time	Drug	Dose	Route	Additional Instructions	Signature / Print Name / Bleep	Time Given	Given by	Pharm.
3d5/07	1900 hrs	OMEPRAZOLE	40 mg	I.V		S.... Bypi23 SK SRITARAN			

VARIABLE PRESCRIPTIONS
(e.g. Steroids, Insulin)

Month ——►
Date ——►

Pharm.	DATE ——►	Start	Change	Change	Change
	TIME ——►	Dose	Dose	Dose	Dose
Drug					
Route					
Additional Instructions					
Signature					
Print Name Bleep No.					

Pharm.	DATE ——►	Start	Change	Change	Change
	TIME ——►	Dose	Dose	Dose	Dose
Drug					
Route					
Additional Instructions					
Signature					
Print Name Bleep No.					

ORAL ANTICOAGULANTS

TARGET INR RANGE

Drug	INR
Time	DOSE
Signature	SIGNATURE
Print Name Bleep No.	
Pharmacy	GIVEN BY

DISCHARGE MEDICATION (TO BE PRESCRIBED ON SEPARATE DISCHARGE & TTO FORM)	Seen by Pharmacist	Given to Patient on Ward (Nurse to sign here)
	Initials	Date

WMD001

REGULAR PRESCRIPTIONS			PATIENT'S NAME:			HOSPITAL No:									

MONTH		YEAR		DATE ———➤											
				TIMES ———											
DRUG (Approved Name)				6											
OXYGEN															
Dose	Route	Frequency	Start Date	12											
15ℓ	Face mask with rebreather Bag	—	30l5l09												
Signature S		Pharmacy	Stop Date	18											
Print Name Bleep No.	K.Srinivasan Bip127														
Additional Instructions			Stopped by	22											

DRUG (Approved Name)				6											
OMEPRAZOLE				⑧											
Dose	Route	Frequency	Start Date	12											
40mg	iv	od	30l5l09												
Signature S		Pharmacy	Stop Date	18											
Print Name Bleep No.	K.Srinivasan Bip123														
Additional Instructions			Stopped by	22											

DRUG (Approved Name)				⑤											
PARACETAMOL															
Dose	Route	Frequency	Start Date	⑫											
1g	iv/or/pr	qds	30l5l09												
Signature S		Pharmacy	Stop Date	⑱											
Print Name Bleep No.	K.Srinivasan Bip123														
Additional Instructions			Stopped by	㉒											

DRUG (Approved Name)				6											
SENNA				⑥											
Dose	Route	Frequency	Start Date	12											
TT	po	od	30l5l09												
Signature S		Pharmacy	Stop Date	⑱											
Print Name Bleep No.	K.Srinivasan														
Additional Instructions			Stopped by	22											

DRUG (Approved Name)				6											
CEFTROXIME				⑧											
Dose	Route	Frequency	Start Date	12											
750mg	iv	tds	30l3l09	⑭											
Signature S		Pharmacy	Stop Date	18											
Print Name Bleep No.	K.Srinivasan Bip123														
Additional Instructions			Stopped by	㉒											

DRUG (Approved Name)				6											
METRONIDAZOLE				⑧											
Dose	Route	Frequency	Start Date	12											
500mg	iv	tds	30l5l09	⑭											
Signature S		Pharmacy	Stop Date	18											
Print Name Bleep No.	K.Srinivasan Bip123														
Additional Instructions			Stopped by	㉒											

REGULAR PRESCRIPTIONS PATIENT'S NAME: HOSPITAL No:

MONTH	YEAR	DATE →														
		TIMES →														
DRUG (Approved Name)			6													
Dose	Route	Frequency	Start Date	12												
Signature		Pharmacy	Stop Date	18												
Print Name																
Bleep No.																
Additional Instructions			Stopped by	22												
DRUG (Approved Name)			6													
Dose	Route	Frequency	Start Date	12												
Signature		Pharmacy	Stop Date	18												
Print Name																
Bleep No																
Additional Instructions			Stopped by	22												
DRUG (Approved Name)			6													
Dose	Route	Frequency	Start Date	12												
Signature		Pharmacy	Stop Date	18												
Print Name																
Bleep No.																
Additional Instructions			Stopped by	22												
DRUG (Approved Name)			6													
Dose	Route	Frequency	Start Date	12												
Signature		Pharmacy	Stop Date	18												
Print Name																
Bleep No.																
Additional Instructions			Stopped by	22												
DRUG (Approved Name)			6													
Dose	Route	Frequency	Start Date	12												
Signature		Pharmacy	Stop Date	18												
Print Name																
Bleep No.																
Additional Instructions			Stopped by	22												
DRUG (Approved Name)			6													
Dose	Route	Frequency	Start Date	12												
Signature		Pharmacy	Stop Date	18												
Print Name																
Bleep No.																
Additional Instructions			Stopped by	22												

NOTES ON THE USE OF THE PRESCRIPTION SHEET

A.   Print legibly in black ink using approved drug names.

B.   The prescription sheet is valid for 2 weeks only. After this time, the chart must be re-written to allow further drug administration to be recorded.

C.   Any changes in drug therapy must be ordered by a new prescription. DO NOT alter existing instructions.

D.   'Regular prescriptions' should be prescribed indicating the frequency and time of administration.

E.   When a drug is not administered record the appropriate number in the administration record box and initial:
1. – Patient away from ward.
2. – Patient could not receive drug (e.g. nil by mouth, vomiting, no venous access).
3. – Patient refusing drug.
4. – Drug not available.
5. – On instructions of doctor.
6. – Patient did not require drug.
7. – Patient self-administering.
8. – Illegible.

F.   Enter dietary regimens in the 'Regular Prescriptions' section. Do not use the intravenous chart.

G.   Discharge drugs. These should be prescribed on the separate Discharge & TTO Prescription Sheet. The pharmacist should indicate on the front of this chart that the Discharge Prescription has been seen by the pharmacy and the nurse should indicate that the patient has been given the discharge drugs.

H.   Sliding scale insulin should be prescribed on the separate insulin prescription chart. Additionally, on the Regular section of this chart a cross-reference to that chart should be added, e.g. "insulin – see sliding scale insulin chart".

PREPARATIONS ADMINISTERED BY REGISTERED NURSE OR MIDWIFE UNDER PATIENT GROUP DIRECTIONS

DRUG (Approved Name)	Dose	Date	Time	Given by	Dose	Date	Time	Given by	Pharm

---

MONTH   YEAR   DATE ────────►

WHEN REQUIRED PRESCRIPTIONS   Tim

DRUG (Approved Name) MORPHINE

Dose	Route	Max Frequency	Start Date
5-10 mg	im/iv	4°	30.5.07

Signature	Pharmacy	Stop Date
S		

Print Name / Bleep No. K. SERURAN

Additional Instructions	Stopped by

DRUG (Approved Name) METOCLOPRAMIDE

Dose	Route	Max Frequency	Start Date
10mg	iv/im/po	tds	30.5.07

Signature	Pharmacy	Stop Date
S		

Print Name / Bleep No. K. SERURAN 81023

Additional Instructions	Stopped by

DRUG (Approved Name)

Dose	Route	Max Frequency	Start Date

Signature	Pharmacy	Stop Date

Print Name / Bleep No.

Additional Instructions	Stopped by

DRUG (Approved Name)

Dose	Route	Max Frequency	Start Date

Signature	Pharmacy	Stop Date

Print Name / Bleep No.

Additional Instructions	Stopped by

DRUG (Approved Name)

Dose	Route	Max Frequency	Start Date

Signature	Pharmacy	Stop Date

Print Name / Bleep No.

Additional Instructions	Stopped by

DRUG (Approved Name)

Dose	Route	Max Frequency	Start Date

Signature	Pharmacy	Stop Date

Print Name / Bleep No.

Additional Instructions	Stopped by

continued overleaf

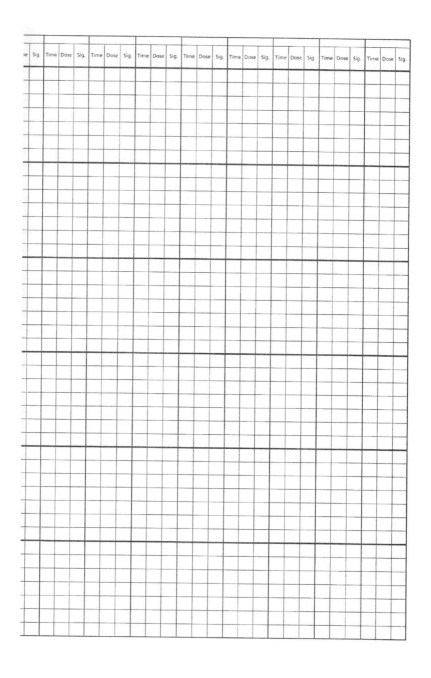

INTRAVENOUS INFUSION THERAPY
Record time of changing syringe pump. Administration of blood products and some medicines require two signatures. See the Trust's Medicines Policy.
Do not use more than 2 continuation sheets.

PATIENT'S NAME

HOSPITAL NUMBER

Date	Time	Intravenous Fluid	Volume	Additives and Special Instructions	Dose	Running Time or Flow Rate	Signature/ Print Name/ Bleep	Unit/Batch Number (Blood Products only)	Time Begun	Administration Signature	Witness Signature	Time Ended	Pharm. Initials
26/5/17	1800	CEDOSIN	500 ml	-		Stat	Simon S.S.27						
26/5/17	1800	BLOOD	1u	-		Stat	Simon Simon						
26/5/17	1800	BLOOD	1u	-		2°	Simon Simon						

Scenario 6

Mr Smith is a 60-year-old man. He has hypertension and is currently taking diuretics (2.5 mg bendroflumethiazide). He is known to suffer from gout. The patient now presents with a swollen right big toe. He is allergic to penicillin (urticarial rash). His date of birth is 30/08/1947 and his identity number is 123567. The consultant is Dr Briggs.

Please write out his drug chart.

Points to note

- The patient must stop the diuretics as they precipitate gout.
- An alternative anti-hypertensive must be prescribed.
- He must be prescribed non-steroidal anti-inflammatory drugs with proton pump inhibitors.
- In the long-term treatment of gout you may be able to use allopurinol 100–300 mg by mouth once a day. However, this drug needs serum urate levels to be monitored. Another drug that can be used is colchicine 1 mg by mouth qds for 4 days.
- You will need to mention the rash in the allergies section and state that it is caused by penicillin. This is usually written in red.

HAMMERSMITH HOSPITALS NHS TRUST
MEDICINE PRESCRIPTION CHART

DRUGS SENSITIVITIES AND FOOD ALLERGIES

PENICILLIN
— Rash

Weight (kg)	AFFIX ADDRESSOGRAPH LABEL HERE
	SURNAME SMITH
Height (m)	FIRST NAME(S) HENRY
Surface Area (m²)	HOSPITAL NUMBER 12357
	DATE OF BIRTH 3018/47

Date of Admission	Ward	Consultant
30|5|09	A&E	DR BRIGGS

ONCE ONLY PRESCRIPTIONS

| | Pharmacy Cost Centre | | | | | | Tick box if Private Patient | | |

Date	Time	Drug	Dose	Route	Additional Instructions	Signature / Print Name / Bleep	Time Given	Given by	Pharm.

VARIABLE PRESCRIPTIONS
(e.g. Sterioids, Insulin)

Month ➤
Date ➤

Pharm.	DATE ➤	Start	Change	Change	Change
	TIME ➤	Dose	Dose	Dose	Dose
Drug					
Route					
Additional Instructions					
Signature					
Print Name Bleep No.					

Pharm.	DATE ➤	Start	Change	Change	Change
	TIME ➤	Dose	Dose	Dose	Dose
Drug					
Route					
Additional Instructions					
Signature					
Print Name Bleep No.					

ORAL ANTICOAGULANTS

TARGET INR RANGE

Drug	INR
Time	DOSE
Signature	SIGNATURE
Print Name Bleep No.	GIVEN BY
Pharmacy	

DISCHARGE MEDICATION (TO BE PRESCRIBED ON SEPARATE DISCHARGE & TTO FORM)	Seen by Pharmacist		Given to Patient on Ward (Nurse to sign here)
	Initials	Date	

WMD001

REGULAR PRESCRIPTIONS   PATIENT'S NAME: HOSPITAL No:

MONTH	YEAR	DATE → TIMES	6									
DRUG (Approved Name) INDOMETHACIN			⑥									
Dose 75mg	Route Po	Frequency bd	Start Date 3/5/07	12								
Signature S		Pharmacy	Stop Date	18								
Print Name Bleep No. K. SRITARAN BP123			②									
Additional Instructions			Stopped by	22								
DRUG (Approved Name) OMEPRAZOLE			6									
			⑧									
Dose 40mg	Route Po	Frequency od	Start Date 3/5/07	12								
Signature S		Pharmacy	Stop Date	18								
Print Name Bleep No. K. SRITARAN BP123												
Additional Instructions			Stopped by	22								
DRUG (Approved Name) PARACETAMOL			6									
Dose 1g	Route Po	Frequency 5ds	Start Date 3/5/07	12								
Signature S		Pharmacy	Stop Date	18								
Print Name Bleep No. K. SRITARAN. BP123												
Additional Instructions			Stopped by	22								
DRUG (Approved Name) BENDROFLUMETHIAZIDE			6									
			⑥									
Dose 2.5mg	Route Po	Frequency od	Start Date 3/5/07	12								
Signature S		Pharmacy	Stop Date	18		STOPPED						
Print Name Bleep No. K. SRITARAN BP123					S	ACTS BADLOE sout.						
Additional Instructions			Stopped by	22								
DRUG (Approved Name)			6									
Dose	Route	Frequency	Start Date	12								
Signature		Pharmacy	Stop Date	18								
Print Name Bleep No.												
Additional Instructions			Stopped by	22								
DRUG (Approved Name)			6									
Dose	Route	Frequency	Start Date	12								
Signature		Pharmacy	Stop Date	18								
Print Name Bleep No.												
Additional Instructions			Stopped by	22								

Scenario 7

Mr Blake is a 40-year-old man who is admitted with raised temperature and cough. He has absent air entry on auscultation of the right lower lobe. His sputum is discoloured. His blood tests show a raised white cell count. Chest X-ray shows lower lobe consolidation. He is taking diazepam to help him sleep. His date of birth is 12/01/1967. His identity number is 67897 and his doctor is Dr Richards.

Please write out his drug chart.

Points to note

- This patient has lower lobe pneumonia.
- Diazepam needs to be stopped, as it is a respiratory depressant.
- This patient needs high-flow oxygen and fluids.
- He needs regular paracetamol.
- He needs antibiotics to cover hospital-acquired and community-acquired bacteria (thus amoxicillin and clarithromycin).
- Nebulised saline and salbutamol may help.

HAMMERSMITH HOSPITALS NHS TRUST **MEDICINE PRESCRIPTION CHART**	Weight (kg)	AFFIX ADDRESSOGRAPH LABEL HERE
DRUGS SENSITIVITIES AND FOOD ALLERGIES	Height (m)	SURNAME BLAKE
		FIRST NAME(S) DAVID
	Surface Area (m²)	HOSPITAL NUMBER 67857
NKDA		DATE OF BIRTH 12|1|67

	Date of Admission 30|5|07	Ward A&E	Consultant DR RICHARDS

ONCE ONLY PRESCRIPTIONS

Date	Time	Drug	Dose	Route	Additional Instructions	Signature / Print Name / Bleep	Time Given	Given by	Pharm.

VARIABLE PRESCRIPTIONS
(e.g. Steriods, Insulin)

Month ➤ Date ➤

Pharm. DATE ➤ TIME ➤	Start Dose	Change Dose	Change Dose	Change Dose						
Drug										
Route										
Additional Instructions										
Signature										
Print Name Bleep No.										

Pharm. DATE ➤ TIME ➤	Start Dose	Change Dose	Change Dose	Change Dose						
Drug										
Route										
Additional Instructions										
Signature										
Print Name Bleep No.										

ORAL ANTICOAGULANTS

TARGET INR RANGE

Drug	INR
Time	DOSE
Signature	SIGNATURE
Print Name Bleep No.	
Pharmacy	GIVEN BY

DISCHARGE MEDICATION (TO BE PRESCRIBED ON SEPARATE DISCHARGE & TTO FORM)	Seen by Pharmacist	Given to Patient on Ward (Nurse to sign here)
	Initials Date	

WMD001

REGULAR PRESCRIPTIONS PATIENT'S NAME: HOSPITAL No:

MONTH	YEAR	DATE →	
		TIMES	

DRUG (Approved Name) AUGMENTIN

Dose	Route	Frequency	Start Date
1.2s	IV	GDS	3d5b7

Signature	Pharmacy	Stop Date

Print Name / Bleep No. K. Sriraman Bp123
Additional Instructions Stopped by

Times column: 6, (E), 12, (14), 18, (22)

DRUG (Approved Name) CLARITHROMYCIN

Dose	Route	Frequency	Start Date
500	PO	BD	3015b7

Signature	Pharmacy	Stop Date

Print Name / Bleep No. K. Sriraman Bp123
Additional Instructions Stopped by

Times column: 6, (8), 12, 18, (0), 22

DRUG (Approved Name) PARACETAMOL

Dose	Route	Frequency	Start Date
Lg	IV/oral	QDS	Jo/5b7

Signature	Pharmacy	Stop Date

Print Name / Bleep No. K. Sriraman Bp123
Additional Instructions Stopped by

Times column: (6), (12), (18), (22)

DRUG (Approved Name) NORMAL SALINE NEBS

Dose	Route	Frequency	Start Date
5ml	neb	QDS	3d5b7

Signature	Pharmacy	Stop Date

Print Name / Bleep No. K. Sriraman
Additional Instructions Stopped by

Times column: (6), (12), (18), (22)

DRUG (Approved Name) OXYGEN

Dose	Route	Frequency	Start Date
15l	Face mask with rebreath	—	3d5b7

Signature	Pharmacy	Stop Date

Print Name / Bleep No. K. Sriraman Bp123
Additional Instructions Stopped by

Times column: 6, 12, 18, 22

DRUG (Approved Name)

Dose	Route	Frequency	Start Date

Signature	Pharmacy	Stop Date

Print Name / Bleep No.
Additional Instructions Stopped by

Times column: 6, 12, 18, 22

REGULAR PRESCRIPTIONS				PATIENT'S NAME:						HOSPITAL No:						
MONTH	YEAR	DATE ⟶ TIMES ⟶														
DRUG (Approved Name)				6												
Dose	Route	Frequency	Start Date	12												
Signature		Pharmacy	Stop Date	18												
Print Name Bleep No.																
Additional Instructions			Stopped by	22												
DRUG (Approved Name)				6												
Dose	Route	Frequency	Start Date	12												
Signature		Pharmacy	Stop Date	18												
Print Name Bleep No.																
Additional Instructions			Stopped by	22												
DRUG (Approved Name)				6												
Dose	Route	Frequency	Start Date	12												
Signature		Pharmacy	Stop Date	18												
Print Name Bleep No.																
Additional Instructions			Stopped by	22												
DRUG (Approved Name)				6												
Dose	Route	Frequency	Start Date	12												
Signature		Pharmacy	Stop Date	18												
Print Name Bleep No.																
Additional Instructions			Stopped by	22												
DRUG (Approved Name)				6												
Dose	Route	Frequency	Start Date	12												
Signature		Pharmacy	Stop Date	18												
Print Name Bleep No.																
Additional Instructions			Stopped by	22												
DRUG (Approved Name)				6												
Dose	Route	Frequency	Start Date	12												
Signature		Pharmacy	Stop Date	18												
Print Name Bleep No.																
Additional Instructions			Stopped by	22												

NOTES ON THE USE OF THE PRESCRIPTION SHEET

A. Print legibly in black ink using approved drug names.

B. The prescription sheet is valid for 2 weeks only. After this time, the chart must be re-written to allow further drug administration to be recorded.

C. Any changes in drug therapy must be ordered by a new prescription. DO NOT alter existing instructions.

D. 'Regular prescriptions' should be prescribed indicating the frequency and time of administration.

E. When a drug is not administered record the appropriate number in the administration record box and initial:
1. – Patient away from ward.
2. – Patient could not receive drug (e.g. nil by mouth, vomiting, no venous access).
3. – Patient refusing drug.
4. – Drug not available.
5. – On instructions of doctor.
6. – Patient did not require drug.
7. – Patient self-administering.
8. – Illegible.

F. Enter dietary regimens in the 'Regular Prescriptions' section. Do not use the intravenous chart.

G. Discharge drugs. These should be prescribed on the separate Discharge & TTO Prescription Sheet. The pharmacist should indicate on the front of this chart that the Discharge Prescription has been seen by the pharmacy and the nurse should indicate that the patient has been given the discharge drugs.

H. Sliding scale insulin should be prescribed on the separate insulin prescription chart. Additionally, on the Regular section of this chart a cross-reference to that chart should be added, e.g. "insulin – see sliding scale insulin chart".

PREPARATIONS ADMINISTERED BY REGISTERED NURSE OR MIDWIFE UNDER PATIENT GROUP DIRECTIONS

DRUG (Approved Name)	Dose	Date	Time	Given by	Dose	Date	Time	Given by	Pharm

MONTH	YEAR	DATE ──────►	

WHEN REQUIRED PRESCRIPTIONS

DRUG (Approved Name) SALBUTAMOL			
Dose 5mg	Route neb	Max Frequency PRN.	Start Date 3olska
Signature S		Pharmacy	Stop Date
Print Name Bleep No. K. SRITARAN BMp123			
Additional Instructions with wheeze			Stopped by

DRUG (Approved Name) TEMAZEPAM			
Dose 10mg	Route po	Max Frequency nocte	Start Date 3olska
Signature S		Pharmacy	Stop Date
Print Name Bleep No. K. SRITARAN Bp23			
Additional Instructions			Stopped by

DRUG (Approved Name)			
Dose	Route	Max Frequency	Start Date
Signature		Pharmacy	Stop Date
Print Name Bleep No.			
Additional Instructions			Stopped by

DRUG (Approved Name)			
Dose	Route	Max Frequency	Start Date
Signature		Pharmacy	Stop Date
Print Name Bleep No.			
Additional Instructions			Stopped by

DRUG (Approved Name)			
Dose	Route	Max Frequency	Start Date
Signature		Pharmacy	Stop Date
Print Name Bleep No.			
Additional Instructions			Stopped by

DRUG (Approved Name)			
Dose	Route	Max Frequency	Start Date
Signature		Pharmacy	Stop Date
Print Name Bleep No.			
Additional Instructions			Stopped by

continued overleaf

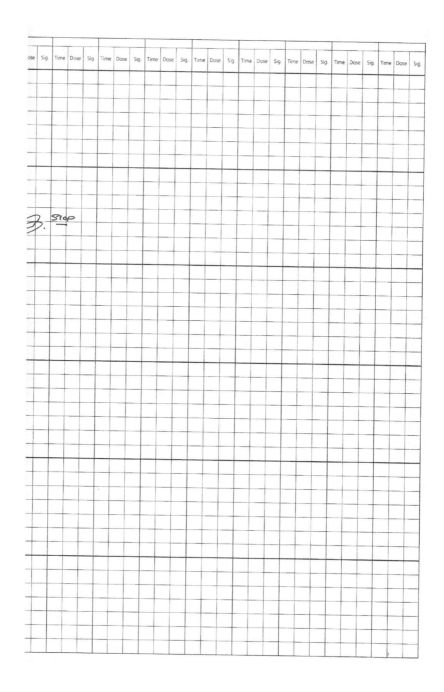

ose	Sig.	Time	Dose	Sig.	Time	Dose	Sig.	Time	Dose	Sig.	Time	Dose	Sig.	Time	Dose	Sig.	Time	Dose	Sig.	Time	Dose	Sig.

INTRAVENOUS INFUSION THERAPY
Record time of changing syringe pump. Administration of blood products and some medicines require two signatures. See the Trust's Medicines Policy.
Do not use more than 2 continuation sheets.

PATIENT'S NAME

HOSPITAL NUMBER

Date	Time	Intravenous Fluid	Volume	Additives and Special Instructions	Dose	Running Time or Flow Rate	Signature/ Print Name/ Bleep	Unit/Batch Number (Blood Products only)	Time Begun	Administration Signature	Witness Signature	Time Ended	Pharm. Initials
Yesterday	approx.	0.9% Normal Saline	Le	2oml KCl		Go	*(signature)* Bleep 023						
Today		STH DEXTROSE	Le	2o ml KCl		6-80	*(signature)* Bleep 23 (F. Samuel)						

100 Writing a GP prescription

Scenario

Mr Summers has come into his GP practice and would like a repeat prescription. You are asked to write the prescription, and he will tell you what medication he is taking.

GP prescriptions

In general (see *British National Formulary*):

- write legibly in ink
- avoid writing more than four items per prescription.

The following should be stated:

- date of prescription
- patient's full name, address and ideally also their age and date of birth
- generic name of drug unless trade names have specific preparations
- dose of the drug:
  - do not unnecessarily use decimal points (e.g. write 2 mg not 2.0 mg, or 200 mg not 0.2 g)
  - 'micrograms,' 'nanograms' and 'units' should not be abbreviated
  - 'as required' drugs need a minimum dose (e.g. Gaviscon 5 ml as required)
  - controlled drugs need the dose to be written in both words and figures
- formulation of the drug (e.g tabs (tablets), caps (capsules))
- frequency with which the drug should be taken:
  - English is preferred (e.g. 'once a day')
  - Latin abbreviations are acceptable
- total quantity – either in days (usually 28 days for repeat GP prescriptions) or the total number (e.g. '2 inhalers')
- special instructions (e.g. take before food).

Finally, sign and date the prescription (ask a registered doctor to countersign it).

Pharmacy Stamp	Age	Title, Forename, Surname & Address
	D.o.B	

Please don't stamp over age box
Number of days' treatment
N.B. Ensure dose is stated

Endorsements

CLOPIDOGREL FC tab 75mg. Mitte (56) tab
TAKE ONE ONCE DAILY

DIGOXIN tabs 250micrograms. Mitte (28) tab
TAKE ONE EACH MORNING

MONTELUKAST (AS SODIUM SALT) tabs 10mg.
Mitte(56) tab TAKE ONE DAILY

AMIODARONE tabs 200mg. Mitte (56) tab
TAKE ONE DAILY

Signature of Prescriber	Date

For
dispenser
No. of
Prescns.
on form

NHS

Figure 26   Sample prescription.

101 Writing a discharge summary

Discharge summaries

- Most hospitals have their own standardised discharge summary or TTA (to take away) form.
- These are usually the only form of communication between the GP and the hospital following a patient's admission to hospital, *and therefore they need to be completed fully, promptly and legibly.*
- Most discharge summaries also act as a prescription.
- A copy of the discharge summary is usually given to the patient, a second copy is sent to the GP and a third copy is kept in the patient's hospital notes.

The following information should be included.

- Patient's name, address, date of birth and hospital number (patient labels may be used, but need to be stuck on all three copies).
- GP's name and address.
- Admission date.
- Reason for admission, and diagnosis.
- Investigations while in hospital.
- Procedures and complications (e.g. post-operative wound infection).
- Outstanding issues and management plan, for example:
  - wound infection – needs antibiotics for 5 days
  - stitches *in situ* – district nurse to remove at day 10 post-op
  - dressing changes – district nurse to change daily.
- Follow-up:
  - has an outpatient department appointment been made? If yes, state date and time
  - consultant, specialty and clinic.
- Medication:
  - drug name, dose, frequency and duration (usually a maximum of 2 weeks only can be prescribed)
  - whether the drug should be continued, and if so, for how long.
- Sign and print name and designation, contact number and date.

Scenario

Mr Meacher is a 24-year-old man who was admitted 3 days ago with acute appendicitis. He subsequently underwent an uncomplicated emergency appendicectomy. He has insoluble stitches *in situ*. You have been asked to discharge him home on a proton pump inhibitor, paracetamol and tramadol.

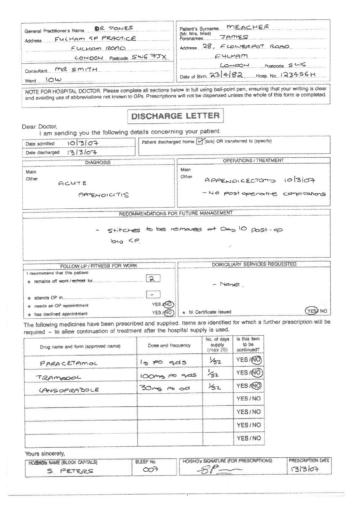

Figure 27   Specimen discharge summary.

102 Writing a transfer letter

A transfer letter should be written by the referring team to the receiving medical team when transferring any patient from one medical unit or hospital to another. Patients are often transferred and reach the accepting hospital out of hours, so the information in the letter is often the only information available to the on-call team.

Importantly, the following information should be written legibly in any transfer letter.

Where?

Address the letter to the receiving consultant, mentioning their specialty.

Who?

Patient details should include full name, age, sex, date of birth, and full address. Hospital numbers aren't always useful, as they differ between trusts.

When?

State date of admission to the referring hospital and date when the decision for transfer was made.

Why?

- Category of transfer (i.e. emergency or elective).
- Reason for transfer (i.e. repatriation or tertiary referral – imaging, medical or surgical management).
- Type of transfer (i.e. one-way or return).

Background

- A brief history, examination and summary of investigations should be included. This may be the first time that the accepting team will be meeting the patient, so assume that they have no prior knowledge.
- Current medication, as this does not usually correlate with those taken prior to admission. Include allergies.
- Outline the management of the patient during their hospital admission.
- Mention any complications that have arisen.
- Summarise any outstanding medical, surgical or social issues.

Finally:

- Include your name, position and contact details.
- A copy of the notes, recent imaging (e.g. X-rays, CT scans) and current blood results should also accompany the patient.

[Adapted from Sritharan K, Elwell VA. Tips on ... writing a transfer letter. *BMJ Careers*. 2006; **332**: 221 and *BMJ Careers*. 2006; **333**: 183.]

103 Referring a patient

There are essentially two ways in which a patient may be referred to a specialist for an opinion – by writing a referral letter or by contacting the specialist (or a member of the team) directly. The latter approach should be reinforced by a letter of referral.

All referral letters should incorporate the following information.

- Patient's name, date of birth, address (and possibly hospital number).
- Patient's location (i.e. inpatient or outpatient – if inpatient, state ward).
- Consultant/specialist to whom the referral is intended, including their department/specialty.
- Reason for referral (the question that needs to be answered).
- Salient features of the history and examination relating to the reason for referral (e.g. if referring a patient with leg ulcers to a vascular surgeon, the risk factors for peripheral vascular disease should be stated).
- Pertinent investigations and their results.
- Past medical history, highlighting comorbidity and general health.
- Medication.
- Outstanding issues which may influence management (e.g. *Clostridium difficile* diarrhoea, lower respiratory tract infection, MRSA grown from leg wound).
- Degree of urgency of referral – if it is urgent, the secretary or registrar of the team should be contacted in addition.
- Finally, date and sign the referral letter giving your name, designation and contact details.

104 Completing an X-ray request form

The responsibilities for any medical radiation exposure are shared between the referring clinician, the practitioner and the operator (usually the radiographer). It is therefore paramount that all X-ray forms are completed in full and that as a referrer sufficient clinical information is provided to allow the practitioner to justify the procedure. In addition, the patient's consent (verbal or written) should be obtained.

The effective dose of radiation varies with the type of examination. A simple chest X-ray will give the patient an effective radiation dose of 0.05 mSv, and an abdominal X-ray will give them an effective dose of 3.5 mSv. In contrast, a spiral CT scan gives a radiation dose equivalent to 80 chest X-rays. Where possible, procedures that do not utilise ionising radiation (e.g. ultrasound or MRI) should be used in preference to those which require ionising radiation.

Information to be included on all X-ray request forms

- Patient's details:
  - name
  - date of birth
  - hospital number
  - address.
- Patient's location (e.g. ward or outpatient department).
- Special requirements:
  - transport
  - interpreter.
- Allergies to contrast media.
- Infection risk (e.g. MRSA, *Clostridium difficile*).
- In female patients:
  - during pregnancy, ionising imaging should be avoided due to the risk of childhood cancers and mental retardation; where imaging is necessary, the dose is capped at 1 mSv for the entirety of the pregnancy
  - all X-ray examinations of the lower abdomen which are not urgent should be limited to the first 10 days following the onset of the last menstrual period (LMP), due to the low risk of pregnancy.
- Imaging history.
- Justification for X-ray:
  - relevant clinical history
  - question to be answered.

- Urgency of request:
  - if urgent, discuss the case with the radiologist on call.
- Referrer's details:
  - doctor's name
  - contact number
  - designation
  - if the referrer is a medical student, the form needs to be countersigned by a clinician.

Finally, sign and date the request form.

IMAGING (X - RAY) DEPARTMENT REQUEST FORM

IF ALL BOXES ARE NOT FULLY COMPLETED THIS EXAMINATION WILL NOT PROCEED

Surname: JONES	Ward / Dept. 10A	
Forename: THOMAS		
D.O.B. 23/4/1946 (M) F		
Hospital No: 123456A	Consultant (Please Print Full Name) MR SMITH.	
Address 23, DUKES AVENUE LONDON W2 4QS	Date of last Imaging Examination 5/12/2006	
	Date of L.M.P. N/A	
	LMP can affect the timing of many procedures	
(NHS) / PRIVATE / RESEARCH	Walking / Chair (Bed) Ward Mobile / Theatre	
RISK FACTORS Please identify significant risk factors. e.g. diabetes / allergy / MRSA / ventilated, etc. NONE.	Is this patient being isolated / barrier nursed? YES /(NO) If yes, state reason:	

Examination Requested

ERECT CHEST X-RAY.

Clinical Findings and Information

- Increasing Shortness of Breath + cough . Temp. 38°
- post-op day 5 open cholecystectomy

O/E: decreased air entry @ Base
- Sats = 90%   ? Consolidation / atelectasis

Referrers Signature	Referrers Name (print)	Referrers Bleep No	Date
EBlanc	E. BLANO	007	23/1/2007

Figure 28   Specimen X-ray request form.

Explaining operations

105 Obtaining informed consent

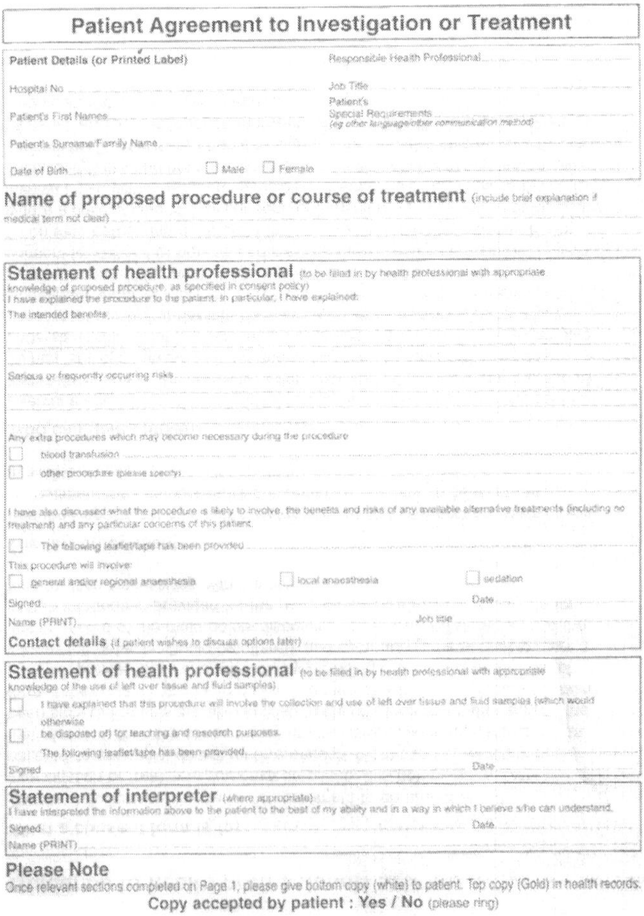

Patient Agreement to Investigation or Treatment

Patient Details (or Printed Label)

Hospital No ....

Patient's First Names ....

Patient's Surname/Family Name ....

Date of Birth .... ☐ Male ☐ Female

Responsible Health Professional ....

Job Title ....

Patient's Special Requirements ....
(eg other language/other communication method)

Name of proposed procedure or course of treatment (include brief explanation if medical term not clear) ....

Statement of health professional (to be filled in by health professional with appropriate knowledge of proposed procedure, as specified in consent policy)

I have explained the procedure to the patient. In particular, I have explained:

The intended benefits ....

Serious or frequently occurring risks ....

Any extra procedures which may become necessary during the procedure

☐ blood transfusion ....

☐ other procedure (please specify) ....

I have also discussed what the procedure is likely to involve, the benefits and risks of any available alternative treatments (including no treatment) and any particular concerns of this patient.

☐ The following leaflet/tape has been provided ....

This procedure will involve:

☐ general and/or regional anaesthesia ☐ local anaesthesia ☐ sedation

Signed .... Date ....

Name (PRINT) .... Job title ....

Contact details (if patient wishes to discuss options later) ....

Statement of health professional (to be filled in by health professional with appropriate knowledge of the use of left over tissue and fluid samples)

☐ I have explained that this procedure will involve the collection and use of left over tissue and fluid samples (which would otherwise

☐ be disposed of) for teaching and research purposes.

The following leaflet/tape has been provided ....

Signed .... Date ....

Statement of interpreter (where appropriate)

I have interpreted the information above to the patient to the best of my ability and in a way in which I believe s/he can understand.

Signed .... Date ....

Name (PRINT) ....

Please Note

Once relevant sections completed on Page 1, please give bottom copy (white) to patient. Top copy (Gold) in health records.

Copy accepted by patient : Yes / No (please ring)

Figure 29 (a) Sample consent form.

Statement of patient

Please read this form carefully. If your treatment has been planned in advance, you should already have yo own copy, which describes the benefits and risks of the proposed treatment. If not, you will be offered a copy now. If you have any further questions, do ask – we are here to help you. You have the right to change your mind at any time, including after you have signed this form.

I agree to the procedure or course of treatment described on this form.

I understand that you cannot give me a guarantee that a particular person will perform the procedure. The person will, however, have appropriate experience.

I understand that I will have the opportunity to discuss the details of anaesthesia with an anaesthetist befor the procedure, unless the urgency of my situation prevents this. (This only applies to patients having genera or regional anaesthesia.)

I understand that any procedure in addition to those described on this form will only be carried out if it is necessary to save my life or to prevent serious harm to my health.

I have been told about additional procedures which may become necessary during my treatment. I have listed below any procedures **which I do not wish to be carried out** without further discussion.

_____

_____

_____

I agree/disagree to the collection and use of left over tissue and fluid samples described on this form.

Patient's signature_____ Date_____

Name (PRINT)_____

A witness should sign below if the patient is unable to sign but has indicated his or her consent. Young people/children may also like a parent to sign here (see notes).

Signed_____ Date_____

Name (PRINT)_____

Confirmation of consent (to be completed by a health professional when the patient
is admitted for the procedure, if the patient has signed the form in advance)

On behalf of the team treating the patient, I have confirmed with the patient that s/he has no further question and wishes the procedure to go ahead.

Signed_____ Date_____

Name (PRINT)_____ Job title_____

Important notes: (tick if applicable)
- ☐ See also advance directive/living will (e.g. Jehovah's Witness form)
- ☐ Patient has withdrawn consent (ask patient to sign/date here)_____

Figure 29   (b) Sample statement of patient.

To be able to consent a patient for a procedure, you must be able to perform the procedure yourself or have been appropriately trained to seek consent. Informed consent can only be obtained from patients who have the mental capacity to give consent, and patients under the age of 16 years need their parent's informed consent.

Informed consent may be either verbal or written, and relies on the patient being given a full explanation of the procedure/investigation (including any prior work-up and their management post-procedure) and its expected benefit and risks. The patient should be able to understand the procedure and be able to reason. It is therefore important to avoid using medical jargon, to ensure that the patient has understood what they have been told by constantly checking, and to give the patient sufficient time both to ask questions and to finally reach a decision. Where alternative options are available, the patient should be made aware of these.

General approach

- Introduce yourself to the patient, giving your full name and grade.
- Tell the patient that you would like to discuss their operation (signpost).
- Assess the patient's prior knowledge of the procedure.
- Explain the preparation required.
- Explain the procedure.
- Explain what the patient should expect in the post-procedure phase.
- Outline both the risks and the benefits of the procedure.
- Discuss the alternative options.
- Summarise the key points in the discussion.
- Ensure that the patient's concerns are addressed.
- Give the patient time and reach a mutually agreeable decision.
- Leave the patient your contact details in case they have any further questions.
- If possible, give the patient an information sheet to take away.

Importantly:

- *Use language that the patient will understand.*
- *Constantly check to ensure that the patient has understood.*
- *Be open to questions, and elicit any concerns the patient may have.*
- *Be empathic.*

Note: An interpreter may be required.

106 Laparoscopic cholecystectomy

Scenario

Mrs Brodie is an obese 45-year-old woman who has had multiple admissions in the past for acute cholecystitis. An ultrasound scan has demonstrated multiple gallstones in the gallbladder, and she has been scheduled for a laparoscopic cholecystectomy. You have been asked to see Mrs Brodie in the pre-admissions clinic and to explain the procedure to her.

Introduction

- Introduce yourself to the patient, giving your name and grade.
- Tell the patient that you would like to give her more information about her operation.
  I would like to tell you a bit more about what the procedure entails, including its risks and benefits and any alternative options. If you don't understand anything, you want more detailed information or you have any questions, please ask.
- Check the patient's knowledge of the operation.

Explain

- The gallbladder is a small sack which sits below the liver under the ribs on the right-hand side of your body.
- Its role is to store bile – a green liquid produced by the liver which drains via a tube into the gallbladder (draw a diagram). The bile then drains via another tube (the bile duct) into the intestine, where its function is to digest fats.
- Stones commonly form in the gallbladder. Sometimes they do not cause any problems but, as in your case, they can cause pain, infection (including pancreatitis) and blockages which can make you become jaundiced (yellow).
- Laparoscopic cholecystectomy is an operation which aims to remove the gallbladder using keyhole surgery.

Preparation for procedure

- In pre-admissions clinic today we will take a full history and examine you and also perform some basic investigations, such as blood tests.

- The procedure will be performed under a general anaesthetic, which means that you will be sound asleep. The anaesthetist will talk to you in detail about the anaesthetic later on today/on admission.
- On admission, you will also be seen by the surgical team who will be performing the procedure. They will be able to answer any further questions that you may have, and will ask for you to sign the consent form for the operation.

Procedure

- You will be sound asleep during the procedure.
- While you are asleep a urinary catheter (tube) will be inserted into your bladder to help to drain the urine.
- You will also have a nasogastric tube inserted into your nose to decompress/drain your stomach.
- We will make approximately four small (about 1 cm) incisions over your tummy (abdomen) – one at the umbilicus (belly button) and the others in the upper abdomen. Through these incisions we can pass specialised surgical instruments as well as a small camera which will allow us to see on a television screen the inside of your abdomen as we work.
- We will also need to inflate your abdomen with carbon dioxide to give us more room to operate inside the abdomen.
- Surgical clips will be used during the operation.
- During the procedure it may also be necessary to place a small tube into the bile duct, inject dye and take X-rays so that we can make sure there are no gallstones within the duct.
- The incisions will be closed with dissolvable stitches.
- The procedure usually takes around 60–90 minutes.

After the procedure

- You will be woken up in the recovery room and when you have completely come round you will be transferred back to the ward. You may feel groggy, sleepy or nauseous.
- You will have a line (cannula) in your arm, and you will be given fluids via a drip until you are ready to eat and drink.
- You can start drinking approximately 4 hours after the operation, and you can start eating shortly after this.
- You should be able to eat a normal diet.
- If you feel sick or are in pain, tell the nursing staff and they will be able to give you medication to control this.

- The nasogastric tube and catheter will be removed when you can tolerate oral fluids.
- A blood test will be performed, looking in particular at your liver function tests (including amylase).
- Most people stay in hospital overnight. However, everyone is different, and you may need to stay a little longer. This is determined by your overall health.
- It usually takes 1–2 weeks to recover (stay off work) and about 2–4 weeks to resume all your normal activities.
- In the event that keyhole surgery is not possible, you are likely to be hospital for longer (4–5 days). The recovery time at home will also be longer (6–8 weeks).
- You should avoid strenuous exercise and lifting until you have recovered, but gentle exercise is encouraged.
- Avoid driving until you are confident that you can perform an emergency stop without pain.
- Before you are discharged, the medical staff will advise you as to the type of stitches that have been used to close the skin. Non-absorbable sutures or skin slips will need to be removed 10 days after the operation. Absorbable sutures do not need to be removed.
- In addition, you will be given a date to return for follow-up in the outpatient clinic.

Specific risks of the procedure

- Conversion to an open procedure (3% of cases) due to technical difficulties, when a larger incision (10–20 cm) will be made under the ribcage.
- Damage to the common bile duct (1 in 400 cases).
- Pain (shoulder tip pain due to pneumoperitoneum, which usually settles within 24 hours).
- Bleeding.
- Wound infection.
- Paraumbilical/incisional hernia.
- Stones in the common bile duct and jaundice.
- Post-cholecystectomy syndrome (bloating, abdominal pain and diarrhoea).
- General complications include urinary tract infection, chest infections, deep vein thrombosis and pulmonary embolism.

Benefits

- The body can manage without a gallbladder.
- Removal of the gallbladder should relieve the symptoms that you have been experiencing due to gallstones (e.g. pain, infections).
- Because of the smaller incisions that are used, keyhole surgery has the advantages of a quicker recovery and a shorter hospital stay. Patients also report less pain post-operatively and experience fewer complications such as chest and wound infections, adhesions and hernias.

Risks of not performing the procedure

- Without the operation it is likely that you will continue to have episodes of acute cholecystitis, in which the gallbladder becomes inflamed and infected, causing pain and fever. However, the frequency of these episodes cannot be predicted.
- There are no alternative options currently available.

Possible concerns of the patient

- Is this procedure safe for a fat person? In fact it is ideal for an overweight person, as there are fewer wound complications.
- When can I return to work?
- What are the chances of converting to an open procedure?
- How long does the operation take?

Closure

- Outline the key points in the discussion.
- Ensure that any concerns have been elicited and addressed.
- Give the patient an information leaflet and possibly also a consent form to read prior to being admitted.
- Give the patient your contact details (e.g. bleep number) should they have any more questions.

Patients who are considered poor candidates

- Patients with cardiac disease and chronic obstructive pulmonary disease.
- Patients who have undergone previous upper abdominal surgery.
- The elderly, who are less likely to tolerate a pneumoperitoneum.

---

107 Open inguinal hernia repair

Scenario

A 75-year-old man with a right inguinal hernia is on the waiting list for an open inguinal hernia repair. Explain the operation to him.

Introduction

- Introduce yourself to the patient, giving your name and grade.
- Tell the patient that you would like to give him more information about his operation.
- Check the patient's knowledge of the operation.

Explain

- An inguinal hernia is a protrusion of tissue through a weakness in the lower abdominal wall.
- It is common. One in 20 men will develop an inguinal hernia, and these hernias are more common in men than in women.
- Patients can present as you did, with a lump or pain.

Preparation

- In pre-admissions clinic today we will take a full history and examine you as well as performing some basic investigations, such as blood tests.
- The procedure can be performed under either general anaesthetic (where you will be put to sleep) or local anaesthetic.
- If a general anaesthetic is required, the anaesthetist will discuss this with you later on today/on admission.
- On admission, you will also be seen by the surgical team who will be performing the procedure. They will be able to answer any further questions that you may have, and will ask for you to sign the consent form for the operation.
- Local anaesthetic may be injected into the wound at the end of the operation and will last for 4–6 hours, after which you may experience more pain.

The procedure

- A small incision will be made over the site of the hernia, and the weakness in the abdominal wall will be repaired and reinforced using a non-absorbable mesh.

After the procedure

- You will be woken up in recovery (if under general anaesthetic) and transferred back to the ward when you are stable.
- You may experience grogginess and nausea from the anaesthetic, and pain at the incision site. If you experience nausea or pain, tell the nursing staff and they can give you medication to manage these symptoms.
- You can start to drink and then eat almost immediately.
- The surgery may be performed as a day case so that you can go home afterwards, provided you are eating and drinking and have passed urine without problem.
- Before you are discharged the medical staff will advise you as to the type of stitches used to close the skin. Non-absorbable sutures or skin slips will need to be removed 10 days after the operation. Absorbable sutures do not need to be removed.
- The wound should be dressed with a waterproof plaster until it has healed completely (for 5 days after surgery).
- You can shower normally the day after surgery with the plaster on, but baths should be avoided until the wound has healed (i.e. a scar has formed).
- Gentle exercise is encouraged, and walking will reduce the risks of deep vein thrombosis and pulmonary embolism.
- Avoid smoking and coughing, avoid heavy lifting for 6 weeks and avoid driving for 1–2 weeks (until you can comfortably perform an emergency stop).
- It usually takes around 2–3 weeks to recover following surgery.
- Contact your GP if you experience any excessive wound discharge/ bleeding, redness or increasing pain at the wound site, fever, nausea or vomiting.
- You will not necessarily be followed up in clinic afterwards.

Specific risks

- Bleeding: scrotal and wound haematoma (this should settle with time).

- Acute urinary retention (common in the elderly, in whom there is a 1 in 100 risk) requiring catheterisation.
- Injury to the vas deferens.
- Damage to the ilioinguinal nerve resulting in numbness or parasthesia over the medial aspect of the thigh.
- Pain or shrinkage of the testes due to damage to the testicular artery.
- Hernia recurrence (1% incidence with mesh repair) with further surgery.
- Incisional hernias.
- Wound or mesh infection.
- Scarring.
- Adhesions.
- General complications include atelectasis, chest infection, deep vein thrombosis, pulmonary embolism and death (rare).

Benefits

- The hernia is repaired and the lump and pain are eradicated in a planned, safe manner.
- Complications of incarceration and strangulation are avoided.

Alternative options

- The hernia may be managed using a truss.
- The hernia may also be repaired laparoscopically. This is determined by both surgeon preference and patient factors (e.g. bilateral or recurrent hernias).
- If untreated, the hernia may grow bigger, cause more pain or lead to obstruction and strangulation if bowel becomes trapped within the hernia sack. If the latter occurs, the segment of bowel involved may become ischaemic/gangrenous (i.e. it may die) and will need to be removed as part of an emergency procedure.

Concerns of the patient

- How did I get the hernia?
- Will the hernia come back?
- What will happen if a complication occurs?
- Will my fertility be affected?

Closure

- Outline the key points in the discussion.
- Ensure that any concerns have been elicited and addressed.
- Give the patient an information leaflet and possibly also a consent form to read prior to being admitted.
- Give the patient your contact details (e.g. bleep number) should they have any more questions.

108 Transurethral resection of the prostate (TURP)

Scenario

Mr Gibson is a 72-year-old man with benign prostatic hyperplasia who has had a number of admissions for acute urinary retention. He is being seen in the pre-admissions clinic, and you are asked to explain the procedure to him.

Introduction

- Introduce yourself to the patient, giving your name and grade.
- Tell the patient that you would like to give him more information about his operation.
- Check the patient's prior knowledge of the operation.

Explain

- The prostate gland is only found in men.
- Its function is to produce secretions which make up semen. However, it does not produce any hormones.
- The gland is found at the outlet of the bladder and surrounds the urethra (the tube which runs through the penis and carries urine from the bladder as well as semen during sexual intercourse).
- The valve or sphincter which controls urine flow from the bladder sits below the prostate.
- The prostate tends to get bigger with age, and in a proportion of men this enlargement can lead to problems passing urine. These problems can include a poor stream, difficulty initiating urination, the sensation of incompletely emptying the bladder and even an inability to any pass urine (urinary retention).

- You may also find that you need to strain when you pass urine, that you are needing to pass urine more frequently and that you are waking up several times at night because you need to pass urine.
- In addition, since the bladder does not empty completely, you may experience recurrent urinary infections and stones.
- TURP is an operation which aims to relieve these problems with passing urine by surgically removing the inner part of the prostate gland using an instrument which is passed through the penis.

Preparation

- In the pre-admissions clinic today we will take a full history and examine you as well as performing some basic investigations, such as a midstream urine (MSU) specimen and blood tests (to check renal function).
- If you are taking any blood-thinning agents, such as warfarin, aspirin or clopidogrel, you will need to stop these 2 weeks before the operation, because of the increased risk of bleeding.
- The procedure will be performed under a general anaesthetic, which means that you will be sound asleep. It can also be performed under spinal anaesthesia, and the anaesthetist will talk to you in detail about the anaesthetic later on today/on admission.
- On admission, you will also be seen by the surgical team who will be performing the procedure. They will be able to answer any further questions that you may have, and will ask for you to sign the consent form for the operation.
- You will not be able to eat or drink for 6 hours before the operation.

Procedure

- The patient is placed in the lithotomy position.
- A rigid telescope (cystoscope) will be passed into your penis/urethra, past your prostate and into your bladder. This allows us to examine the prostate and bladder and to check whether anything has changed.
- A resectoscope sheath (an instrument with an electrical cutting attachment and a telescope) will then be passed into the penis, and as we resect/remove parts of the prostate we will be able to visualise where we are operating on a television screen.
- The bladder will be continually irrigated with glycine solution during the operation.
- A urinary catheter will be inserted at the end of the operation.
- The operation takes approximately 1 hour.

After the procedure

- You will be woken up in recovery (if under general anaesthetic) and transferred back to the ward when you are stable.
- You may experience grogginess and nausea from the anaesthetic, and pain. If you experience nausea or pain, inform the nursing staff and they can give you medication to manage these symptoms.
- It will take about 7–10 days to recover, and you will be in hospital for approximately 4 days.
- You can start to drink initially and then eat almost immediately after the operation. If you feel nauseous, inform the nurses and they will be able to give you anti-sickness medication.
- The catheter that was inserted during your operation will be connected to irrigation fluid which will wash out any clots out from your bladder.
- The catheter will be removed when the irrigation fluid is minimally bloodstained. This is usually about 2–3 days after the operation.
- You may experience problems controlling the passing of urine and a burning sensation when the catheter is first removed. This should settle over the next couple of days.
- Some patients are unable to pass urine. If this is the case, a catheter will be reinserted and may remain in place for up to 1–2 weeks.
- Driving should be avoided for 4 weeks after the operation.
- Sexual intercourse should be avoided for 6 weeks after the operation.
- It takes about 6 weeks to recover completely, and heavy lifting should be avoided for 3 months. However, gentle exercise is encouraged and reduces the risk of deep vein thrombosis and pulmonary embolism.
- Once you have been discharged, contact your GP if you experience fever, difficulty in passing urine, inability to pass urine, or large amounts of per urethral bleeding.
- You will be followed up in clinic approximately 6 weeks after the procedure, and the nursing staff will advise you as to the date and time of the appointment before you leave.

Specific risks

- Bleeding:
    - may require a blood transfusion
    - may lead to clot retention requiring catheterisation
    - if delayed may occur up to 6 weeks post-operatively.
- Urinary tract infection – treated with antibiotics.

- Urethral or bladder neck stricture – may lead to difficulty in passing urine.
- Retrograde ejaculation.
- Erectile dysfunction.
- Reduced fertility.
- Urinary incontinence – may require catheterisation or medication (anti-cholinergic).
- General risks include chest infections, deep vein thrombosis, pulmonary embolism, myocardial infarction and death.

Benefits

- This procedure relieves the urinary symptoms caused by the enlarged prostate gland.

Alternatives

- If nothing is done, 1 in 3 patients report that their symptoms worsen. However, symptoms may not change or improve.
- Medication can be used to relax the bladder neck (e.g. tamsulosin, an alpha-blocker) and shrink the prostate.
- Open prostatectomy is indicated when the prostate is too large for TURP, or in early prostate cancer.

Closure

- Outline the key points in the discussion.
- Ensure that any concerns have been elicited and addressed.
- Give the patient an information leaflet and possibly also a consent form to read prior to being admitted.
- Give the patient your contact details (e.g. bleep number) should they have any more questions.

109 Laparoscopic nephrectomy

Scenario

A 57-year-old man has been diagnosed with renal-cell carcinoma, and on CT scan has a 2-cm mass on the left kidney that is confined to the kidney (T1) with no distant spread. He has been booked for a laparoscopic left nephrectomy.

Introduction

- Introduce yourself to the patient, giving your name and grade.
- Tell the patient that you would like to give him more information about his operation.
- Check the patient's prior knowledge/understanding of the operation.

Explain

- There are two kidneys. One kidney can safely be removed, as the other kidney should be able to take over its function.
- The kidneys are located at the back of the abdomen (retroperitoneum), and laparoscopic nephrectomy is a procedure that uses keyhole surgery to remove the diseased kidney.

Preparation

- In the pre-admissions clinic today we will take a full history and examine you as well as performing some basic investigations, such as an ECG, chest X-ray and baseline blood tests (full blood count, renal function, etc.).
- We will need to have a list of your medication, as there are some drugs, such as warfarin (a blood-thinning agent), which will need to be stopped.
- More specialised tests such as lung function tests and an echo-cardiogram may also be required.
- The procedure will be performed under a general anaesthetic, which means that you will be sound asleep. The anaesthetist will talk to you in detail about the anaesthetic later on today/on admission.
- On admission, you will also be seen by the surgical team who will be performing the procedure, and the side to be operated on will be marked. They will be able to answer any further questions that you may have, and will ask for you to sign the consent form for the operation.
- You are advised to stop smoking.

Procedure

- While you are under the general anaesthetic, you will be positioned on your right side.

- A urinary catheter (tube) will be inserted into your bladder to help to drain the urine, and a nasogastric tube will be inserted into your nose to decompress/drain your stomach.
- Four incisions approximately 2 cm in length will be made. One incision will be at the umbilicus (belly button) and the other three will be strategically positioned over the remainder of the abdomen.
- Through these incisions we can pass specialised surgical instruments as well as a small camera which will allow us to see on a television screen the inside of your abdomen as we work.
- We will also need to inflate your abdomen with carbon dioxide to give us more room to operate inside the abdomen.
- The kidney will be freed up from its surrounding structures and, using special titanium clips, the ureter and blood vessels which supply the kidney will be clipped and cut.
- The kidney will then be placed as a whole in a plastic bag and delivered through the incision at the umbilicus.
- A drain (plastic tube) will be left in the abdomen, and the incisions will finally be closed using dissolvable stitches.
- The operation usually takes about 3 hours.
- For technical reasons it may not always be possible to perform the operation using keyhole surgery, and the surgeon may need to convert and perform an open procedure during which a larger incision will be made.

After the procedure

- You will be woken up in recovery and transferred back to the ward when you are stable.
- You may experience grogginess and nausea from the anaesthetic, and pain. If you experience nausea or pain, inform the nursing staff and they can give you medication to manage these symptoms.
- You will be given fluids via a drip in one of your veins, and this will continue until you start drinking sufficiently.
- You should be able to start initially drinking sips and then eating approximately 6 hours after the operation.
- The nasogastric tube which was inserted during the operation will be removed once you start drinking fluids (usually the following day), and the catheter will be removed after that.
- You should be fully mobile 24 hours after the operation, and you can expect to remain in hospital for about 3 days.

- You will be seen in the outpatient department clinic 6 weeks after the operation, and you will be given the time and date of the appointment before you are discharged.

Specific risks

- Conversion to an open procedure (1 in 20 risk).
- Bleeding – may require blood transfusion or further surgery.
- Infection (wound, retroperitoneal abscess or collections) – may require antibiotics or drainage.
- Acute urinary retention requiring catheterisation.
- Damage to bowel requiring further surgery.
- Ileus.
- Constipation requiring laxatives.
- Adhesions causing bowel obstruction in the future.
- Development of hypertension.
- Renal failure – may require renal dialysis or transplant.
- General risks include chest and wound infections, deep vein thrombosis, pulmonary embolism, myocardial infarction and death (all of these risks are increased in smokers).

Alternatives

- Not removing the kidney is likely to result in spread of the tumour, which would then become inoperable. The life expectancy at 5 years is less than 5% once spread has occurred.
- Partial nephrectomy (removal of part of the kidney) is usually only considered in solitary or bilateral tumours, and is not the optimal treatment in this case.
- Open nephrectony is a procedure that involves making a larger incision in the upper part of the abdomen and removing part of one rib. However, this procedure is associated with increased post-operative pain and a higher risk of complications such as chest infection, chronic wound pain and incisional hernia.

Closure

- Outline the key points in the discussion.
- Ensure that any concerns have been elicited and addressed.
- Give the patient an information leaflet and possibly also a consent form to read prior to being admitted.
- Give the patient your contact details (e.g. bleep number) in case they have any more questions.

Explaining radiological procedures

110 Upper gastrointestinal endoscopy

Scenario

Mrs Rickman is a 30-year-old woman with a history of dyspepsia and epigastric pain. She has been scheduled for an upper gastrointestinal endoscopy, and you are asked to explain the procedure to her.

Introduction

- Introduce yourself to the patient and establish a rapport.
- Ask the patient for permission to discuss the investigation.
- Check the patient's prior understanding of the procedure.

Explain

- A long flexible tube with a camera and a light source is passed into your mouth down your oesophagus (food-pipe) and into your stomach to allow us to visualise the inner lining of your food-pipe, stomach and duodenum (first part of the small bowel).
- The images can be seen on a television screen in the room.
- We are performing this test because of the symptoms of epigastric (abdominal) pain that you are experiencing, and to see if we can identify a cause.
- The test can show areas of narrowing, inflammation, ulcers and tumours which would be unlikely in your age group.
- A biopsy (sample of tissue) from the stomach lining may be taken during the procedure which could aid us in achieving a diagnosis.

- In addition, we can dilate any narrowing in your food-pipe and treat areas which are bleeding if necessary.

Preparation

The following precautions need to be taken in the situations outlined below.

- If the patient is on warfarin or heparin this needs to be stopped and a blood test needs to be performed on the morning of the procedure to ensure that the clotting is within the normal range.
- If the patient has a heart condition (e.g. valve replacement), antibiotics will need to be given before the procedure.
- Diabetics should request a morning appointment and omit their diabetic medication on the morning of the procedure.
- Aspirin and other anti-platelet agents such as ibuprofen should be stopped 2 weeks before the procedure.
- The night before:
  - do not eat or drink from after midnight until after your procedure
  - continue to take your regular medication with a sip of water.
- On the day of the procedure, on arrival:
  - you will need to change into a hospital gown
  - a cannula (line) will be inserted into a vein in your arm
  - you will be seen by the clinician performing the procedure, who will explain the procedure and its risks and benefits, after which you will be asked to sign a consent form
  - you should advise the doctor of any medication (especially warfarin or anti-platelet medication) that you are taking, and also any allergies
  - you should tell the doctor if you have a heart condition (e.g. heart valve), as you will need antibiotics before the procedure and also if you have a pacemaker or are diabetic.

Procedure

- You will be positioned on your side.
- Any dentures will need to be removed.
- The back of your throat will be sprayed with a local anaesthetic to numb the area, and this can taste unpleasant.
- You may also be given a sedative through your cannula to relax you.

- Your heart rate and saturations will be monitored throughout the procedure, and you may be given oxygen via a face mask or nasal prongs.
- Once you are sedated, the telescope will be passed to the back of your mouth and you will be asked to swallow to help it to pass into your oesophagus. It will then be passed into your stomach and duodenum.
- Air and water may be pumped into the stomach to help to get a better view, and you may feel bloated.

After the procedure

- You will be monitored regularly until you have come round from the sedation.
- You may have a hoarse voice or a sore throat due to the tube, and you may feel bloated.
- You can drink once you are able to swallow.
- You will be able to go home afterwards, but you should not drive, drink alcohol or make any major decisions for 24 hours, due to the effect of the sedation impairing your judgement.
- Ensure that there is someone to drive you home and to look after you for 12 hours after the procedure.
- You can go back to work 1–2 days after the procedure.
- The doctor may or may not discuss the results of the investigation.
- The results of the investigation should be available at your next appointment and will also be sent to your GP. Biopsy results can take a few weeks.

Risks

- Bleeding at a biopsy site.
- Aspiration and/or chest infection.
- Perforation (uncommon).
- Allergic reaction to the sedation.
- Complications from pre-existing heart or lung disease.
- Death (rare).

Benefits

- The procedure aids the diagnosis of the patient's symptoms.

Alternative investigations

- Barium meal – this can be used to assess the oesophagus and stomach, but it has the disadvantage of using X-rays. Furthermore, biopsies cannot be taken.

Closure

- Ask the patient whether they have any questions.
- Thank the patient.
- Give them your bleep number and name in case they have any further questions.
- Give them an information leaflet from the hospital which explains the procedure in more detail.

111 Colonoscopy

Scenario

Mr Ryan has been referred for a colonoscopy. You are the doctor on duty and you are asked to talk to the patient about the procedure.

Introduction

- Introduce yourself to the patient and establish a rapport.
- Ask the patient for permission to discuss the investigation.
- Check the patient's prior understanding of colonoscopy.

Explain

- Colonoscopy is a procedure in which we look at the inside of your large bowel and the lower end of yout small bowel by passing a tube/ telescope into your back passage.
- You have been referred for this procedure because you may be experiencing some problems when opening your bowels (such as bleeding), a change in your bowel habits, unexplained anaemia or weight loss, or you may have a family history of bowel cancers, and your doctor would like us to take a look at the bowel to see if we can find a cause for the symptoms or any abnormalities.

Preparation

- To be able to successfully visualise your bowel, we need it to be as empty as possible, so the procedure requires some preparation.
- Two days beforehand we ask that you have a small light dinner, and on the day before the procedure, before coming into hospital, you will need to take a laxative (a medication which will clear the bowel).
- The laxative comes in the form of a drink which we will supply you with, and you will need to take more of this on the morning of the procedure. The laxative is quite strong, and you may need to take time off work to allow you to stay at home to make frequent visits to the toilet. You may also experience tummy cramps.
- On the day of the procedure, we also ask that you remain nil by mouth – don't eat or drink anything.
- Elicit any important past medical history which may affect the preparation or procedure (e.g. diabetes, coagulopathies, heart conditions) and also medication (e.g. aspirin, warfarin, insulin).
- Ask the patient whether they have any questions or concerns at this stage. It is important that you are prepared to tackle any questions or anxieties that may arise (see box below).

Patient's concerns

- Could it be bowel cancer? Their parents may have died of cancer.
- Will I die?
- Will I be awake?
- Will I bleed?
- Is it painful?

Complications

- Haemorrhage
- Perforation
- Drug reactions
- Death

- You may want to say that at this stage you cannot predict what the findings will be, but reassure the patient that if there is anything that looks suspicious for cancer, a biopsy (sample of tissue) will be taken during the procedure. Tell the patient that the results will be available at their next clinic appointment.

- You will be seen by the clinician who will be performing the procedure, who will explain the procedure and its risks and benefits, after which you will be asked to sign a consent form.

Procedure

- You will be asked to change into a gown and you will be positioned on your left side.
- The procedure should take about 30 minutes.
- You will be sedated through a vein in your arm to make you sleepy and relaxed and to relieve the discomfort.
- The sedation should last until the procedure has finished, but the sedative effect can last for longer.
- While you are sedated a small tube with a light at the end will be passed through your back passage.
- There will be a camera attached to the tube, and the bowel can then be seen on a television screen in the room.
- Small samples of the bowel may be taken during the procedure.
- Ask the patient whether they are taking warfarin or have a prosthetic heart valve. Warfarin will need to be stopped for a biopsy, and antibiotic prophylaxis is required in patients with a prosthetic heart valve.
- You may experience some discomfort during the procedure, but if you tell the doctor they can give you a painkiller.

After the procedure

- You may notice some spotting of blood and aching from the back passage, but this should stop within a few hours.
- You will be able to go home straight after the procedure, but you should not drive, drink alcohol or make any major decisions for 24 hours, due to the effects of the sedative.
- Ensure that there is someone to drive you home and look after you.

Risks

- The main risks are bleeding, perforation of the bowel, drug reactions and death (rare). The risk is low, but if any of these were to happen we would manage each appropriately with, for example, a blood transfusion if bleeding is severe, or surgery and antibiotics in the case of a perforation.

- The risk of complications is higher when there is inflammation or disease affecting the bowel wall, or if a polyp is removed.

Alternatives

- Other alternatives are available, such as a barium enema or CT pneumocolon, and each of these has its risks and benefits. However, a biopsy cannot be taken during either of these procedures.

Closure

- The results of the investigation should be available at your next appointment, and will also be sent to your GP.
- Ask the patient if they have any questions.
- Thank the patient.
- Give them your bleep number and name in case they have any further questions.
- Give them an information leaflet from the hospital which explains the procedure in more detail.

112 Barium enema

Scenario

Mr Smith is a 65-year-old man who has lost 2 stone in weight over 2 months and has also noticed a change in his bowel habits. He has been referred for a barium enema, and you are asked to explain the procedure to him.

Introduction

- Introduce yourself to the patient and establish a rapport.
- Ask the patient for permission to discuss the investigation.
- Check the patient's prior understanding of the procedure.

Explain

- A barium enema uses barium, which shows up on X-ray, to look at the architecture of the colon (large bowel) wall.
- Barium is introduced into the back passage and a series of X-rays are taken. This may be technically difficult if your mobility is poor.

- The ionising radiation dose received is about 13 mSv, which is viewed as an acceptable dose. Note that a barium enema cannot be performed in pregnancy because of the use of ionising radiation.
- We are performing this test because you have been experiencing symptoms of weight loss and a change in bowel habits. You may also be having abdominal pain or bleeding from the back passage.
- This investigation will help us to try and find a cause for your symptoms.
- A barium enema can demonstrate the presence of diverticula (outpouchings of the large bowel wall), strictures (narrowings), colitis (inflammation), polyps and, importantly, cancers.

Preparation

- In order to get the best results, the bowel needs to be as empty as possible. You are therefore required to prepare the bowel by:
  - eating a low-residue diet 24 hours before the procedure
  - drinking a laxative (Picolax) the evening before the procedure
  - using a suppository on the morning of the procedure.
- The enema and suppository will be prescribed.
- You will be seen by the clinician performing the procedure, who will explain the procedure and its risks and benefits. You will then be asked to sign a consent form.

Procedure

- The procedure will be performed by a radiologist (a doctor who specialises in radiology).
- You will be positioned on your left side on a table designed to facilitate the use of X-rays.
- A digital rectal examination (examination of the back passage using a finger) will be performed, and a tube will then be passed 5–6 cm into your rectum (back passage).
- A small balloon will be inflated to prevent the tube from falling out, and the tube will be connected to a bottle of barium (a white opaque solution).
- Air will also then be introduced into the rectum (double contrast), and you will be asked to assume a number of different positions to allow the air and barium to mix and travel up the bowel. The table can also be tilted to facilitate this, and a series of X-ray images will be taken.

- Occasionally the bowel can go into spasm, and you may then experience abdominal cramps. An injection of the drug Buscopan can be given to treat these.
- You may feel uncomfortable or bloated during the procedure, due to the introduction of barium and air into your bowel, but this should settle afterwards.

After the procedure

- You may experience abdominal cramps, pain and bloating, which should settle.
- You can eat and drink normally straight after the procedure, and you should drink plenty of fluids.
- You will pass the barium on opening your bowels for a few days after your procedure.
- If you feel unwell, contact your GP.

Risks

- The preparation of the bowel can lead to dehydration and electrolyte disturbances.
- Tenesmus (sensation of wanting to open your bowels).
- Bowel perforation with or without peritonitis.
- Air or barium embolus (rare).
- Colitis (inflammation of the bowel).
- Bleeding that requires transfusion.
- Bowel obstruction.
- Inadequate procedure.
- Death (rare).

Benefits

- This is a sensitive investigation which may aid diagnosis.

Alternatives

- CT pneumocolon, in which a CT scan is used. However, this delivers a higher dose of ionising radiation.

Closure

- The radiologist will interpret the X-rays and write a formal report which will be sent to your GP.
- Ask the patient whether they have any questions.
- Thank the patient.
- Give them your bleep number and name in case they have any further questions.
- Give them an information leaflet from the hospital which explains the procedure in more detail.

113 Endoscopic retrograde cholangiopancreatography (ERCP)

Scenario

Mrs Jones is an obese 40-year-old woman with a history of gallstones. She has jaundice, and an ultrasound scan has demonstrated multiple stones within the gallbladder and a dilated common bile duct. She is scheduled for an ERCP, and you are asked to explain the procedure to her.

Introduction

- Introduce yourself to the patient and establish a rapport.
- Ask the patient for permission to discuss the investigation.
- Check the patient's prior understanding of the procedure.

Explain

- A long flexible tube with a camera and a light source is passed into your mouth down your oesophagus (food-pipe), into your stomach and into the duodenum (first part of the small bowel).
- The images can be seen on a television screen.
- The entrance (papilla) to the common bile duct which is located in the duodenum is identified, and a special contrast which can be seen on X-ray is injected.
- A series of X-rays are then taken, and this demonstrates whether there is an obstruction or a narrowing within the common bile duct or the other interconnected ducts of the liver, pancreas and gallbladder.

- We are performing this test because you are jaundiced, and this can be caused by an obstruction or narrowing of one of these ducts (tubes). This investigation will therefore aid our diagnosis.
- In addition, if an obstruction or narrowing is seen we will be able to treat this at the same time.

Preparation

- Do not eat or drink for 8 hours before the procedure.
- Regular medication should not be omitted, but taken with a sip of water.
- You will be seen by the clinician performing the procedure, who will explain the procedure and its risks and benefits. You will then be asked to sign a consent form.
- Tell the doctor if you:
  - are diabetic
  - are taking anti-platelet medication (this needs to be stopped 2 weeks before the procedure)
  - are taking warfarin (clotting needs to be corrected before the procedure)
  - have allergies to shellfish or contrast media
  - have a pacemaker, joint replacement or prosthetic heart valve (you will need prophylactic antibiotics).

Procedure

- You will need to change into a hospital gown.
- You will be positioned on a table designed to facilitate the use of X-rays.
- Any dentures will need to be removed.
- The back of your throat will be sprayed with a local anaesthetic to numb the area, and this can taste unpleasant.
- You may also be given a sedative through your cannula, which will be inserted into one of the veins of your hand, to help you to relax.
- Your heart rate and saturations will be monitored throughout the procedure, and you may be given oxygen via a face mask or nasal prongs.
- Once you are sedated, the telescope will be passed to the back of your mouth and you will be asked to swallow to help it to pass into your oesophagus. It will then be passed into your stomach and finally into the duodenum.

- Contrast will then be injected into the entrance of the common bile duct and a series of X-rays will be taken.
- If a blockage is seen, the doctor may enlarge the opening to the common bile duct to facilitate the passage of any stones (i.e. perform a sphincterotomy). This is done by making a small cut using a specialised wire that is passed down the endoscope.
- If a narrowing is seen, a small plastic tube (stent) can be inserted into the duct to brace it open.
- The procedure should take around 45–60 minutes.

After the procedure

- You will be monitored regularly until you have come round from the sedation.
- You may have a hoarse voice or a sore throat due to the tube.
- You can drink once you are able to swallow (usually after 2 hours), but you should not drink milk products, as these stimulate gall-bladder contraction and bile secretion.
- You can eat the following day.
- You will be able to go home the same day unless an intervention such as a sphincterotomy has been performed, in which case you will be kept in overnight and have a blood test performed to check your liver function tests.
- You should not drive, drink alcohol or make any major decisions within 24 hours of the procedure, as the sedative can impair your judgement.
- If you are discharged, ensure that there is someone to drive you home and to look after you for 12 hours after the procedure.
- The doctor may discuss the results of the investigation with you, or they may discuss them at a follow-up appointment.
- Contact your GP or go to Accident and Emergency if you become unwell afterwards.

Risks

- Bowel, stomach or oesophageal perforation – requires surgery.
- Bleeding (1 in 100 risk) – may require blood transfusion or surgery.
- Aspiration pneumonia.
- Reaction to sedation.
- Pancreatitis (inflammation of the pancreas) (1 in 20 risk).
- Cholangitis (infection of the collection of communicating ducts).
- Inadequate procedure or failure of procedure.

Benefits

● This procedure aids diagnosis and allows treatment at the same time.

Alternatives

● Magnetic resonance cholangiopancreatography (MRCP) may be used. This is a non-invasive procedure which utilises MRI to visualise the biliary tract. However, procedures such as sphincterotomy cannot be performed using this method.

Closure

● Ask the patient whether they have any questions.
● Thank the patient.
● Give them your bleep number and name in case they have any further questions.
● Give them an information leaflet from the hospital which explains the procedure in more detail.

114 Bronchoscopy

Scenario

Mr Mannering is a 55-year-old man who was referred to the respiratory team with haemoptysis. He is due to have a flexible bronchoscopy as an outpatient, and you are asked to explain the procedure to him.

Introduction

● Introduce yourself to the patient and establish a rapport.
● Ask the patient for permission to discuss the procedure.
● Check the patient's prior understanding.

Explain

● This is a safe and quick procedure that enables visualisation of the airways in the lung using a long thin flexible tube.
● We are performing this procedure to try to identify a cause for the haemoptysis (bleeding) that you are experiencing.
● In addition to looking at your airways, a biopsy (tissue sample) and mucus sample can also be taken, and this can aid diagnosis.

- This technique can also be used to remove foreign objects and growths that are obstructing the airways, to give medication and to control bleeding.

Preparation

- Do not eat for 8–10 hours before the procedure.
- Regular medication should not be omitted, but taken with a sip of water.

On arrival at the clinic

- You will be seen by the clinician performing the procedure, who will explain the procedure and its risks and benefits. After this you will be asked to sign a consent form.
- You should tell the doctor about the following:
    - any medication (e.g. aspirin, clopidogrel, warfarin)
    - any allergies
    - diabetes
    - risk of pregnancy.
- Your breathing will be tested using a hand-held device known as a spirometer/PEFR meter.
- You may be given medication via a face mask to assist your breathing (nebuliser).

Procedure

- The procedure takes around 15–20 minutes.
- You will need to change into a hospital gown, and dentures and contact lenses should be removed.
- You will be either seated upright or lying on a table.
- The back of your throat will be sprayed with a local anaesthetic to numb the area, and this can taste unpleasant.
- You may also be given a sedative through your cannula, which will be inserted into one of the veins of your hand, to help you to relax.
- Your heart rate and saturations will be monitored throughout the procedure, and you may be given oxygen via a face mask or nasal prongs.
- Once you are sedated, the bronchoscope (thin tube) will be passed through your mouth or nose and you may be asked to make a high-pitched sound to help the tube advance past your vocal cords into your trachea (windpipe) and finally the smaller airways in your lungs.

- A sputum and/or biopsy sample may be taken during the procedure. The biopsy can be performed with either a brush or a needle passed through the bronchoscope.
- Saline (salt water) may also be passed through the bronchoscope to wash the lungs. The washings will then be immediately suctioned and collected, and they can be analysed for any abnormal cells (this is known as bronchial alveolar lavage).
- The procedure should not be painful, but you may experience discomfort/pressure and feel the need to gag/cough.

After the procedure

- You will be monitored regularly until you have come round from the sedation (this takes approximately 2 hours), and will remember little of the procedure.
- You may experience:
  - hoarseness and a sore throat – throat lozenges and gargling warm water will help to relieve these symptoms
  - haemoptysis (coughing up blood) if a biopsy was taken – this should settle within 24 hours.
- You can drink once you are able to feel the back of your throat.
- You will be able to go home afterwards, but you should not drive, drink alcohol or make any major decisions for 24 hours, due to the effects of the sedative impairing judgement.
- Ensure that there is someone to drive you home and to look after you for 12 hours after the procedure.
- You can go back to work 1–2 days after the procedure.
- The doctor may or may not discuss the results of the investigation.
- Contact your GP or go to Accident and Emergency if you experience heavy bleeding, if you develop breathing problems or if you have a fever.

Risks

- Bronchial spasm affecting breathing.
- Arrhythmias ('abnormal heart beat').
- Chest infection with fever (16% of cases).
- Persistent hoarseness.
- Shortness of breath.
- Surgical emphysema ('air that crackles under the skin').
- Failure of procedure.
- Death (rare).

- Following biopsy:
  - pneumothorax (< 1% of cases) requiring a chest drain
  - haemoptysis with major bleeding.

Benefits

- This procedure aids diagnosis.

Alternatives

- Rigid bronchoscopy – this requires a general anaesthetic, and may be used if the above procedure fails.
- Percutaneous biopsy – in which a tissue sample is obtained by passing a needle into the chest wall under local anaesthetic. This procedure is associated with a higher risk of pneumothorax.

Closure

- The results of the investigation should be available at your next appointment, and will also be sent to your GP. Biopsy results typically take around 1 week to be processed.
- Ask the patient whether they have any questions.
- **Thank the patient.**
- Give them your bleep number and name in case they have any further questions.
- Give them an information leaflet from the hospital which explains the procedure in more detail.

115 Renal biopsy

Scenario

Mr Hanson is a 46-year-old man with unexplained renal failure. He has been advised to have a renal biopsy, and you have been asked to explain the procedure to him.

Introduction

- Introduce yourself to the patient and establish a rapport.
- Ask the patient for permission to discuss the investigation.
- Check the patient's prior understanding of the procedure.

Explain

- You have two kidneys, which are located in the right and left flank/loin.
- Renal biopsy is a method of obtaining a sample of tissue from the kidney by introducing a biopsy needle (possibly several times) through the skin overlying the affected kidney.
- Ultrasound will be used to guide the needle into the kidney.
- The tissue sample obtained will be tested to try to identify a cause (e.g. scarring, infection, abnormal deposits) for the symptoms experienced (e.g. renal failure, haematuria, proteinuria, transplant rejection) and to determine the best course of management.

Preparation

- Do not eat for 8–10 hours before the procedure.
- Regular medication should not be omitted, but taken with a sip of water.
- On arrival, a blood test will be performed and a urine sample will be requested.
- You will be seen by the clinician performing the procedure, who will explain the procedure and its risks and benefits, after which you will be asked to sign a consent form.
- You should tell the doctor about:
  - all current medication
  - any allergies.

Procedure

- The procedure will take approximately 1 hour.
- You will need to change into a hospital gown, and will be positioned on your stomach (or on your back for transplanted kidney biopsies).
- You will be given a sedative through your cannula, which will be inserted into one of the veins of your hand, to help you to relax.
- In addition, you will be given a local anaesthetic via an injection over the biopsy site, which will numb the area.
- An ultrasound probe will be used to help to guide the needle into the kidney. You will be asked to hold your breath as the needle is inserted through the skin, and you may feel pressure as the needle enters the kidney. A few attempts may be needed to obtain a good sample of tissue.

After the procedure

- You should lie in bed (absolute bed rest) for 6–12 hours after the procedure, and you may be kept in overnight.
- You will be advised to drink plenty of fluids, and your blood pressure and heart rate will be monitored at regular intervals while you are in hospital.
- It is normal to feel discomfort at the injection site and to pass blood in your urine (haematuria) after the procedure. This usually settles after 24 hours.

Risks

- Pain (common).
- Bleeding at the biopsy site and haematuria may require blood transfusion (1 in 30–60 cases) and possibly a further procedure, including nephrectomy.
- Proteinuria.
- Damage to adjacent structures (rare).
- Death.
- Risks associated with the local anaesthetic include pain, bruising and/or bleeding at the injection site, and allergic reactions.

Benefits

- A tissue sample is obtained which may aid diagnosis and management.

Alternatives

A tissue sample can be obtained by two other methods:

- open surgery under a general anaesthetic
- via a transjugular approach (through a blood vessel).

Both of these alternatives have a higher risk of complications such as bleeding.

Closure

- You should contact your doctor if you experience prolonged blood loss in your urine, or if you are unable to pass urine, develop a fever or experience increasing pain.

- The results of the investigation should be available at your next appointment, and will also be sent to your GP.
- Ask the patient whether they have any questions.
- Thank the patient.
- Give them your bleep number and name in case they have any further questions.
- Give them an information leaflet from the hospital which explains the procedure in more detail.

116 Coronary angiography

Scenario

Mr Morgan is a 65-year-old banker who was admitted with unstable angina. He has been admitted with chest pain and is scheduled for an angiogram and possible angioplasty. Explain the procedure to him.

Introduction

- Introduce yourself to the patient and establish a rapport.
- Ask the patient for permission to discuss the investigation.
- Check the patient's prior understanding of the procedure.

Explain

- Arteries in your heart can become narrowed with atheroma (deposits of lipid, fibrous tissue and calcium). This can reduce the blood supply to your heart muscle, leading to angina (chest pain) and/or a heart attack.
- An angiogram is a procedure that enables us to assess whether the blood vessels in your heart are diseased.
- This will help us to establish a diagnosis for the chest pain that you have been experiencing, and at the same time, if a blockage is found, it may also be treated.

Preparation

- Do not eat from midnight onwards on the morning before the procedure.
- Regular medication should not be omitted, but taken with a sip of water.

- On arrival you will be seen by the clinician performing the procedure, who will explain the procedure and its risks and benefits, after which you will be asked to sign a consent form.
- You should tell the doctor about:
  - all current medication
  - any allergies, including previous contrast reactions.

Procedure

- The procedure will take approximately 30–45 minutes.
- You will need to change into a hospital gown, and will be positioned lying flat.
- A sedative will be given through a cannula, which will be inserted into a vein in your hand. This will help you to relax, but you will still be awake.
- Local anaesthetic will be used to numb the skin in your groin.
- A tube will then be passed into one of the arteries via a small incision or needle puncture over the anaesthetised area in the groin, and this tube will be carefully steered into each of the coronary arteries (the arteries which supply the heart).
- Contrast medium (dye which shows up on X-ray) will then be injected into the vessels and a series of X-ray images will be taken. This will give us a map of your coronary arteries and show any narrowing within them.
- If a narrowing/blockage is seen, it may be possible to introduce a small balloon (on the end of the tube) into the artery via the groin and to use the balloon to widen the narrowing. It is also possible to place a small tube (stent) within the artery to try to hold the vessel open.
- In addition, contrast can be injected into the left ventricle (main chamber) of your heart, and X-ray images can then give us information about how well the heart is pumping/working.
- Your heart rate and saturations will be monitored throughout the procedure, and you may be given oxygen via a face mask or nasal prongs.

After the procedure

- You will be monitored regularly until you have come round from the sedation (this takes approximately 2 hours), and you should lie in bed (absolute bed rest) for 4–6 hours after the procedure.

- You will be able to go home afterwards. However, you may be kept in overnight if the bleeding from the groin site is excessive or an intervention has been performed.
- You should not drive, drink alcohol or make any major decisions for 24 hours, due to the effects of the sedative on your judgement.
- Ensure that there is someone to drive you home and to look after you for 12 hours after the procedure.
- The doctor should discuss the results of the investigation with you once the effects of the sedation have worn off.
- Contact your GP or go to Accident and Emergency if bleeding from the groin is excessive or if you develop any other side-effects.

Risks

- These depend on the patient's age and on the severity of cardiac disease (e.g. previous coronary artery bypass graft, myocardial infarction, heart failure and comorbidity).
- They include:
  - arrhythmias (1 in 100 cases)
  - bleeding with or without haematoma
  - pseudoaneurysm of the femoral artery
  - radiation damage to the skin
  - stroke (long-term disability)
  - myocardial infarction
  - contrast reaction leading to an asthma attack, convulsions, renal failure or death (rare)
  - lower limb ischaemia (compromised blood supply to the leg) that requires surgery
  - emergency coronary artery bypass grafting.

Benefits

- This procedure aids both the diagnosis and future management of a patient with symptoms suggestive of ischaemic heart disease.

Closure

- Ask the patient whether they have any questions.
- Thank the patient.
- Give them your bleep number and name in case they have any further questions.

- Give them an information leaflet from the hospital which explains the procedure in more detail.

117 Ultrasound scan

Introduction

- Introduce yourself to the patient and establish a rapport.
- Ask the patient for permission to discuss the investigation.
- Check the patient's prior understanding of the procedure.

Explain

- Ultrasound uses high-frequency sound waves to produce images of the body.
- It does not use ionising radiation (i.e. X-rays), and is therefore a safe, fast and simple diagnostic and therapeutic procedure.
- Images can be captured in two or three dimensions and also in real time, and can therefore be used to assess blood flow (e.g. Doppler ultrasound).

Ultrasound is useful for diagnosing pathology in the following soft tissue structures:

- heart
  - transoesophageal/transthoracic echo
  - demonstrates valve architecture, thrombus, hypertrophy, gives functional data
- blood vessels
  - carotid artery for stenosis
  - abdominal aorta for aneurysmal disease, etc.
- liver – size, cystic and solid masses, portal vein pathology
- gallbladder – stones, thickening, dilation of common bile duct, size
- pancreas – cystic and solid structures/masses
- kidneys – hydronephrosis, size, calculi
- bladder – stones, tumours, size, residual volume
- uterus, ovaries, fetus
- eyes
- thyroid and parathyroid glands – size, masses
- scrotum – cysts, hydrocele, size, necrosis, tumours.

In addition, it can be used to guide the following procedures:

- needle biopsies (e.g. breast, thyroid)
- aspiration of fluid
- drainage of collections.

Preparation

- Specific to procedure: varies from not eating or drinking for up to 12 hours (biopsies) to drinking various amounts of water while avoiding passing urine, in order to fill the bladder (renal tract ultrasound).
- On arrival, you will be seen by the clinician performing the procedure, who will explain the procedure and its risks and benefits, after which you may in some cases be asked to sign a consent form.
- You should tell the doctor/radiographer about:
  - all current medication (e.g. anticoagulants such as warfarin, aspirin, which will affect whether a biopsy is performed)
  - any allergies, including previous contrast reactions.

Procedure

- You may need to change into a hospital gown, and will usually be positioned lying flat (depending on the area to be imaged).
- A clear water-based gel will be applied over the area of interest to improve the contact with the ultrasound transducer probe, which will then be placed firmly on your skin.
- The probe generates inaudible high-frequency sound waves which bounce off surfaces within the body. The returning signal is recorded by the probe and used to generate an image of the structure of interest.
- Once the procedure is complete the gel will be wiped from your skin.
- In some procedures the transducer will be placed into internal openings within the body rather than on the skin – for example, the oesophagus in transoesophageal echo (to view the heart), the rectum in transrectal ultrasound (to view the prostate gland) and the vagina in transvaginal ultrasound (to view the uterus and ovaries).
- The procedure should not be painful (although you may feel pressure), and it takes around 30–60 minutes, the time varying according to the area investigated.

After the procedure

- You should be able to go home after the procedure and resume all normal activities.
- The ultrasound images obtained will need to be reported by the radiologist, and you may or may not be given a verbal preliminary report.
- The results of the investigation should either be available at your next clinic appointment, or will be sent to your GP.

Risks

- There are no risks unless ultrasound is used to facilitate a procedure (e.g. biopsy).
- Ultrasound is reflected by air and gas, and is therefore *not* useful when imaging the following:
  - bowel
  - stomach
  - may produce inadequate views of the pancreas or aorta if bowel is overlying.
- It is also not ideal for imaging bone.
- The images obtained are operator dependent.

Benefits

- Non-invasive.
- Cheap.
- Safe (non-ionising radiation) and can be repeated several times without risk, so it is the investigation of choice in women and children.
- Good soft tissue definition.
- Gives real-time information.

Closure

- Ask the patient whether they have any questions.
- Thank the patient.
- Give them your bleep number and name in case they have any further questions.
- Give them an information leaflet from the hospital which explains the procedure in more detail.

118 MRI scan

Introduction

- Introduce yourself to the patient and establish a rapport.
- Ask the patient for permission to discuss the investigation.
- Check the patient's prior understanding of the procedure.

Explain:

- The principles of MRI are complex.
- The patient is placed in a strong magnetic field and intermittently exposed to a series of inaudible radio pulses.
- A large proportion (70%) of the human body is composed of water, and the hydrogen ions which form each water molecule respond to the radio pulses and themselves emit radio pulses which are detected and used to generate an image.
- Establish and explain the indication for the procedure.

Preparation

- Since the creation of a magnetic field is integral to the investigation, metallic objects are not allowed in the MRI machine. On arrival you will therefore be asked to complete a questionnaire to ensure that you do not have the following:
  - pacemaker
  - metal prostheses
  - implants
  - surgical clips
  - injury from shrapnel or grinding instruments
  - metal in the head or eyes.
- In addition, you will need to remove all metallic objects on your person (e.g. jewellery, watch, glasses, keys, wallet, credit cards), as they can be de-magnetised.
- The safety of MRI in pregnancy has not been established, and therefore MRI using contrast is not recommended in cases where pregnancy is either confirmed or suspected.

Procedure

- You may be asked to change into a hospital gown, and will be positioned lying flat on a padded bed which will then be moved into a horizontal narrow cylinder. You will effectively be lying in a magnetic field, and the cylinder is necessary to acquire the MRI images.

- You will be provided with a headset to reduce the noise from the MRI machine. However, you will be able to hear and communicate with the technician who is performing the scan, and you can ask for the procedure to be stopped at any time.
- You need to lie still throughout the study, which varies in duration according to the area to be imaged, and can last for up to 1 hour.
- The procedure is not painful, although some patients feel claustrophobic inside the MRI machine.

After the procedure

- You should be able to go home after the procedure and resume all normal activities immediately.
- The MRI images obtained will need to be reported by the radiologist, and you may or may not be given a verbal preliminary report.
- However, the results of the investigation should either be available at your next clinic appointment or will be sent to your GP.

Risks

- Anxiety caused by claustrophobia, leading to early termination of the procedure.
- Injury or death (rare) due to the accidental admission of patients with metal within their bodies (e.g. prostheses, pacemaker) or on their persons (e.g. watch, jewellery).

Disadvantages

- Expensive.
- Exclusion criteria.

Benefits

- Good soft tissue definition is achieved.
- Useful for imaging bone, brain tissue and joints.

Closure

- Ask the patient whether they have any questions.
- Thank the patient.

- Give them your bleep number and name in case they have any further questions.
- Give them an information leaflet from the hospital which explains the procedure in more detail.

119 CT scan

Introduction

- Introduce yourself to the patient and establish a rapport.
- Ask the patient for permission to discuss the investigation.
- Check the patient's prior understanding of the procedure.

Explain

- This is a simple non-invasive painless investigation.
- It uses X-rays (ionising radiation) to obtain multiple images of 'slices' of the body.
- In addition, CT scans can be performed with contrast (X-ray dye) which can highlight specific structures, such as bowel or blood vessels.
- The typical ionising dose for a chest, abdominal or pelvic CT scan is 10 mSv.
- Check and justify the indication for the CT scan.

Preparation

- Depending on the scan, you may be required not to eat or drink beforehand.
- You will be seen by the clinician who will be performing the procedure, who will explain the procedure and its risks and benefits, after which you may in some cases be asked to sign a consent form.
- You should tell the doctor/radiographer about the following:
  - pregnancy
  - diabetes
  - all current medication
  - any allergies, including previous contrast reactions.
- All jewellery should be removed, as it may interfere with the results of the scan.
- For a CT scan of the head, hearing aids, dentures, glasses and earrings should be removed.

Procedure

- The procedure will take around 30–90 minutes, depending on the area being imaged, and is performed by a radiographer (a technician who specialises in radiography).
- You may need to change into a hospital gown, and will be positioned lying flat on a movable table linked to the doughnut-shaped CT scanner.
- If contrast is used, it will be injected through a cannula inserted into a vein in your arm.
- The area to be imaged will then be positioned in the centre of the large doughnut, which contains the X-ray tube.
- Prior to the start of the investigation, all staff will leave the scanning room. However, you will be observed through a window and will be able to communicate with the radiographer via an intercom.
- The X-ray tube will then rotate around you, and the X-ray beams which emerge from your body will be detected and recorded to create a two-dimensional cross-sectional image. The table will move a short distance every few seconds in order to generate a series of 'slices' through your body, and these will be put together by a computer to create a three-dimensional image of the area of interest.

After the procedure

- You should be able to go home after the procedure and resume all normal activities.
- If contrast has been used you should drink plenty of fluid.
- The CT images obtained will need to be reported by the radiologist, and you may or may not be given a verbal preliminary report.
- However, the results of the investigation should either be available at your next clinic appointment with the referring doctor or will be sent to your GP.

Risks

- Contrast allergic reaction, which may result in an asthma attack, renal failure or death.
- Radiation exposure:
  - there is a 1 in 100 chance of developing cancer from a single 10 mSv exposure
  - CT scans should be avoided where possible in children, pregnant women, and adults under 40 years of age.

Benefits

- CT scanning provides information that can aid diagnosis and management.

Closure

- Ask the patient whether they have any questions.
- Thank the patient.
- Give them your bleep number and name in case they have any further questions.
- Give them an information leaflet from the hospital which explains the procedure in more detail.

Management

Patient management consists of the organisation of care in the context of either managing a disease or treating it in a variety of settings, from hospital wards to clinics and family medicine. You should always familiarise yourself fully with the patient's notes, paying particular attention to past investigations and treatment regimens and recent test results.

The consultation is also an opportunity for you to discuss their current problems and address any lifestyle or compliance issues that the patient may have. You should also offer supportive advice and information concerning the patient's illness, as this will help to empower the patient with regard to the management of their own illness.

Each of the scenarios below identifies the key points that you need to address during a consultation.

120 Managing diabetes

Scenario

You are a doctor in family medicine. Mrs Patel is a 65-year-old woman with type 2 diabetes. She has come to her family practice for general advice about her diabetes. You are asked to advise her about managing her diabetes.

Preparation for the consultation

Obtain and read through the medical notes and, importantly, review previous blood glucose measurements and blood tests (including HbA_{1c} and renal function).

Introduction

- Introduce yourself to the patient, confirm her identity and establish a rapport.
- Sit opposite the patient in order to allow good eye contact.
- Ascertain why she has presented to clinic, and identify her concerns and her expectations of the consultation.

The consultation

- Explain that you would like to discuss her diabetic control and management.
- Ask to see any records (e.g. a BM diary).

Complications of diabetes

Explain to the patient the possible repercussions of poor long-term diabetic control:

- eyes – retinopathy, glaucoma and cataracts
- kidneys – glucose in the urine damaging the internal structures in the kidneys, leading to renal failure which may require dialysis in the future
- nerves – peripheral neuropathy
- feet – ulceration is common, and these ulcers may become infected
- vasculature – the blood supply to the head, heart and peripheral nerves is susceptible to damage which can lead to stroke, ischaemic heart disease, myocardial infarction and limb amputation.

Education and information

Advise the patient about the following:

Diet

- Be aware that a patient's ethnicity may influence their dietary habits.
- Advise the patient to:
  - avoid long periods of starvation which can lead to hypoglycaemia
  - avoid saturated fats and sugar which can lead to hyperglycaemia
  - include complex carbohydrates, such as bread, potatoes and pasta, in their diet, and explain that wholemeal flour is always preferable to white flour
  - avoid onion, garlic and bitter gourd (kaerela) when cooking, due to their hypoglycaemic effects.
- Herbal remedies for the treatment of diabetes should not be used, especially in conjunction with conventional medical treatment, without medical advice.
- Refer the patient to a dietitian if appropriate.

Exercise

Regular exercise with weight reduction will reduce the body's insulin requirement.

Foot care

- Highlight the importance of foot care.
- Inform the patient that a chiropodist is available.

Eyes

- Explain the importance of regular eye tests for early detection of disease.
- The DVLA needs to be informed about insulin-treated diabetics and also informed if their eyesight deteriorates.

Medical treatment

- A wide range of treatment regimes are available.
- Ensure that the patient is on the following medication. If they are not, ascertain whether there are any contraindications to starting these medications:
  - insulin – short or long acting
  - oral hypoglycaemics (e.g. metformin, gliclazide)
  - ACE inhibitors
  - aspirin
  - statins.
- Blood tests should be performed every 3 to 6 months.

General support

- Give the patient literature on diabetic control.
- Advise them about available support groups, such as the Diabetic Society.
- Tell the patient that they should make regular appointments with the diabetic nurse and doctor.

Support at home

- Give the patient a BM diary.
- Ask them to record their blood sugar levels before each meal.

- Ask them to bring the diary to each visit so that their diabetic control can be monitored.

Closure

- Outline the key points of the consultation.
- Ensure that any concerns have been elicited and addressed.
- Ask the patient whether they have any questions.
- Give the patient your contact details in case they have any more questions.
- Arrange a follow-up appointment.
- Thank the patient.

121 Sectioning a patient and the Mental Health Act

Scenario

You are a student in family medicine. The GP has asked you to accompany him to see Mr DiNozzo, a 35-year-old, mentally ill patient. Familiarise yourself with the Mental Health Act beforehand.

The patient suffers from schizophrenia and has had an acute delusional episode. He is now threatening to kill himself, as he believes there are voices telling him to do so. Summarised below are the important points that one should know about the Mental Health Act 1983.

Mental Health Act 1983

There are three important acts that doctors should be aware of:

- Section 2: Admission for assessment
- Section 3: Admission for treatment
- Section 4: Emergency admission for assessment.

Section 2

- Compulsory admission and detention at a hospital for 28 days.
- Not renewable.
- Indications: patient needs to be detained for their own health/safety or to protect others; patient suffers from a mental disorder that requires assessment for a limited period.

- The application consists of the written recommendations of two registered medical practitioners (not from the same hospital or practice).
- Doctors need to examine the patient.

Section 3

- Admission for treatment for no longer than 6 months.
- The exact nature of the mental disorder must be stated.
- Detention is renewable for a further 6 months.
- Indications: mental illness; severe mental impairment; psychopathic disorder or mental impairment and mental disorder of a nature or degree that requires medical treatment in a hospital; admission is necessary for the health or safety of the patient or for the protection of other individuals.
- The application consists of the written recommendations of two registered medical practitioners (not from the same hospital or practice).
- Application is valid for 2 weeks.

Section 4

- Admission for 72 hours only.
- Indications: urgent necessity; mental disorder requiring admission; the patient is a danger to him- or herself or others.
- Application made by relative or approved social worker or approved senior nurse or medical practitioner who has seen the patient within the last 24 hours.
- Usually converted to Section 2 on arrival at hospital.

Note: Sectioning a patient does not allow you to treat a concurrent physical condition unless it is life-threatening.

Therefore with regard to Mr DiNozzo:

- under the Mental Health Act the GP can apply for a Section 2 for assessment, and then the psychiatrists can take over the patient's care
- if the patient refuses to go, the GP will have to take out a Section 4, and this will be converted to Section 2 on admission.

122 Managing epilepsy, including driving and childhood epilepsy

Scenario

You are a doctor in family medicine. Mr Adams, a 30-year-old builder, has been diagnosed with epilepsy. He is understandably concerned about this diagnosis, and the GP has asked you to talk to him about it.

Preparation for the consultation

● Familiarise yourself with Mr Adams' notes, paying particular attention to the type of seizures that he has been suffering.
● Past medical history, occupation and family history of diseases are also important.

Introduction

● Introduce yourself to Mr Adams.
● Explain that you are the junior doctor at the surgery and that the GP has asked you to see him to discuss his recent diagnosis.
● Ascertain what Mr Adams has been told so far, and establish his understanding of the disease.
● Ask him if there is anything he is not sure about and whether he requires any further information.
  – Mr Adams asks you to tell him more about the disease.
  – Explain that in epilepsy the neurochemistry of the brain is altered, which leads to heightened electrical activity. This is associated with loss of consciousness, jerky movements of the limbs, lip smacking, lip biting, incontinence or daydreaming (absent seizures).
● There are two main types of epilepsy:
  – partial seizures
  – generalised (tonic–clonic seizures).
● Ask the patient to describe his seizures.
  – Mr Adams tells you that he loses consciousness and falls to the ground, often also wetting himself.
● Ask him whether he experienced any such events as a child.
  – He replies that he had a few seizures in childhood, but these went away.

- Explain that children may have febrile convulsions at a young age and soon grow out of them, and that very young children may have infantile spasms known as 'salaam attacks.'

Treatment

- Explain that treatment revolves around inhibiting neuronal activity associated with the neurotransmitter glutamate (excitatory), and potentiating that associated with the neurotransmitter GABA (inhibitory) in an attempt to reduce the heightened neuronal activity.
- When treating epilepsy, it is important to adopt a stepwise approach. This may be achieved by titrating doses upwards to achieve seizure control, then allowing for additional anticonvulsants or tapering the first drug down to allow for substitution of other drugs.
- Use of one drug is sufficient in many patients, although when polypharmacy is involved one must consider the serious side-effects and toxicity profiles of each drug, and the possibility of drug interactions.

Drug	Effect of drug	Uses
Sodium valproate	Enhances GABA activity	All types of seizures
Carbamazepine	Prevents neuronal firing, membrane stabiliser	Partial and generalised seizures; not for myoclonus or absence seizure

Occupation and social aspects

- Mr Adams works as a scaffolder. You must tell him that his job is unsafe, as he spends significant amounts of time at a considerable height from the ground, and if he has a seizure he risks serious injury or death.
- Explain that he may need to go on sick leave for a while and look for another job.
- Inform him of the financial assistance available to him until he finds a more suitable occupation.

Driving

- Mr Adams drives, so you must explain to him that by law he must refrain from driving and inform the DVLA (or equivalent driving/licensing authority) of his condition.
- If you believe that the patient is not willing to do this him- or herself, it is your responsibility to inform the driving/licensing authority.
- DVLA restrictions state that in order to drive you must be seizure free for 1 year.
- Also warn the patient that while he is on anti-epileptic medication he may not operate machinery, and that he should seek medical advice with regard to potential drug interactions before taking any additional medication (prescription or otherwise).

Closure

- Ask the patient whether he has any further questions.
- Give the patient an information leaflet about epilepsy.
- Advise the patient of any support that is available to him.
- Make a follow-up appointment with the patient.
- Confirm that he has understood everything you have discussed.
- Thank the patient.

123 Managing asthma done

Scenario

You are a doctor in general practice. Miss Jones, a 25-year-old ballet dancer, comes to see you for advice about keeping her asthma under control, particularly during performances.

Preparation before consultation

- Find the patient's notes and familiarise yourself with her past medical history.
- Assess her asthma control and review her past peak flow readings.
- Check for previous hospital admissions for asthmatic events and establish whether any of these were life-threatening.
- Look at her past prescriptions and ascertain what medications she is taking.

Introduction

- Introduce yourself to Miss Jones and establish a rapport.
- Tell Miss Jones that you understand that she would like some advice about how to control her asthma better, and ask her whether she has any other concerns.
  - Miss Jones explains that her asthma is hindering her ability to perform ballet.
  - She is also unwilling to take any form of steroids, as they cause weight gain, which makes her feel uncomfortable when wearing a tutu.
- Ask her what inhalers she is taking.
  - She says that she is not taking the brown inhaler, but takes the blue inhaler whenever her asthma flares up. She mentions that a month ago she was hospitalised with an acute asthma attack.
- At this point you should realise that there are compliance issues that you must tackle.

Treatment and management

- Ask the patient how many times she takes her inhalers a day.
- Explain that the brown inhaler is a preventive inhaler, and that she must take two puffs twice a day, and that the blue one is to be taken whenever she experiences chest tightness or feels an attack is imminent.
- Give her a dummy inhaler from a training pack and assess her inhaler technique.
  - She fails miserably.
- Explain that one of the ways you can improve control of asthma is by improving inhaler technique.
- Demonstrate the correct inhaler technique:
  - First stand up and take a few deep breaths in and out.
  - Then take three deep breaths in and out, and on the third inspiration press the inhaler, hold your breath and gently release. Repeat this again.
  - Ask Miss Jones to repeat this technique.
  - Again she fails to use the inhaler correctly.
- Explain that most of the drug is currently being released into the air, and tell her that you will make an appointment with the practice nurse for inhaler training.
- Suggest the use of a spacer device and demonstrate one to her.
  - Miss Jones is not too keen on this idea.

- Tell her about the variety of other drugs on offer, such as Seretide, a combination of Becotide and a long-acting β_2-agonist, or another long-acting β_2-agonist such as salmeterol. You can explain that this is a type of blue inhaler which works for longer.
- Explain that, failing this, a short course of steroids may be used in an acute attack. Tell the patient that she needs to be aware of the signs of acute asthma because it is life-threatening, she needs hospitalisation and she may need artificial ventilation.
- Explain that steroids will only be used in an acute setting, and that if she wants to avoid them then her asthma needs to be under much better control. Tell her that weight gain is one of the many possible side-effects, but that the side-effects vary from person to person.
- Other side-effects include skin thinning, easy bruising, development of osteoporosis and diabetes.
- Tell the patient that steroids are only given for short periods and will be withdrawn slowly with gradual dose reduction.

Additional support and lifestyle issues

- Give her a few lifestyle management tips on diet, i.e. recommend swimming.
- Give the patient a prescription for a peak flow meter and explain that she must take a reading every day and record it. She must bring the record of the readings to every appointment.
- Refer the patient to the hospital for spirometry and lung function tests, and explain that if her asthma remains poorly controlled you will have to send her to see a lung specialist at the hospital.
- Provide the patient with additional literature about asthma, local support groups and website addresses.

Closure

- Arrange to see Miss Jones again in a few weeks to check on her control, and enquire whether she has any other problems or questions before she leaves.
- Thank the patient.

Additional notes on childhood asthma

Controlling childhood asthma is similar. However,

- more emphasis is needed on inhaler technique and the use of spacers
- many children suffer from poor compliance
- it is best to use short-acting β_2-agonists and inhaled corticosteroids
- additional therapy includes:
  - long-acting β_2-agonists (e.g. salmeterol)
  - slow-release tablets
  - leukotriene-receptor antagonists (e.g. montelukast).

124 Managing hypertension

Scenario

You are a student in general practice, and are asked to see Mr Obewi, a 56-year-old man who has been seen by the practice nurse and appears to have had elevated blood pressure on his previous three visits, despite being treated with anti-hypertensive drugs. He is of African descent and has been on a calcium-channel antagonist for the past 2 years.

Preparation before consultation

- Obtain the patient's notes and familiarise yourself with his past medical history.

Introduction

- Introduce yourself and establish a rapport.
- Explain that the practice nurse has asked you to see him.
- Ask him if he is aware of why.

Consultation

- Explain that on his previous three visits to the surgery his blood pressure has appeared to be slightly elevated.
- Ask the patient if he has any idea why this might be.
- Ask him whether there are any stresses or strains at home or if he has been at work.
- Question Mr Obewi further about his life at home, diet, exercise and work.

Management

- Ascertain whether he has been compliant and has been taking his medication.
- Ask if there are times when he has forgotten to take his medication or run out of pills (the date of a patient's latest prescription will be on record).
- Ask the patient to describe in his own words which medication he takes, when he takes it and how.
- Ascertain whether the patient is aware of the possible consequences of not taking his prescribed medication.

Complications

- Explain that uncontrolled hypertension can lead to problems with:
  - eye sight
  - kidneys
  - heart
  - lungs.
- Explain that it can increase the risk of stroke.
- Explain that it can cause headaches.

Monitoring

- Ask the patient whether he checks his own blood pressure.
- Advise him on the range of blood pressure monitors available, and recommend one for him to use.
- Tell the patient that blood pressure varies during the day, and that the best time to take his medication would be first thing in the morning.
- Ask him if he has any family history of blood pressure, strokes, loss of vision, eyesight problems or kidney problems. You need to be aware that some patients of Afro-Caribbean descent are genetically pre-disposed to elevated blood pressure.

Lifestyle issues

- Ask the patient about his occupation.
- Ask him about diet and exercise, and encourage him to lose weight.
- Encourage him to undertake cardiovascular aerobic exercise three times a week, and to ensure that his diet contains at least 5 portions of fruit and vegetables a day.

- Recommend stress-reducing exercises (e.g. yoga).
- Ask him about smoking and alcohol consumption, and give smoking cessation and alcohol reduction advice.
- Advise the patient that you may need to increase the dose of his current medication or change his medication if his blood pressure remains high.
- Tell him that you would like to send him for some tests (e.g. blood tests, echocardiogram).
- Review the Hypertension Society guidelines for blood pressure management (A+B or C+D). Note that beta-blockers have been removed.

Closure

- Warn the patient that if his blood pressure remains high you may need to refer him to a specialist at the hospital.
- Give the patient a leaflet (e.g. *Blood Pressure* published by the British Heart Foundation) and the website addresses of self-help groups and the British Hypertension Society.
- If the patient was elderly, you might suggest a dosette box to aid compliance.
- Remind him that if he suffers any dizziness, faintness, paralysis, loss of consciousness or slurred speech he must seek medical attention immediately.
- Reaffirm the salient points from the consultation.
- Confirm that the patient has understood everything that has been discussed.
- Make a follow-up appointment for the patient.
- Thank the patient and remind him to get in touch if he has any questions or problems.

125 Managing high cholesterol

Scenario

You are a doctor in general practice and you have been asked to speak to Mr Williams, a 55-year-old man who has just been given the results of his serum cholesterol and triglyceride levels. Please speak to him about his test results and give him appropriate advice.

Preparation before consultation

- Obtain the patient's notes and familiarise yourself with his past medical history.
- Of particular note are any coexisting medical conditions, his weight and any family history of diabetes, hypercholesterolaemia or ischaemic heart disease.
- Look for references to his smoking habits, alcohol intake, occupation, and family and social situation.

Introduction

- Introduce yourself.
- Explain that you have been asked to talk to him about his recent blood test results and in particular his cholesterol level results.
- Ask him if he understands what the blood tests were for, and check his understanding of their significance.
- Inform the patient of his results.
  - The results for his serum cholesterol and triglycerides are elevated.
- Discuss the results with the patient, comparing them with his previous blood results.

Management

- Explain to the patient that ideally his cholesterol level should be below 5 mmol/l.
- Explain what cholesterol is and that when its levels are elevated it can increase the risk of:
  - ischaemic heart disease
  - myocardial infarction
  - pancreatitis
  - strokes and aneurysms.
- Explain that cholesterol levels can be reduced by addressing the following risk factors:
  - smoking (needs to stop) and alcohol consumption (needs to be reduced)
  - dietary fat intake (needs to be reduced)
  - lack of exercise (regular exercise should be started).

Lifestyle issues

- Increase exercise.
- Give dietary advice about reducing saturated fat intake and increasing intake of polyunsaturated fats.
- Address the need for high-impact aerobic exercise of at least 20 minutes' duration, three times a day.

Aim of treatment

- Explain that the therapy for cholesterol involves the use of drugs such as statins, fibrates and nicotinic acid derivatives.
- Most commonly used are statins (e.g. atorvastatin, simvastatin), which act by inhibiting the production of cholesterol by the liver. Common side-effects include muscle weakness.
- Tell the patient that you would like to monitor his cholesterol levels, but he must address his risk factors.

Closure

- Ask the patient whether he has any questions or concerns.
- Reaffirm the salient points of the consultation.
- Finish by arranging a follow-up appointment, and tell the patient to feel free to come back in the mean time if he has any questions.

126 Managing warfarin

Expected knowledge

- What warfarin is
- How it works
- Indications for its use
- Side-effects and complications
- How to prescribe warfarin
- How to monitor warfarin levels

Warfarin

Warfarin is an anticoagulant (blood-thinning agent) which belongs to the coumarin family of drugs. It prevents blood clot formation by inhibiting vitamin-K-dependent clotting factors, namely factors II, VII, IX and X. Other drugs to be aware of include clopidogrel, heparin, streptokinase and tissue plasminogen activator (tPA). These drugs have a different mode of action to warfarin.

Explaining warfarin

- Introduce yourself to the patient and establish a rapport.
    - Tell them your name and who you are.
    - *Hello, my name is John Smith and I'm a final year medical student.*
- Signpost what you would like to discuss and assess the patient's understanding of his condition.
    - *I would like to talk to you about a medication called warfarin that we have started. Do you know what it is for or why we have started it?*
- Explain the need to be on warfarin as described below.

Scenario 1

Pulmonary embolism and deep vein thrombosis prophylaxis

Explain the need for anticoagulation to a patient who has had a pulmonary embolism.

- You have a clot on your lungs, which is why the doctors have started you on a drug called warfarin. This will help to thin your blood and dissolve the clot, as well as preventing any new clots from forming.
- It is the clot on your lungs which has caused the sudden chest pain and shortness of breath that you have been experiencing, and it would also explain the blood that you've coughed up.
- You will need to be on warfarin for life.

Scenario 2

Atrial fibrillation

Explain the need for warfarin therapy to a patient who has just been diagnosed with atrial fibrillation, and who may require warfarin for up to

3 months prior to attempting DC cardioversion to get the heart back into sinus rhythm.

- Your heart is not beating properly, and as a result blood is being pooled in the heart, and you are at risk of blood clots forming in the heart.
- These clots, once formed, can travel to different parts of the body – for example, to the brain where they can cause a stroke and to the legs where they can disrupt the blood supply and cause pain.
- They may even get stuck in the blood vessels that supply the kidney, and cause kidney failure. We have started you on warfarin to prevent these clots from forming in the first place.

Indications for using warfarin

- Prophylaxis for deep vein thrombosis (DVT).
- Treatment for DVT and pulmonary embolism.
- Prophylaxis for prosthetic heart valves.
- Atrial fibrillation.
- Anti-arrhythmia therapy.

About the drug

- You will need to take warfarin, which comes in 1 mg, 3 mg and 5 mg tablets, on a daily basis.
- The dose or amount of warfarin that you need to take will depend on how thin your blood is, and this is assessed by a blood test which measures your INR (international standardised ratio). The higher the INR is, the thinner your blood is and therefore the less likely it is to clot.
- The INR value that we are aiming for varies for each patient, and is dependent on the indication for warfarin. In patients with atrial fibrillation and pulmonary embolism an INR between 2 and 3 is needed. Patients with prosthetic heart values will require INR values of between 3 and 4.
- Warfarin doses will be adjusted according to your INR value.
- While you are in hospital your doctor will advise you of the dose of warfarin you have to take, and also how much warfarin you will have to take once you are at home and until your next blood test.

- When you are being discharged from hospital you will be given a standard yellow warfarin therapy book. You should keep this with you at all times and check that your name, address and other details are correct. Please read through the book, as it gives you vital information such as the dos and don'ts of warfarin therapy.
- Once you are at home, you will need to attend a warfarin clinic on a regular basis to have a blood test to measure your INR. The clinic will then advise you, based on the test result, what dose of warfarin to take.
- You must keep regular appointments with the warfarin clinic at the hospital and report any abnormal bleeding.

Additional advice for patients

- You need to know your warfarin dose and wear a Medi-alert bracelet at all times.
- As a warfarin patient you will be advised not to take any non-steroidal anti-inflammatory drugs (NSAIDs), such as aspirin, ibuprofen and sodium diclofenac.
- You must inform your family practitioner/general practitioner that you are taking warfarin. In addition, you must inform your dentist, as they will need to take precautions while treating you.
- Warfarin is not recommended in pregnancy.
- In women the menstrual bleed may be heavier than usual.
- Warfarin should not be taken with alcohol.
- Warfarin should be stopped prior to any form of surgery, due to the risk of bleeding. It must also be stopped before pacemaker insertion.

127 Managing obesity and measuring BMI

Scenario

You are a student on placement in general practice. Mr Jones, a 35-year-old man, would like his body mass index (BMI) measured. Comment on the significance of the measurement.

Introduction

- Introduce yourself and develop a rapport with the patient.
- Ask Mr Jones if he knows why he is here, and tell him you would like to measure his BMI.

- Explain that the measurement will tell you whether he is the correct weight for his height.

Measuring BMI

- Ask the patient to remove his coat, empty his pockets and remove his shoes and socks. Then stand him with his legs apart and heels to the edge of the upright ruler. Measure the patient's height by lowering the slider to the top of the head.
- Take the measurement to the nearest centimetre. Record this measurement.
- Then ask the patient to stand on the weighing scale, and obtain the weight in kilograms.
- Calculate the patient's BMI by using the following formula: BMI = weight (kg)/height squared (m^2).

BMI defined:

- BMI < 17: anorexic
- BMI 18–20: low normal
- BMI 20–25: normal
- BMI 25–30: overweight (Grade 1)
- BMI 30–40: obese (Grade 2)
- BMI > 40: morbidly obese (Grade 3).

Lifestyle issues

- You will need to encourage:
  - weight reduction
  - exercise
  - a reduction in sugar and fat intake
  - high-fibre diet
  - cutting down or stopping smoking
  - reducing or stopping alcohol consumption
  - including 5 portions of fruit/vegetables a day in the diet
  - an overall balanced diet
  - increased aerobic exercise.
- Explain the need to expend more calories than are consumed.
- Explain that the risk of heart disease is proportional to abdominal circumference.
- Explain the need for overall weight reduction.
- Explain that there are drugs that can be used in the very overweight, with medical support.

Support

- Provide the patient with information leaflets.
- Encourage him to use the local gym.
- Give details of local support groups.

Closure

- Advise the need for referral to a dietitian.
- Check that the patient understands the significance of having an increased BMI.
- Tell him that you would like to run a few blood tests for thyroid function, urea and electrolytes, fasting cholesterol and blood glucose and a full blood count.
- Repeat the salient points from the consultation and confirm that the patient has understood them.
- Make a long-term follow-up appointment to check on progress.
- Let Mr Jones know that he will need regular appointments with the practice nurse to monitor his weight and overall health.
- Thank the patient.

128 Explaining antipsychotic therapy

Scenario

You are a doctor in family medicine, and you are asked to see Mr Potter, a 19-year-old university student. He has been brought in by his mother, who tells you that he is behaving rather 'oddly.'

Preparation for consultation

- Obtain the patient's notes and familiarise yourself with his past medical history.
  - You find that he has not had an episode like this before.
  - Other than a few viral infections as a child, his medical records are unremarkable.

Introduction and consultation

- Introduce yourself to Mr Potter and his mother, and establish a rapport.

- Ask Mr Potter what has brought him into the surgery today.
  - The patient says that there is 'an alien invasion' and that he is going to destroy the whole place and its inhabitants. He then falls silent.
- Ask the patient's mother what changes in behaviour she has noticed in her son.
  - She tells you that sometimes he says there are voices telling him to kill people.
  - She says that it all began after he started university the previous year.
  - She believes that he got into 'the wrong crowd' and has been taking drugs.
- Mr Potter is unable to communicate coherently at this time and to confirm or deny possible drug use.
- Observe the patient, and ask him what he is thinking right now.
  - Mr Potter tells you that there are spiders crawling on the carpet.
  - He then tells you to shut up because he is hearing voices talking about him.
- Ask the patient if the voices are talking directly at him or about him.
  - He says that the voices are talking about him.
- Question the mother about the patient's childhood and his development stages.
- Ask Mr Potter if he knows where he is, and carry out a Mini Mental State Examination (MMSE).
  - The patient is unable to complete the MMSE.
  - He appears to be elated.

Screening for other psychiatric disease

- Ask the patient if he feels life is worth living and if he has ever thought about or tried killing himself (suicidal ideation).
  - Mr Potter says he had never previously done so, but since he's been hearing these voices he has thought about suicide.
- All of Mr Potter's symptoms suggest that he has an acute psychotic disorder, and it would be advisable to have him admitted as he is a danger to himself and those around him.

Management

Immediate

- Exclude or treat any organic pathology by performing blood tests (i.e. drug and alcohol levels, white cell count, C-reactive protein, glucose, liver function tests), urinary drug screen and an ECG.
- Remove predisposing, precipitating or maintaining factors.
- Assess the risks with or without:
  - hospital admission
  - referral to a psychiatrist or psychiatric liaison nurse
  - medical treatment (i.e. antipsychotic medication).

Long term

- Identify and modify risk factors.
- Review social support (i.e. finance, housing and employment).
- Ensure drug compliance.

Background information on antipsychotic therapy

- Seek specialist advice.
- A delay in starting therapy can render patients dangerous.
- Start antipsychotic therapy before admission.
- First-line antipsychotics include:
  - amisulphide
  - olanzapine
  - risperidone.
- First-line treatments should be commenced at the lowest recommended dose to reduce extrapyramidal side-effects (e.g. acute dystonia, parkinsonism, akathisia, tardive dyskinesia).
- If compliance is poor, consider the use of depot injections.
- Advise the patient of the DVLA (or equivalent driving/licensing authority) restrictions while taking antipsychotics.

Closure

- Summarise the key points of the consultation.
- Address any questions and concerns that the patient and his mother may have.
- Ensure that the patient is in a place of safety during this acute episode.
- Arrange a follow-up appointment.

- Confirm that the patient has understood everything you have discussed.
- Thank the patient.

129 Managing depression

Scenario

You are a medical student in general practice. Miss Lambert, a 23-year-old mother of three, would like to talk to you about her low mood.

Preparation before consultation

- Familiarise yourself with the patient's notes. Including her past medical history, medication (including recreational drug use) and compliance, and social history (i.e. employment, social network, life stressors, dependents).
  - You see that she had her first child at the age of 16 years and has since had two more children, all by different fathers.
  - She lives in a council flat, is unemployed and lives on benefits.
  - In the past she had a problem with alcohol and was a known heroin addict. She has since given up alcohol and is taking methadone for heroin rehabilitation.

Introduction

- Introduce yourself to the patient and establish a rapport.
- Ask Miss Lambert what has brought her to the surgery today.
  - She tells you that she is feeling sad, and starts to cry.
  - She tells you that she has just broken up with her boyfriend after having an abortion last week.
  - She has no friends or family to turn to.
- Identify the patient's key concerns. Be empathic and encourage questions.
- Take a detailed history (screen for depression).
- Offer to examine the patient.

DSM-IV criteria for diagnosing a major depressive disorder

One of the following must be present for > 2 weeks:

- Depressed mood, or anhedonia.

Plus five of the symptoms listed below:

- Feelings of overwhelming sadness and/or fear, or the inability to feel emotion.
- Lack of interest in daily activities.
- A change in appetite with significant weight gain or loss.
- Disturbed sleep patterns, i.e. insomnia or hypersomnia.
- Psychomotor agitation or retardation.
- Mental or physical fatigue.
- Guilt, nervousness, helplessness, hopelessness, worthlessness, iso-lation/loneliness or anxiety.
- Lack of concentration.
- Recurrent suicidal ideation.
- Feeling of abandonment.

Management

- Advise the patient that she has 'clinical depression' and that support is available.
- Explain that there are a number of antidepressants available.
  - Selective serotonin release inhibitors (SSRIs), i.e. citalopram.
    (i) Drug of choice where there is a risk of overdose.
    (ii) Side-effects: anxiety, agitation and stomach upsets, i.e. nausea and vomiting.
  - Tricyclic antidepressant drugs.
    (i) Side-effects: drowsiness, dry mouth, blurred vision, urinary retention, constipation and cardiac toxicity.
  - Monoamine oxidase (MAO) inhibitors.
    (i) Not to be used in combination with other therapies.
- Commence Miss Lambert on a suitable medication, i.e. citalopram.
- Advise the patient of the possible side-effects and to seek medical advice should they occur.
- Advise the patient that the beneficial effects will not be seen immedi-ately but will take approximately six weeks.
- Management may also include:
  - referral to a counsellor or psychiatrist
  - hospital/day unit admission

- psychotherapy
- electro-convulsive therapy (ECT)
- exercise
- social support
- social services, i.e. issues surrounding child protection.

Closure

- Summarise the key points of the consultation.
- Address any questions and concerns.
- Provide information leaflets on depression and details of support groups.
- Arrange a follow-up appointment.
- Advise the patient that should their symptoms deteriorate or they experience side-effects to the medication, they must seek immediate medical attention.
- Confirm that the patient has understood everything you have discussed.
- Thank the patient.

130 Discussing contraception

Scenario

You are a doctor in general practice. Miss Marsh, a 16-year-old girl, has just started dating a boy who is 2 years older than her, and would like to start a sexual relationship with him. She has come to see you for advice about contraception. Please discuss this with her and give her appropriate advice.

Preparation before consultation

- Familiarise yourself with the patient's notes.

Introduction

- Introduce yourself to the patient and establish a rapport.
- Ask Miss Marsh what has brought her to the surgery.
  - She explains to you that she has met a boy and has started to have a relationship with him, and would like some advice about contraception.

- Take a detailed history. Include hypertension, deep vein thrombosis, sexual history and medication.
- Offer to examine the patient, including blood pressure measurement.
- Advise that this is a major step to take in a relationship, and ascertain whether she has thought about it, is fully informed and aware of the possible consequences.
- Explain that there are a number of different contraceptives available.

Oestrogen-progesterone combined oral contraceptive

- You take oral contraceptive pills for 21 days, and stop on day 22.
- Bleed is experienced during seven-day 'break period'.
- Side-effects include nausea, vomiting, headache, breast tenderness, fluid retention, weight gain and risk of developing blood clots.
- It can interact with medication to reduce efficacy, i.e. antibiotics.

Progesterone-only pill

- Taken continuously, i.e. for 28 days.
- Menses is experienced in the fourth week.
- This is a weak form of contraception, and additional protection may be required.

Depot contraceptives

- Progesterone implant.
- Placed subcutaneously, i.e. in the arm.
- It is renewed every 3 months.
- Risk of amenorrhoea.

Condoms

- A device made out of latex or polyurethane and is used during sexual intercourse.
- It is placed on a man's erect penis and physically blocks the ejaculated semen from entering the body of a sexual partner.
- It is used to prevent pregnancy and the transmission of sexually transmitted diseases.

Additional information

- Mutually agree and prescribe the most appropriate contraceptive.
- If the OCP is the contraceptive of choice, advise:
  - once contraception is stopped it may take months for menstruation to return to normal
  - a blood test is required to check liver function
  - regular blood pressure checks are required
  - discontinue four weeks prior to major elective surgery due to the risk of DVT/PE
  - stop the OCP if there is development of sudden chest pain, shortness of breath, calf pain or leg swelling.

Closure

- Summarise the key points of the consultation.
- Address any questions and concerns.
- Provide information leaflets on contraception.
- Arrange a follow-up appointment to check blood pressure.
- Confirm that the patient has understood everything you have discussed.
- Thank the patient.

131 Managing a patient with acne

Scenario

You are a doctor in family medicine. Miss Gurney, a 16-year-old girl, would like to speak to you about her skin problem. The GP prescribed coal tar soap on a previous occasion, which has proved to be rather smelly and she has since stopped using it. Her skin problem is now beginning to worry her and is interfering with her life.

Preparation before consultation

- Obtain the patient's notes and familiarise yourself with her condition and her medical history.

Introduction and consultation

- Introduce yourself to the patient and establish a rapport.
- Ask her what has brought her to the surgery today.

- Ascertain what her problems and concerns are.
  - She tells you that she has 'awful' spots on her face, chest and back.
  - Her skin is always greasy and there is white pus coming out of the spots that is worrying her and has caused her stress both at school and at home.
  - She has no friends, and other schoolchildren often tease her because of her appearance.
  - Finally she tells you that the coal tar soap is very smelly and did not help.
- You must listen to her carefully and be sure that she has said everything she wanted to tell you before offering your advice.
  - She then adds that she is eager to start the oral contraceptive pill, as a friend at school had the same problem until she started taking the pill.

Management

- Empathise with the patient.
- With regard to treatment options, tell her that there are a few more possibilities in addition to coal tar soap and the pill.
- Ask her whether she is in a sexual relationship or has a boyfriend.
- If the answer is no, tell her that you would rather start her on antibiotics, e.g. oxytetracyclines.
- Advise her that if the antibiotics do not work you will consider giving her an oral contraceptive pill, known commercially as Dianette.
- Explain that if this treatment does not work, you will refer her to the hospital to see a dermatologist for a treatment known as Roaccutane.
- You must emphasise that this is a trial-and-error process and that it may take some time to find the most effective treatment for her.
- Be aware that Roaccutane is teratogenic and that Dianette alone should not be considered sufficient contraceptive protection.

Complications

- Blood clots.
- Weight gain.

Lifestyle issues

- Advise the patient to reduce her confectionery intake and to keep to a low-fat diet.
- Weight reduction is often helpful.
- Regular face washing with non-perfumed soap can also help.
- The use of oil-free make-up and foundation is another possibility.

Closure

- Ask the patient whether she understands everything you have discussed.
- Explain that you would like to try her on antibiotics first.
- Make an appointment to see her again in 10 days to assess whether there has been any improvement or if another treatment should be tried.
- Give her an information leaflet on acne management.
- Ask her whether there are any other issues she would like to discuss.
- Thank the patient.

132 Giving sun protection advice

Scenario

You are a doctor in family medicine and Mr Lucas comes to see you. He has a large red patch across his back and shoulders which he says is painful to the touch.

Introduction and consultation

- Introduce yourself to the patient and establish a rapport.
- Ask the patient what has brought him to see you today.
  - He explains that he returned the previous day from a week's holiday in the south of France, and that while he was out there he noticed that his skin was burning. He had applied plenty of sunscreen.
- Take a brief history, concentrating on the following:
  - the amount of time spent in the sun
  - whether he used any sunscreen and, if so, what sun protection factor it contained
  - which areas of his body were exposed.
- Mr Lucas says that he was sunbathing.
- Explain that he has sunburn.

Management and treatment

- Explain that for now the patient should use calamine lotion, but that if the skin blisters and there are any signs of infection, he may need to be prescribed some antibiotic cream to apply to the affected areas.

Advice

- Offer the patient sun protection advice.
- Advise him to wear loose white clothing, a hat, sunglasses, etc. during the summer months.
- Tell him to avoid exposure to the sun between midday and 4pm, when the sun is at its height.
- Be aware that even during winter people are still vulnerable (e.g. skiers).
- Inform the patient of the need to use sun protection (i.e. sunscreen with a high sun protection factor).
- Ask about any occupation-related sun exposure (e.g. he may be a holiday representative or a lorry driver).
- Advise him to avoid sun beds and not to work in the sun.
- Advise him of the risks of sun damage and the fact that it can lead to the development of skin cancers. Emphasise the importance of regular mole checks.
- Give him some leaflets about sun protection and the risks of sun damage.

Closure

- Ask the patient whether he has any questions.
- Check his understanding of everything you have discussed.
- Tell him to return in a few days after applying calamine lotion if the skin has not settled.
- Thank the patient.

Discharging patients

Discharge almost universally occurs in a hospital setting. It is of paramount importance that you ensure that the patient feels well enough to return home. It is equally important to ascertain their ability to cope with their current living situation, and that they are aware of any changes in medication or treatment that have occurred since they were last at home. Try to advise lifestyle changes that may be helpful to the patient, and warn of any foreseeable impact that their recent hospitalisation may have on their lifestyle. Finally, when concluding the consultation, make sure that you have addressed the patient's **ICE** during the consultation:

- Ideas
- Concerns
- Expectations.

133 Discharging a post-MI patient

Scenario

You are a doctor on a busy cardiology firm. Mr Simons, a 56-year-old man, is about to go home following a non-ST-elevation myocardial infarction (NSTEMI). Before he leaves he would like to ask you a few questions about his recent illness and whether there are any precautions that he must now take, especially with regard to his new relationship with a woman 20 years his junior.

Preparation before consultation

- Review the patient's notes, paying particular attention to how long ago he had the NSTEMI and whether he has had any previous episodes.
- Take a look at his prescription chart and TTA to see what drugs he is going home with.

Introduction and consultation

- Introduce yourself and establish a rapport.
- Explain that you understand the patient is returning home today, and ask him how he feels about this and whether he feels well enough to go home.
- Ask him if he has any dizziness or chest pain at the moment.
- Ask whether he has made arrangements for someone to pick him up from the hospital.
- Inform the patient that a follow-up appointment has been made with the consultant to see him in the outpatient clinic in 3 months' time.
- Warn him that the DVLA has issued a statement that anyone who has had a myocardial infarction is not to drive for 3 months.
- Tell him that he will need an echocardiogram and treadmill test, which we will organise as an outpatient, in order to ascertain the strength and function of his heart.

Social aspects

- Ask the patient about his employment situation.
- Tell him that you are issuing him with a certificate of illness for the length of his stay in hospital and up to 6 weeks thereafter, but following this period he will need to obtain one from his GP.
- Question the patient about his living situation.
  - Does he live in a flat or a house?
  - How many stairs are there?
  - If he lives in a flat, is there a reliable, working lift?
  - Who does he live with?
- At this stage he says that he is living with his girlfriend and is worried about his sexual relationship with her, as he is aware that sexual activity will put a strain on his heart.
- You need to address this issue with tact and professionalism.
- Explain that his MI does not mean he will not be able to have a sexual relationship but that, for the time being at least, he will need to take it easy.

Lifestyle issues

- Discuss the need to optimise his risk factors for ischaemic heart disease.
- Give advice on smoking cessation and reducing alcohol consumption.

- Advise the patient to take regular exercise.
- Give him dietary advice:
  - reduce intake of saturated fats
  - increase intake of polyunsaturated fats.

Management

Discuss and explain the new drugs he has been prescribed:

- statin – to reduce cholesterol
- ACE inhibitor (e.g. ramipril/enalapril) – to increase the strength of the heart muscle and decrease blood pressure
- aspirin – to thin the blood
- clopidogrel – to thin the blood to prevent clot formation
- beta-blocker (e.g. atenolol) – to reduce the contractility of the heart and thereby reduce the workload
- glyceryl trinitrate spray – to be sprayed under the tongue when the patient feels chest pain or tightness
- paracetamol – for general pain relief.

Additional information

- Warn the patient that his blood pressure will need to be monitored, as it is a major risk factor for MI.
- Remind him that he must seek medical attention immediately if he experiences persistent chest pain or tightness and pain radiating to the jaw or left arm.
- Ask him whether he has any questions.

Support

- Give him an information leaflet, or booklets from the British Heart Foundation.
- Give him the contact details of the local heart attack support group.
- Give him the contact details of the DVLA (or equivalent driving authority), and remind him that if he drives against regulations he will be putting not only his own life at risk but also the lives of members of the public.
- Ensure that a comprehensive discharge plan is in place.

Closure

- Arrange the patient's outpatient appointments and tests.
- Tell him that a full explanatory letter will be sent to his GP to ensure continuity of care.
- Wish him well and say goodbye.

134 Discharging a patient with COPD on steroids and oxygen therapy

Scenario

You are a doctor on a respiratory firm. Mr Andrews, a 68-year-old man with chronic obstructive pulmonary disease (COPD), was admitted with acute exacerbation of his COPD and is about to be discharged with home oxygen. He has also been given a prescription for treatment with oral steroids. Discuss his condition with him before he leaves.

Preparation

- Obtain the patient's notes and familiarise yourself with his past medical history.
  - He was assessed for home oxygen and the domiciliary team are to install it in a few days' time. In the mean time he has a portable oxygen cylinder.
  - The occupational therapist's written notes about him state that he is independent and has no problems with washing and dressing.
  - His drug chart shows that he will be taking prednisolone for a few weeks, and also a course of antibiotics.
- Speak to the nurse and the physiotherapist who are looking after him to find out about his progress and mobility.
  - His chest infection is clearing up and his mobility has improved.

Introduction

- Introduce yourself to the patient and establish a rapport.
- Ask him if he is feeling well enough to go home.
  - He tells you that he cannot wait to get home.
- Explain that now he is going to have oxygen at home, no one should smoke in the house as it is a fire risk.
  - He assures you that he has stopped smoking.

- Also tell him that he is to wear the oxygen prongs when he is sitting down and relaxing, and that the local branch of the British Oxygen Company (BOC) will deliver oxygen to him when his supply runs out.

Management

- Explain that in addition to his usual inhalers he has been given a short course of steroids. Warn him that he is not allowed to stop this drug himself, but that the GP will gradually taper off the medication.
- In the mean time he should be aware that steroids:
  - cause skin thinning
  - depress the immune system.
- Tell him that he will require the flu vaccine.

Lifestyle

- Explain that he may put on weight, so must take regular exercise and eat sensibly.
- More importantly, the patient must carry a steroid patient card and wear a Medical Alert bracelet to warn medical personnel that he is on steroids.
- Tell him that he must also inform his dentist about his medication before undergoing even minor dental procedures.
- He must stop smoking and avoid secondary smoke.
- Confirm that he has understood everything you have told him, and give him any relevant literature.

Social aspects

- Enquire into his living situation.
  - Who does he live with?
  - Can he cook or does he have meals on wheels?
  - Who does his shopping?
  - Are there any stairs at home? If so, how many?
  - Has his home been modified by the occupational therapists?
- Determine the level of his independence.
  - Can he wash, dress and feed himself?
  - Is he continent?
- Ascertain the level of support he receives from family and friends.

Closure

- Ask the patient whether he has any questions or concerns.
- Tell him that the consultant will see him in clinic in 3 months' time, but that he should visit his GP if he has any problems in the mean time.
- Tell him that a full explanatory letter will be sent to his GP to ensure continuity of care.
- Wish him well and say goodbye.

135 Discharging an elderly patient

Scenario

You are a doctor in elderly care. Mr Alfred, an 85-year-old man, was admitted with confusion and unsteadiness and is due to return home today. Discuss his discharge plans and home situation before letting him leave.

Preparation

- Obtain the patient's notes and familiarise yourself with his past medical history.
- Read the minutes from the multi-disciplinary team meeting concerning Mr Alfred.
- Talk to the nurse and the physiotherapist who have been looking after him about his progress and mobility.
- Review Mr Alfred's drug chart and note down the drugs that he will be taking home with him. You may also wish to look through the *British National Formulary* to familiarise yourself with the possible side-effects that he may experience, especially with any drugs he has been started on since admission.

Introduction and consultation

- Introduce yourself to the patient and establish a rapport.
- Explain that before he is discharged you would like to discuss his care at home.
- Find out about his living situation (e.g. council flat, top floor, living alone, nursing home, presence of ramps, rails, commode, etc.). If appropriate, ask him if he would consider moving somewhere else.

- Assess the patient's cognitive capacity by conducting a Mini Mental State Examination:
  - patient's name
  - month and year
  - location
  - remember address
  - name three objects
  - dates of World Wars I & II
  - name of Prime Minister
  - count down from 20, etc.

Social aspects

- Enquire about the social aspects of the patient's living situation.
  - Who does he live with?
  - Can he cook or does he have meals on wheels?
  - Are there any stairs at home? If so, how many?
  - Has his home been modified by the occupational therapists?
- Determine his level of independence.
  - Can he perform activities of daily living such as shopping and cleaning?
  - Can he wash, dress and feed himself?
  - Is he continent?
- Ascertain the level of support he receives from family/friends.
- Ask whether he has any worries about returning home.
- ICE: Address each.
- Discuss Mr Alfred's medication and determine whether he is compliant. Consider a dosette box prescription.
- Ensure an adequate package of care is in place:
  - GP, occupational therapist, physiotherapists and social services
  - meals on wheels
  - carers.
- Arrange a follow-up appointment in clinic in 3 months' time and inform the patient that a letter will be sent to his GP to ensure continuity of care.

Closure

- Ask the patient whether he has any questions.
- Ask him if he has someone coming to pick him up or whether hospital transport needs to be arranged.
- Wish him well and say goodbye.

136 Discussing nursing home placement with the patient's relatives

Scenario

You are a doctor in elderly care. Mr Lambeth is an 86-year-old man who is hemiplegic, doubly incontinent and partially sighted. He is a widower with two adult children. He was admitted following a fall. Previously he was living at home on his own with a carer. During the fall he sustained a hip fracture and his mobility has deteriorated. At the multi-disciplinary team meeting it was felt that Mr Lambeth would benefit from, and would be an ideal candidate for, a nursing home placement. Please discuss this with members of his family.

Preparation

- Obtain the patient's notes and familiarise yourself with his past medical history.
- Read the minutes from the multi-disciplinary team meeting concerning Mr Lambeth.
- Gather brochures and leaflets about local nursing homes.
- Contact the social services/welfare officer and talk to them about nursing home placement.

Introduction

- Introduce yourself to the patient and establish a rapport.
- Determine which members of the patient's family are present.
- Explain that you have been looking after Mr Lambeth during his stay at the hospital, and that he is recovering well.
- Ask his relatives whether they have any questions.

Explanation

- Explain that Mr Lambeth's overall health has deteriorated and he is now unable to look after himself as he did previously.
- Tell them that since his stroke he is only able to move and functionally use one side of his body, and therefore his mobility has been significantly reduced.
- Tell them that at the multi-disciplinary team meeting it was decided that he would be an ideal candidate for a nursing home placement.
- Ask the family their opinion.

Information and support

- Explain the different options with regard to provision of care:
  - own home with carer
  - respite care – temporary while carer gets leave
  - sheltered accommodation with warden
  - residential home with no nursing facilities
  - nursing home with full-time care with nursing staff.
- Inform the family that a nursing home would be most appropriate to Mr Lambeth's needs, and ask them if they would be happy with this.
- Tell them that Mr Lambeth does not have the capacity to make this decision and that, as his next of kin, it is their responsibility now.
- Give them leaflets and brochures about local nursing homes.
- Tell them that a meeting will be arranged with social services, and that Mr Lambeth will remain on the ward until a placement can be found.
- Give them the name and contact details of the discharge nurse who will be in touch with them about the placement.

Closure

- Ask them to look through the leaflets and to contact you if they have any questions or queries.
- Thank them.

Communication skills

Breaking bad news

This is obviously a sensitive issue that requires empathy and professionalism. You must ensure that you are sufficiently well versed in the subject matter to be ready to answer swiftly and confidently any questions the patient may pose. Be ready to offer support in terms of help groups, leaflets and advice, and you may even consider it appropriate to include the hospital chaplain. Presented below are a number of different scenarios in which you may have to break bad news, but remember that these are only guidelines, and in these situations your professional judgement and ability to empathise are what will really dictate how you deal with these situations.

137 Gym instructor diagnosed with multiple sclerosis (MS)

Scenario

You are a doctor in family medicine. Miss Davis, a 28-year-old gym instructor, has a follow-up appointment with you regarding an MRI scan she has had at the district general hospital. While she was there nerve conduction studies were carried out and cerebrospinal fluid was taken for electrophoresis. She has recently been complaining of blurred vision and tingling in her hands. She is understandably anxious and worried. Her notes unfortunately show that the results have all come back suggesting that she has multiple sclerosis. It is your responsibility to break this news to her in a considerate, professional manner.

Preparation before consultation

- Take some time to familiarise yourself with the patient's notes and to establish clearly in your mind what you are going to say to her.
- Discuss the situation with one of your seniors before you go and see the patient.
- It may be useful to access the local primary care trust's policy on drugs for multiple sclerosis.
- Tell the practice manager or receptionist that you will be in a separate room, and ask them not to disturb you. It may be helpful to ask the practice nurse to be on standby so that she can offer her support.
- Remember that these are only suggestions and you must exercise your better judgement according to the situation.

Introduction

- Introduce yourself to the patient and establish a rapport.
- Ascertain how much she already knows and understands about her illness.
- Take a brief history from her to establish whether the symptoms are still present, have worsened or have regressed.
- Ask her whether she has any questions.

Explanation

- Now begin to acknowledge the gravity of her situation to her gradually.
  - For example, *Your results are back and unfortunately they do not look promising.*
- Again, allow her time to ask any questions before continuing.
- Now tell her that, unfortunately, the results indicate that she has multiple sclerosis.
- Ascertain how much she knows about MS and what experience, if any, she has of the disease.
- Explain to the patient in layman's terms exactly what MS is, remembering to adjust the level at which you pitch the explanation according to the patient's background and understanding. In this case the following would be suitable:
  - *MS is a disease where a varying degree of nerves in the body are affected. Nerves are like wires going from your brain to your muscles. What happens in MS is that the insulating material around the nerves breaks down at specific points and so prevents*

the nerves from working properly. That's why you have been experiencing blurred vision and tingling in your hands. This damage is caused by your own immune system. However, we don't yet fully understand what causes this to occur. This is why we don't yet have a cure for MS. However, we do have drugs available that can control the symptoms of the disease and shorten the length of relapses.

- Empathise with the patient's fears for the future not only with regard to her health but also with regard to her social situation. In this scenario this is particularly pertinent, as the patient is a gym instructor – an occupation which certainly requires her to be physically able. Try to explain how MS may or may not affect her:
  - *With this condition there are various degrees to which people are affected. At one end of the spectrum are the people who go for long periods without any symptoms whatsoever, but on occasion suffer relapses of their symptoms. At the other extreme are people whose MS progresses without periods of remission, resulting in their symptoms becoming steadily worse.*
  - *But it is so early on in your case that we can't yet tell where exactly you fit into this spectrum. We're going to keep an eye on you with regular check-ups to make sure we know exactly what's going on with the MS. With regard to your job, I'm afraid I can make no guarantees. As the MS progresses you will certainly find it difficult to continue as a gym instructor.*
- Be prepared to explain the test results. In this case, for example:
  - *The MRI scan looks at soft tissues and found plaque-like structures along your spinal cord, which are characteristic of MS.*
  - *The tests on your cerebrospinal fluid showed oligoclonal bands in electrophoresis, and delayed nerve conduction was found, all of which are characteristic of MS.*
- Empathy is important, but make sure that you are realistic and do not give the patient any false hope.
- *May I ask whether you have support at home from family or friends?*
  - If the patient answers yes: *That's good because it can really help to talk to about what's going on and what will happen in the future.*
  - If the patient answers no: *I'll help you to get in touch with the MS support group as soon as possible. Social services and occupational therapists will also help out if necessary.*
- Ask the patient whether she has any questions about what she has been told so far.

- Explain that for the time being her GP will be treating her, but she may be referred to a neurologist at the district general hospital when the need arises.
- Explain that there are no set treatment regimes for MS, but that your aim will revolve around symptom control. For example, for an acute flare-up you will be using steroids, but in the later stages you will be using drugs such as immune modulators (e.g. baclofen) for symptom control, and muscle relaxants.

Closure

- Summarise what you have discussed with the patient, highlighting the salient points.
- Confirm that the patient has understood everything you have told her, and take time to clarify any concerns she may raise.
- Give the patient any relevant literature concerning MS, as well as the contact details of the Multiple Sclerosis Society and the primary care trust's MS nurse.
- Tell the patient that you understand she may be feeling overwhelmed by the volume of information she has received, and make another appointment to see her the following week.
- Recommend that if there is someone close to her whom she will be relying on for support, that she brings them to her next appointment.
- Finally, remind the patient that you and her GP are there to help her, and that she can contact you for help and advice at any time.

138 End-stage renal failure requiring dialysis

Scenario

You are a doctor on a medical firm. Mr Anderson, a 35-year-old man, was admitted with acute renal failure. His symptoms have not improved and he is showing signs of end-stage renal failure. You will need to counsel him and break the bad news that he may require dialysis in the next few days.

Preparation before consultation

- Take some time to familiarise yourself with the patient's notes and to establish clearly in your mind what you are going to say to him.
- Turn off your bleep for the duration of the consultation.

Introduction

- Introduce yourself to the patient and establish a rapport.
- Pull the curtains around the bed.
- Ask him how he is feeling.
- Tell him that you have been looking after him on the ward.
- Break the gravity of his situation to him slowly. Tell him that you have some bad news.
- Tell him that his blood tests show that his kidneys are failing.
- In addition, his catheter is not draining very much urine.
- Give him some time for the news to sink in.
- Ask him whether he has any questions.
- Ask him whether you can continue or if there is anyone he wishes to telephone or to have with him.

Explanation

- When he allows you to continue, tell him that it looks as if he may need to have dialysis until his kidney function improves.
- Explain that this will mean his blood will flow from one of the veins in his arm to a dialysis machine and back into his body, and that the machine will effectively do what his kidneys are currently failing to do, and 'clean' his blood.
- Dialysis will last for 3 hours, three times a week.
- Warn the patient that it will be important to restrict his fluid and salt intake.
- Give him a leaflet explaining dialysis in more detail.
- Ask him whether he has any questions.
- Tell him that his kidneys are failing, but that dialysis may give his kidneys sufficient respite to recover.
- He may ask you what will happen if his kidneys fail completely, and you will have to address the fact that transplantation may be necessary. Assure him that at this stage transplantation is not yet a concern.
- Tell him that you would like to biopsy his kidney later this week. Explain that this involves taking a small sample of kidney tissue, and that it will allow you to gain a clearer understanding of what is going on.

Social aspects

- Ascertain how great an impact this will have on the patient's ability to work.
- Tell him that you will arrange suitable transport to and from the hospital for his dialysis.

Support

- Offer the patient information leaflets.
- Offer to call the hospital chaplain.
- Give the patient the contact details of local support groups.

Closure

- Ask the patient whether he has any questions or if he requires you to talk to members of his family.
- Encourage him to think about what has been discussed, and tell him that you will come back to talk to him about it later.
- Thank the patient, and tell him that the consultant will also be available later if he has any more questions.

139 Diagnosis of rheumatoid arthritis

Scenario

You are a medical student in family medicine. Mrs Abrahams, a 38-year-old woman, asks to see someone about her diagnosis of rheumatoid arthritis (RA). The practice manager asks you to have a word with her, as the GP is busy.

Preparation before consultation

- Obtain the patient's notes and familiarise yourself with her past medical history.
- Check when she was diagnosed with RA and the course of her disease to date.
  - You find in her notes that she is a ballet teacher.

Introduction and consultation

- Introduce yourself to the patient and establish a rapport.

- Ask the patient what has brought her to the surgery and what she would like to discuss.
  - She asks you to tell her about RA and the prognosis of the disease, and how long she will be able to continue to work.
- Explain that RA is an immune reaction against the joints of the body, and that common ailments include early-morning stiffness and joint swelling and pain.
- As the disease advances the affected joints may become loose (this is known as subluxation), and eventually require replacement or cause mobility problems.
- Allow time for her to digest this information, and ask her if she understands everything you have said and whether she has any questions.

Support

- Give the patient any pertinent literature to take away and read.
- Give her the contact details of the local support groups.

Management

- Explain that treatment includes painkillers, steroids and special drugs known as disease-modifying anti-rheumatoid arthritis drugs (DMARDS), such as methotrexate.
- Explain that initially you will prescribe painkillers and anti-inflammatory drugs and give steroids for acute episodes and maintenance. In the longer term the patient may progress to the use of DMARDS.
  - She asks whether the disease can be cured.
- Explain that treatment revolves around symptomatic control because there is no known cure. Therefore, as time goes by, her joint function will decrease and she may need stronger drugs. Tell her that there are new drugs that are coming on to the market, but it depends on her reaction to the other drugs.
  - The patient asks about anti-TNF therapy.
- Explain that anti-TNF treatment is only available for patients with advanced disease, so she is not yet eligible.
- Tell her that the GP will manage her for the time being, and that if her symptoms worsen she may be referred to a rheumatologist at the district general hospital.

Closure

- Repeat the salient points of the consultation and confirm that the patient has understood everything you have discussed.
- Ask the patient whether she has any further questions.
- Thank her and say goodbye.

140 Below-knee amputation

Scenario

You are a doctor on a vascular surgery firm. Mrs Cookson, a 67-year-old diabetic woman, has had a failed femoral-popliteal bypass graft and needs to be told that she now requires a below-the-knee amputation. Please convey this information to her and discuss her options.

Preparation before consultation

- Obtain the patient's notes and familiarise yourself with her past medical history.
- Discuss the situation with the firm's registrar.

Introduction and consultation

- Introduce yourself to the patient and establish a rapport.
- Ask her how she is feeling and how she feels the surgery went.
- Tell her that you have some bad news about her leg.

Management

- Tell her that the graft that was put in to try to reperfuse her leg and help to heal her foot ulcer has failed.
  - She asks whether you are planning to try again.
- Tell her that unfortunately that will not be possible, and that her leg will need to be amputated from below the knee.
- At this point the patient will almost certainly be distressed.

Support

- At this stage offer her comfort, give her some tissues and ask her if she would like some time on her own.
  - She asks you to continue.

- Explain that following her amputation she will remain in hospital until the wound has fully healed.

Alternative
donoring
→ blood passing
→ death

Social aspects

- Explain that she will be wheelchair bound initially, but that the majority of patients are suitable candidates for a prosthetic limb and that with the help of physiotherapy and some modifications made to the home, which an occupational therapist will co-ordinate, she will be relatively independent.
- Ask whether there is anyone who could come and support her at this difficult time.
- Ask her whether she lives alone.
- Ask about her living situation (stairs, etc.).
- Tell her that full social, medical and financial support is available.

Closure

- Ask the patient whether she wants you to discuss this with family members.
- Give her relevant leaflets and the contact details of support groups.
- Confirm that she has understood everything you have discussed, and ask her whether she has any questions.
- Tell her that the hospital chaplain is available.
- Tell her that you understand she has had to absorb a lot of information, and that the consultant and his team are available if she requires any support or has any further questions.
- Thank the patient.

141 Breast cancer

Scenario

You are a junior doctor on a general surgery firm. Mrs Cohen, a 46-year-old Jewish woman who was admitted for a lumpectomy, has had her histology results back. Unfortunately the tests came back positive for carcinoma of the breast, and her lymph nodes are also positive for disease. At the multi-disciplinary team meeting that was held jointly with oncology it was decided that it would be best for Mrs Cohen to undergo a mastectomy followed by chemotherapy.

Preparation

- Take some time to familiarise yourself with the patient's notes and to establish clearly in your mind what you are going to say to her.
- Read the minutes from the multi-disciplinary team meeting concerning Mrs Cohen.

Introduction

- Introduce yourself to the patient and establish a rapport.
- Tell her that the test results are back and you have some bad news.
- Tell her that, unfortunately, the tests have shown the lump to be cancerous.
- Ask her if there is anyone she would like to be with her at this time.
  - She asks you to continue.
- Explain that the cancer is malignant and appears to have spread to the lymph nodes, but that it does not appear to have spread elsewhere.
- Explain that her breast will have to be removed.
- Allow time for her to absorb this information.
- Attempt to ascertain whether she has understood everything you have told her. The patient will almost certainly be very upset.
- Give her some tissues, comfort her and tell her that you will be back later to discuss the matter further.
- Make sure that you do not leave her alone. If there are no family/friends present, ask the nurses to keep an eye on her.

Later on you will need to discuss a number of issues, including:

- the appearance of the breast after mastectomy
- breast reconstruction
- how long the operation will take

- discussion with an oncologist
- the use of chemotherapy following the mastectomy
- the effects of chemotherapy
- as the patient is Jewish, you may need to address the genetic component as well, as Ashkenazi Jews are often genetically predisposed to breast cancer and so the disease may run in families. Thus it may be advisable for any immediate female relatives to be screened for breast cancer
- offering the services of the hospital chaplain or Rabbi for religious and spiritual support
- giving the patient pertinent literature and asking for the Macmillan breast cancer nurse to come and see her
- discussion of bras and prostheses that are available to maintain body shape following a mastectomy
- discussion of implants and breast reconstruction.

Conclusion

- Ask the patient whether she has any questions, and address any concerns she may raise.
- Document the conversation in the notes.
- Thank the patient.

142 Malignant melanoma

Scenario

You are a dermatologist. Mrs Holmes, a 30-year-old woman, has come to see you in clinic. She had a mole excised from the side of her face 2 weeks ago. Histology results have shown it to be malignant melanoma. However, as the melanoma was cleared with a margin of 2 mm, there was no lymph node involvement and there were no satellite lesions, she has been given the all clear. It is your responsibility to talk to her, explain her results and discuss her future management.

Preparation

- Take some time to familiarise yourself with the patient's notes and to establish clearly in your mind what you are going to say to her.

Introduction and consultation

- Introduce yourself to the patient and establish a rapport.
- Find out what the patient already knows.
- Take a brief history to establish whether there are any risk factors (e.g. sun exposure, regular holiday/business trips to sunny regions) and any family history of skin cancers or cancerous moles.
- Tell the patient that the whole mole was successfully excised.
  - The patient asks whether it was cancerous. You can either tell her directly that it was, or you can give her a warning shot first. For example, *The test result has come back and it is consistent with melanoma* or *Unfortunately the mole we excised was cancerous.*
- Explain that although the mole was cancerous, and so has the potential to spread, it was caught in time. The mole was excised with a clear margin, and the patient's lymph nodes were also sampled and found to be clear of disease.
- Explain that she will need regular check-ups every 6 months.

Advice

- Offer the patient sun protection advice.
- Advise her to wear loose white clothing, a hat, sunglasses, etc. during the summer months.
- Tell her to avoid exposure to the sun between midday and 4pm when the sun is at its height.
- Be aware that, even during winter, people are still vulnerable (e.g. skiers).
- Inform the patient of the need to use sun protection (e.g. sunscreen with a high sun protection factor).
- Ask about any occupation-related sun exposure (e.g. she may be a holiday representative).
- Advise her to avoid sun beds and to avoid working in the sun.
- Advise her of the importance of melanoma surveillance, and suggest that she asks her partner or family members to look for new moles in areas that are hard to see. Explain that she should look out for moles that:
  - are irregularly shaped
  - have a craggy appearance
  - bleed easily
  - are painful
  - change in colour
  - are ulcerating.

- Tell the patient that if she finds any such moles she must contact you immediately, as you would need to biopsy them as soon as possible.

Support

- Give the patient leaflets about melanoma and sun protection, and advice about dealing with malignant melanoma.
- Give her the contact details of local melanoma support groups and any useful Internet resources.

Closure

- Ask the patient whether she has any more questions.
- Tell her to get in touch if she has any further queries, but otherwise you will see her in 6 months' time.
- Thank the patient.

Additional tips

- Avoid giving survival rates or a prognosis, as you are venturing into the unknown.
- Avoid bombarding the patient with information.
- Patients will often bring someone with them for support, usually their partner, who may have their own questions that you will need to answer. They may even ask questions that the patient has forgotten to ask.
- In advanced tumour cases you will need to offer the help of Macmillan cancer nurses, palliative care teams, local hospice help or hospice-at-home services.

143 Abnormal polyps found on colonoscopy

Scenario

You are a doctor in family medicine. Mr Bryan, a 54-year-old man, comes to see you about the results of his recent colonoscopy. The results have shown that there are suspicious polyps which have been found to be cancerous. Please convey this information to him and explain what is to be done next.

Preparation before consultation

- Obtain the patient's notes and familiarise yourself with his past medical history.
- In particular, check why he was originally referred for a colonoscopy.

Introduction and consultation

- Introduce yourself to the patient and establish a rapport.
- Tell him that the results of his colonoscopy are back. Explain that they suggest the bleeding from his back passage was caused by abnormal growths called polyps, and these polyps have been found to be cancerous.
- Allow time for the news to sink in.
- Confirm that he has understood what you have told him, and answer any questions he may have.
- Tell him that the polyps need to be removed, and this is only possible by removing a part of his bowel.

Management

- Tell the patient that an urgent appointment has been made for him at the hospital with a colorectal surgeon, who will advise him further.
  - He asks you what will happen to him.
- Tell him that part of his bowel will be resected, depending on the extent of the polyps. Usually the two ends of bowel are joined together, but in some cases this may not be possible and he may end up with an opening for his bowel movements through the anterior wall of his abdomen. This opening is known as a stoma (*see* Topic 86).
- Tell him that at this stage you cannot be more specific.
- Offer him a leaflet explaining bowel cancer and its associated surgery.
- Tell him that the local Macmillan nurse will be in touch.
- Offer your support and ask him if there is anyone he would like you to explain this to.
- Tell him that you will see him after his appointment with the colorectal surgeon to discuss his situation.

Closure

- Ask the patient whether he has any further questions.

- Repeat the salient points of the consultation and confirm his understanding of what you have discussed.
- Make a follow-up appointment for the patient.

144 HIV counselling

Scenario

You are a doctor in genitourinary medicine. Mr Wilde, a 46-year-old businessman, comes to see you about his 'little problem.'

Introduction and consultation

- Introduce yourself to the patient and establish a rapport.
- Establish the purpose of the consultation.
    - He tells you that he is HIV positive and does not want anyone to know about this.
- You take a brief history and find out that he frequently visits Thailand on business.
- He is married with children.
- He has recently found himself attracted to men and as a result has had a few homosexual relationships.
- He is a devout Christian and is experiencing strong feelings of conflict about his behaviour.
- Be sympathetic but realistic.
- You must stress how important it is that he tells his wife and his sexual partners, as he is putting their lives at risk.
- Be aware that patients in this situation are often afraid of what their partners and children will think of them.
- Encourage the patient to have HIV counselling.

Explanation

- You must tell the patient that there is a 3-month window between becoming infected and seroconversion.
- Emphasise that all of his sexual partners need to be told.
- Explain that although HIV is the virus that causes AIDS, the fact that a person has HIV does not necessarily mean that they develop AIDS.
- Tell the patient that you will need to monitor certain blood markers (e.g. CD4 and viral load), and start him on antiretroviral drugs.

- Tell the patient that he must use barriers (e.g. condoms) during sexual intercourse to reduce the risk of HIV transmission.
- Female patients who are HIV positive should be advised not to get pregnant, as there is vertical transmission of the virus from the mother to the baby.

Support

- Tell the patient that you would be willing to explain the situation to his wife and any of his sexual partners.
- Give him information leaflets and the contact details of any support groups (e.g. Terrence Higgins Trust in the UK).

Closure

- Tell the patient that you would like to see him again, and make another appointment.
- Ask him if he has any further questions.
- Thank the patient.

Working as a doctor

There is a fine line between being a medical student and working as a doctor. The following topics will help you to develop qualities that you will require throughout your medical career:

- dealing with relatives
- explaining procedures
- conveying information, whether it is about a relative, their management, their treatment, or tests that they are to undergo
- respecting confidentiality issues and not giving out too much information.

145 Mother with a post-operative pulmonary embolism

Scenario

You are a doctor on a surgical ward. Mrs Harris is the daughter of Mrs Davis, a 78-year-old woman who has suffered a pulmonary embolism after surgery to fit a dynamic hip screw following fracture of the neck of the femur a few days previously. Mrs Davis has now been warfarinised and her pulmonary embolism is being treated. Mrs Harris is rather confused and upset, and would like to talk to someone about what has happened.

Preparation

- Before you approach Mrs Harris you must find Mrs Davis' notes and familiarise yourself fully with her case.
- You must inform your seniors that you will be talking to Mrs Harris.
- Under no circumstances must you admit that there has been any fault or that someone is responsible.
- Importantly, Mrs Davies has experienced a complication not uncommon in orthopaedic surgery and it has been managed appropriately.
- Make sure that Mrs Davis is aware of the conversation you are about to have, and that she gives her consent for details to be divulged to her daughter. If she does not, you must be prepared to tell Mrs Harris that you cannot discuss the case fully with her.
- Use a private room away from the other patients.

Introduction and consultation

- Introduce yourself to Mrs Harris and establish a rapport.
- Tell her that you understand that she would like to speak to you about her mother, and allow her to explain what it is she would like to know.
- Avoid using phrases such as 'I understand how you feel', because they are almost always untrue and the relative may feel patronised.
- Say that you are sorry for what has happened.
- Acknowledge that Mrs Harris has every right to be upset.
- Avoid being defensive, as this will only make her angry.
- Try to assure her that her mother is being well cared for and that what has just happened will not happen again.

Explanation and negotiation

- Explain that certain people have a predisposition to clot formation, i.e. deep vein thromboses and pulmonary embolism.
- Explain that Mrs Davis is being carefully monitored and being given drugs to dissolve the clot.
- Assure Mrs Harris that her mother has had the appropriate investigations, i.e. blood tests, chest X-ray, ventilation-perfusion (V/Q) scan and CT scan of her lungs and arteries (CTPA).

Closure

- Mrs Harris will almost certainly want to talk to the consultant, so be ready to arrange a meeting.
- Ask her if she has any further questions.
- Give her a patient leaflet explaining pulmonary embolism and the need for her mother to be on warfarin (*see* Topic 126 for further details).
- Finally, offer the support of the hospital chaplain.
  - At this point Mrs Harris says that she would like to make a formal complaint.
- Tell her that she will need to write to or telephone the complaints department.

Background

- You will have to check your own individual hospital or local trust complaint policy. However, when a complaint is made by patients or relatives, all team members are invited to give their opinion and write a short formal letter about their involvement in the care of the patient.
- Responses and replies are legal documents, and thus most trusts will offer a solution or resolution to stop the relatives taking the complaint further.

146 Discussion with a husband whose wife is to be admitted following a head injury

Scenario

You are a doctor in Accident and Emergency. Mrs Stewart, a 34-year-old woman, fell off a ladder and is currently unconscious with a Glasgow Coma Scale of 7. It is your duty to explain the situation to her husband and to tell him about the next steps in her management.

Preparation

- Obtain the patient's notes and familiarise yourself with her past medical history.
- Look at her observation and drug charts.
- Check her most recent test results.

Introduction

- Introduce yourself to Mr Stewart and establish a rapport.

Explanation

- Explain that as a result of the fall his wife is currently unconscious and intubated.
- Tell him that she is due to have a brain scan to look for any causes or injuries, such as fractures, or bleeds which may be causing her current state.
- Warn Mr Stewart that if his wife deteriorates she may have to be moved to a specialist unit or require surgery.
- State that this is not the case at present.

Support

- Offer him the use of a telephone to contact anyone he wishes to speak to.
- Ask him if he would like the support of the hospital chaplain.

Closure

- Ask Mr Stewart if he has any further questions and whether he understands what you have told him.

- Explain that you will be back to speak to him as soon as you know anything more.
- Tell him that in the mean time he can go and sit with his wife if he wishes.
- Thank him.

147 Discussion of a teenage patient's medical management with a parent

Scenario

You are a doctor in family medicine. Mrs Jacobs would like to talk to you about her 17-year-old daughter, Jessica, who has just come to see you. Mrs Jacobs is demanding information about her daughter, who is your patient.

Introduction and consultation

- Introduce yourself to Mrs Jacobs and establish a rapport.
- Ask her what brings her to the surgery today.
  - She tells you that she would like to know why her daughter came to see you and what was discussed in the consultation.
- Explain to her that:
  - without the consent of her daughter you are not allowed to give out any information
  - you only have the legal right to inform the patient's parents if the patient is less than 16 years of age.
- You may give the mother non-specific information such as:
  - *Your daughter did come to see me but I am not at liberty to divulge any information.*
- Common OSCE scenarios include daughters seeing a doctor for contraceptive advice, or with unexpected pregnancies and seeking termination advice.
- You must tell the mother that as her daughter is over 16 years of age she is legally classed as an adult.
- 'Gillick competence' is a phrase you should be aware of. It is coined from the 1985 case *Gillick vs West Norfolk and Wisbech Area Health Authority*. In this case the House of Lords ruled that:

As a matter of law the parental right to determine whether or not their minor child below the age of 16 will have medical treatment terminates if and when the child achieves sufficient understanding and intelligence to enable him to understand fully what is proposed.

Dealing with difficult patients

When dealing with difficult patients you must draw on your skills of negotiation. Each patient is different, and you must be able to gauge the level at which you need to pitch your explanations of treatment. Some patients, usually older individuals, prefer a paternalistic approach from their doctor, whereas others will want all of the details of their illness and treatment explained. You must be sure not to give in to a patient simply because they are being forceful, but without being confrontational in your approach. This is truly a fine art, and one which you will hone with experience.

148 An American patient who wants an MRI

Scenario

You are a doctor in family medicine. Miss Bush, an American patient, presents with frequent severe headaches and is concerned that she may have a brain tumour. She would like an MRI.

Preparation

- Obtain the patient's notes and familiarise yourself with her past medical history.
    - You discover that she has previously been diagnosed as suffering from migraines by a neurologist and has already been prescribed treatment.

Introduction and consultation

- Introduce yourself to the patient and establish a rapport.
- Ask her what has brought her into the surgery today.
    - She tells you that she has been having severe headaches and is worried that she has a brain tumour.
- Explain that from her notes you understand she suffers from migraines.
    - She is adamant that there is something more serious wrong.

- Take a brief history of the presenting complaint.
  - The patient's history points to migraines.
- You tell her this and ask what she would like you to do.
  - She demands an MRI, saying that if she was in the USA she would have had one by now.
- Explain to her that none of her symptoms point to a brain tumour and that you cannot find anything clinically to justify an MRI.
  - The patient now adds that she fell and hit her head on the floor 2 days ago, and on inspection you find a head laceration to support this.
- Explain that at this stage you will be looking for fractures and not soft tissue matches, so a CT scan would be most suitable, and that a CT scan is similar to an MRI.
  - The patient agrees to this compromise.

Closure

- Make arrangements for the patient to attend the local hospital for a head CT scan following discussion with the on-call neurosurgical team.

149 A woman who wants a mammogram

Scenario

You are a doctor at a district general hospital. Mrs Ellis, a 35-year-old secretary of Jewish descent, comes to see you. Her mother was recently diagnosed with breast cancer and she would like you to arrange a mammogram for her.

Preparation

- Obtain the patient's notes and familiarise yourself with her past medical history.
  - There is a letter in her notes from an oncologist advising the patient that she is at risk of breast cancer.

Introduction and consultation

- Introduce yourself to the patient and establish a rapport.
- Take a breast history from the patient and ask her if she has noticed any lumps or discharge from her nipples.

- Mrs Ellis has recently given birth and has generally tender breasts because she is breastfeeding.
- Obtain her verbal consent and carry out a physical examination.
- Explain that as she is breastfeeding a mammogram is not recommended at present, but you can offer her an ultrasound scan.
- Take time to stress that although her mother has developed breast cancer, this does not mean that she will inevitably develop it as well.
- Suggest that once she has stopped breastfeeding she should return for a formal breast examination.

Closure

- Give the patient a leaflet explaining the early symptoms and signs of breast cancer that she should be alert for.
- Thank Mrs Ellis and advise her that if in the mean time she has any questions she should return for another consultation.

150 A male patient who does not want a colonoscopy/ DRE

Scenario

You are a doctor in general practice. Mr Hibbert presents with bright red blood in his stool. It has been recommended that he should have a colonoscopy. You are asked to obtain his informed consent.

Preparation

- Obtain the patient's notes and familiarise yourself with his past medical history.

Consultation

- Introduce yourself to the patient and establish a rapport.
- Ask the patient how he is feeling, and ascertain whether he is still passing blood in his stool.
- Inform the patient that it has been recommended that he has a colonoscopy.
- Ascertain whether the patient knows what a colonoscopy is.

- The patient knows what it is and tells you that he does not want a tube stuck into his back passage, explaining that he had a digital rectal examination and he felt violated.
  - He adds that his cousin had a colonoscopy and had told him that he felt as if he had been raped.
- Explain to the patient that he would be mildly sedated during the procedure.
  - Mr Hibbert replies that he does not want valium.
- Reassure Mr Hibbert that valium will not be used, and advise him that if he does not have a colonoscopy you will be unable to find the cause of his bleeding.

Preparation and precautions

- Warn the patient that before the colonoscopy he will need to have bowel preparation (see procedure below), and that afterwards he may feel bloated because of the air that has been pumped into his bowel.
- He will also not be allowed to operate any heavy machinery or drive afterwards until the effects of the sedation have worn off.

Closure

- Check whether the patient has any further questions or concerns.
  - The patient tells you that he is scared it may be cancer.
- Tell Mr Hibbert that without the colonoscopy you cannot be certain what the cause of the bleeding is, but that any suspicious growths that are found will be sampled.
- Tell the patient that the results should be available within a few days, and obtain his provisional consent.
- Thank the patient and tell him that he will receive a letter in due course informing him of the date of the procedure.

151 A patient who wants an inhaler, having come on holiday to London

Scenario

You are a doctor in family medicine and are asked to see an unregistered patient who has walked in and asked for an emergency appointment.

Introduction and consultation

- Introduce yourself to the patient and establish a rapport.
- Take a brief history of the presenting complaint.
  - The patient tells you he that he is an asthmatic whose salbutamol inhaler has run out. Since he came to London from Birmingham a few days ago he has started to wheeze.
- On examination you find that he has an expiratory wheeze and a PEFR within normal range for his age and height.
- Give him a prescription for a salbutamol inhaler and recommend that he sees his GP when he returns to Birmingham.
- Ask him if he needs anything else.
- Document in your notes the fact that you have seen an unregistered patient.

Closure

- Ask the patient whether he has any questions.
- Remind him to see his own doctor when he returns home.
- Ask him to come back if he feels his symptoms worsening.

152 A patient who is a frequent attender at Accident and Emergency

Scenario

You are a doctor in Accident and Emergency. Miss Bright, a 29-year-old woman, comes to see you. She says that she feels quite ill.

Introduction and consultation

- Introduce yourself to the patient and establish a rapport.
- Find out why she has come to Accident and Emergency and perform a full history and examination.
  - She tells you about a non-specific, common complaint and the examination is unremarkable.
- Ask her whether she has seen her GP.
  - She says that she has, but that he has dismissed her complaint as unimportant.
  - However, when you check her details you find that she is not registered with a GP.

- Ask the patient again.
  - She tells you that in fact she has not seen her GP for years and has since moved to another town.
- Tell the patient that she must register with a GP, and that the GP should be her first point of call.
- Explain that by coming to Accident and Emergency she is taking up the valuable time of a doctor who could be seeing an emergency.
  - In the mean time you run a few tests and find nothing abnormal.

Closure

- Tell the patient that she must register with a GP.
  - She agrees to this.
- Document this in her notes and discharge her.

153 A heroin addict on methadone who attends the GP practice requesting another prescription, claiming to have lost the previous one

Scenario

You are a doctor in family medicine and are asked to see Mr Doherty, a recovering heroin addict, who has come to the surgery to request a repeat prescription of methadone.

Introduction and consultation

- Obtain the patient's notes and familiarise yourself with his past medical history.
- Find out how long he has been in drug rehabilitation.
- Find out when he received his last prescription for methadone.
- Introduce yourself to the patient and establish a rapport.
- Establish why the patient has come to see you today.
  - He says that he has lost his new prescription for methadone.
- According to the patient's notes his last prescription was issued that morning, and this is not the first time he has lost his prescription.
- Attempt to ascertain why the patient keeps losing his prescription, and call the chemist to check whether the prescription has already been received.
  - On this occasion the prescription has not yet been handed in.

Negotiation

- Emphasise to the patient that this cannot keep happening, and explain the option of daily delivery of his methadone dose by his local pharmacy.
  - The patient agrees to this change.

Closure

- Ask the patient whether he has any questions.
- Write a new prescription to cover the patient until the pharmacy can start delivery, and tell him to make an appointment if he has any more problems.

Cross-cultural communication

You must be aware that a patient's cultural origin may dictate their lifestyle and beliefs and have a substantial effect on their health. This section deals with religious beliefs, sexuality and ethnic variations, and how knowledge of these may help a doctor to treat a patient more efficiently. Where appropriate, additional useful background information has been included.

154 Explaining diabetes management to a Muslim patient during Ramadan

'Scenario

You are a doctor in family medicine and Mr Ishmail, a 40-year-old man, comes to see you. He is a type 2 diabetic with poor glycaemic control who has just been switched to insulin, and he would like to fast for Ramadan. His latest blood glucose reading is 12.0. The practice nurse is concerned and would like you to talk to him about his request to fast for Ramadan.

Preparation

- Obtain his notes and familiarise yourself with his past medical history, paying particular attention to his previous HbA$_{1c}$ results.
- Also look out for coexisting conditions and family history of ischaemic heart disease, diabetes or hypertension.

Introduction and consultation

- Introduce yourself to the patient and establish a rapport.
- Explain that you have been asked by the practice nurse to talk to him about his wish to fast for Ramadan, which is a few months away.
- Ask to see his daily blood glucose measurements.

Explanation

- Explain that he has poorly controlled diabetes and that his blood glucose levels are not within an acceptable range, given that he has been on medication for the past 5 years, which is why he has just been transferred to insulin.
- Tell him that you understand he is a Muslim and must fast as part of his religious duties, and that fasting is one of the five pillars of Islam.
- Explain that you do know, however, that if a Muslim is in ill health they are exempt from fasting.
- Tell him that with his current blood glucose reading it is not advisable to fast.

Fasting regime

- Explain that your understanding is that he must fast from dawn to dusk and then have a fairly large meal, followed by another one just before dawn, but in order to fast during the day his blood glucose levels need to be within acceptable limits.
- Ask him about his current eating habits, what he likes to eat and what a typical day's meals include.
- Ask him how this will change during Ramadan. Explain that if he does wish to fast he must recognise when he is hypoglycaemic, and similarly he must recognise when he is hyperglycaemic after the main meal.

Dietary advice

- Tell the patient that he may need to eat more starchy foods so that he can sustain his glucose levels during the day, and instead of using long-acting insulin he may need to switch to taking short-acting insulin just before his main meal.
- Also tell him that he needs to refrain from eating foods that are high in sugar, such as sweetmeats.

- In addition, he will need to refrain from eating onions, garlic and karela (bitter gourd), which are potent hypoglycaemic agents.

III health

- Emphasise that if the patient is feeling unwell he must immediately seek medical attention, as he may develop diabetic ketoacidosis.
- Warn that similarly, in ill health, his insulin requirements will increase and therefore he will need to monitor his blood glucose levels regularly. However, be aware that some Muslims think the drawing of blood is a sign of ill health, and therefore do not permit it during fasting.
- You will also need to tackle the issue of why his glucose levels are not normal at present, and any compliance problems.

Negotiation and support

- As Ramadan is a few months away, tell him that you would like him to take the insulin doses that he has been prescribed and return in a week with a record of his daily glucose levels for assessment.
- Tackle the issues of weight loss and exercise, and dietary advice must also be given in a leaflet about diabetes and diabetes in Ramadan (NHS leaflets are available).
- Suggest that the patient meets with a dietitian to discuss his dietary regimes.
- Tell him to contact his Imam about Ramadan and diabetes and obtain some additional information.
- Ask him whether he requires any further information, and organise a follow-up appointment.

Closure

- Ask the patient whether he has any questions, and draw the consultation to a close.

Background

- Muslims fast on the ninth month of their lunar calendar as part of Ramadan.
- Muslims fast from sunrise to sunset, and dawn is defined as the time when they can visually differentiate between white and black cloth or thread.

- Ramadan ends when the new moon of the following month is visible in Mecca.
- The fast is usually broken with dates.
- A large meal is then consumed and a smaller meal is consumed just before dawn.
- Those who are sick, menstruating, old or nursing are not required to fast.

Other faiths

- The fasting scenario is not just relevant to Muslims. Those of many other faiths (e.g. Hindus) also fast for many religious festivals.

155 Blood transfusion and the Jehovah's Witness

Scenario

You are a doctor on the medical assessment ward. Mrs Davis, a 72-year-old woman, arrives with a presenting complaint of shortness of breath. She looks pale, and blood tests reveal a haemoglobin level of 7.2. Her breathlessness is worsening and she has a per rectal bleed. She also has a past medical history of non-Hodgkin's lymphoma. You decide that she requires an urgent blood transfusion. However, upon looking at her notes you discover that she is a Jehovah's Witness with a do not resuscitate (DNAR) order in place. You have Mrs Davis infused with gelofusin and Hartman's, and she is stable at present. However, if she does not receive a blood transfusion soon she may die. Discuss the situation with her.

- This is a difficult scenario, regardless of experience.
- Remember that you are not alone.
- Discuss the situation with your colleagues and seniors.

Preparation

- Order in your mind the salient features of this case. There are a number of issues that need to be addressed.
    - Without a transfusion and possibly surgery, the patient may die.
    - Jehovah's Witnesses do not allow blood products to be given.
    - A DNAR and living will are in place. Most Jehovah's Witnesses have a living will or advance directive in place.

Introduction and consultation

- Introduce yourself to the patient and establish a rapport.
- Explain that her shortness of breath is a result of the diminished oxygen-carrying capacity of her blood due to reduced haemoglobin levels, and that the only way to rectify this situation is a blood transfusion.
- Stress that her situation has been made worse by the recent blood loss from her bowels.
- Explain that a surgical review would also be necessary, and that surgery will be needed if the bleeding continues. Tell her that for the time being you can maintain her blood pressure by infusing fluids, but that she may also require blood clotting factors such as platelets.
- Ask her whether she would be willing to accept a transfusion, emphasising that without a transfusion she may die.
  - She refuses.

Closure

- Ask Mrs Davis if there is anyone with whom she would like to discuss her situation, such as friends or family, and offer to contact the hospital chaplain.
- Discuss her DNAR status and living will. Unfortunately you have to accept a patient's wishes unless the patient is under 16 years of age or you feel that they are not medically competent to make an informed decision.
- Discuss the issue with any members of the patient's family who are present, too.
- Seek advice from your seniors, and ensure that the patient is making a completely informed decision.

Background information on Jehovah's Witnesses

- No blood transfusions.
- No blood products.
- Transfusion of the patient's own blood during surgery is allowed.
- Fluids are allowed.
- Drugs are allowed.
- All have a living will in place and therefore DNAR.

156 Lesbian couple encountering prejudice while in hospital

Scenario

You are a doctor on a medical ward, and a lesbian couple are facing discrimination on a female-only ward. The sister has asked you to talk to them.

Preparation

Find the patient's notes and familiarise yourself with her case.

Introduction and consultation

- Introduce yourself to the couple and establish a rapport.
- Invite them to a private room and explain that you have been told that they are having a problem on the ward.
- Ask them what has happened.
  - The patient tells you that when her partner came to visit and they embraced in greeting, the female patient in the next bed became agitated and started verbally abusing them.
  - They ask you for a side room.
- Explain that side rooms are generally reserved for patients who require isolation, have diarrhoea, have MRSA or are dying.
- Suggest that they pull the curtain around the bed when the partner is visiting.

Negotiation

- Tell them that you will talk to the bed manager and ask for the patient to be moved to another bed or ward, but explain that beds are scarce and that this may take some time.
- Tell them that you will have a word with the other patients and staff members on the ward in the mean time.

Closure

- Ask the couple if they have any questions and whether they understand what you have told them.
- Document your conversation in the patient's notes, and notify your seniors and the ward sister.

Inter-professional and intra-professional communication

As a doctor you will increasingly find that a multi-disciplinary approach needs to be taken, and this will require you to communicate not only with nurses but also with physiotherapists, occupational therapists, pharmacists and clerical staff. This is true for both hospitals and primary care settings. Each of the following scenarios will allow you to familiarise yourself with situations that, although reasonably common, are rarely addressed.

157 Dealing with underperforming colleagues

Scenario

You are a doctor on a busy medical firm and you notice that one of your colleagues, a fellow doctor, has been underperforming. He is frequently late for ward rounds, not very committed to his work, and on one or two occasions he has written up lethal doses of morphine for his patients. You have rectified his mistakes and covered for him on ward rounds, telling the consultants that he is working elsewhere on the ward when in fact he has not turned up. You have now decided to have a word with him.

- Approach your colleague and ask him if he is having any problems with work.
  - He replies that everything's fine.
- Point out that he has not only missed ward rounds, but he has also written up potentially lethal doses of morphine, and that you have been covering for him on both counts.
  - He again insists there is nothing wrong.
- Tell him that if he has any problems he must face them and get help, as he is putting both his career and the lives of his patients at risk.
- Assure him that you will be there to provide support for him if he needs it, and suggest that he seeks help from colleagues such as the registrar, the consultant or the Sub-Dean and the hospital welfare officer.
- In parting, impress upon him the gravity of the situation and what is at risk. Suggest that he takes some time off to reassess his situation.

158 A senior colleague wants you to hold his bleep

Scenario

You are a junior doctor on a very busy medical team, and a senior colleague has asked you to hold his bleep while he studies for exams. You have held his bleep for the past couple of days, normally during lunch hours, but you are becoming increasingly fed up with this arrangement. You also know that instead of studying, your senior colleague has been spotted in the nearby pub. You are also worried that there may be a time when you are bleeped and you are too inexperienced to carry out the necessary procedure or treat a patient. During the early-morning ward round you told your colleague that you would like to see him about the bleep situation. He agrees to see you in the hospital café after the round. You go to the café and find him. You intend to return his bleep and have an amicable conversation about this issue.

Introduction

- Meet the senior doctor.
- You may be inclined to call him by his first name, but it is not professional to do so, this depends on how you normally address him. In exam situations it is best to be professional.
- Establish that you would like to talk to him about his bleep.
- Allow him time to ask you why.
- Reply politely and say that you would like to return his bleep as you feel uncomfortable holding it.
- Let him know that you are aware that he is studying for his membership exams, but that patient safety is paramount.
- Ask him whether he has asked the consultant and educational supervisor for time off.
  - Your colleague tells you that he has no study leave left, as this is his third or fourth attempt, and he is not able to attend courses either, as his educational grants have run out.
  - He also tells you that his parents are doctors and that he is worried he is going to let them down.
- Be sympathetic, but suggest that he holds his bleep and answers it from the library, and delegates jobs to the FY1 if he believes they are capable.

- You may need to tackle the issue of drinking while on duty and jeopardising patient care.
- Also tell your colleague that you are afraid that you may feel pressurised into something that you are not confident or supposed to do, for example:
  - administer streptokinase
  - sign a DNAR form
  - admit a patient from Accident and Emergency
  - write a prescription for theophylline
  - insert chest drains
  - perform non-invasive ventilation
  - perform a lumbar puncture
  - request CT/MRI scans
  - make decisions about blood transfusions and patient management.
- You also ask him to tell the nurses to bleep the junior doctor for simple procedures such as:
  - prescribing pain relief
  - prescribing laxatives
  - prescribing proton pump inhibitors
  - prescribing fluids
  - inserting cannulas.
- The nurses are not to bleep the junior doctors for DNAR orders, arrests, or speaking to relatives about the advanced management of patients.

Closure

Offer your support, say that you are willing to help in any way you can, and end the conversation in an amicable manner.

159 The multi-disciplinary team (MDT) meeting

Scenario

Mr Grace, an 87-year-old man who was admitted with an upper respiratory tract infection, has been on the ward for 3 weeks. He is recovering, and a discharge plan has been drawn up. He is discussed in the MDT meeting.

Multi-disciplinary team (MDT) meeting

- This is usually a round table meeting with members of the multi-disciplinary team.
- The following individuals are present:
    - consultant (medical or surgical)
    - registrar
    - senior and junior doctor
    - physiotherapist
    - occupational therapist
    - nurse in charge of ward
    - discharge coordinator
    - family members.
- Each patient is discussed individually.
- The MDT meeting usually covers matters such as medication changes, treatment, placements (i.e. housing), and mobility (i.e. activities of daily living).
- This meeting allows each team member (medical and non-medical) to discuss each patient's prognosis, and enables the team to draw up mutually agreed treatment plans.
- Cases are discussed in confidence and confidentiality is a top priority.

160 Dispute with sister in charge over a patient's discharge

Scenario

You are a doctor on an elderly care firm. Mr Saunders, an 80-year-old man, is returning home tomorrow after a urinary tract infection. He is doubly incontinent and has no home help. The sister in charge would like to discuss his discharge.

Introduction and discussion

- Establish a rapport with the sister and tell her that you understand that she wants a word with you about Mr Saunders' discharge.
    - She tells you that she considers he is not fit to go home because he lives on his own, is doubly incontinent and has no help at home to look after him. She is convinced that he will be a failed discharge.
- Explain that the decision was made by the consultant.

- The sister remains adamant and insists that Mr Saunders requires social service input with regard to being placed in a home.
- Ask her to document this in the patient's notes, and tell her that you will inform the consultant.
- Ask one of your seniors, such as the registrar, for their opinion.
- Inform the consultant of the situation and ask him whether the entire team can meet with the nursing staff and sister to discuss Mr Saunders' discharge.
- Alternatively, the consultant may delay the discharge until after the MDT meeting that week.
- This is an MDT issue and it must be rectified at the MDT meeting.
- Do not make a scene with the nursing staff.

161 Interruption during a post-take ward round

Scenario

You are a doctor on a post-take ward round. A nurse approaches you and tells you that a patient's drug chart needs to be altered. She is adamant that it needs to be done immediately, and will not agree to you coming back to do it later. She is being difficult, but you do not want to make a scene. Discuss the situation with her and come to an amicable agreement.

Preparation

Ensure that you take time to calm down, and avoid making a scene.

Introduction

- Apologise first.
- Then you should begin by saying that you are on a post-take ward round, you have a number of patients to see, and you will return when all of the urgent cases have been seen.

Negotiation

- Explain that you understand that the patient needs his drugs, but suggest that the nurse gives him his medication and signs a paper to

say that she has given it, and later she and the doctor can sit down and sign the new chart.
  – The nurse is not prepared to do this.

Closure

- Offer to make the most urgent changes (i.e. for the drugs that the patient must take that morning), and promise to return after the ward round to write up the rest.
- Thank the nurse and resume your post-take ward round.

162 Secretary taking a referral

Scenario

The consultant's secretary takes a referral and accidentally forgets to inform you, the doctor, that the patient will be arriving in hospital. The sister from the medical assessment unit bleeps you to say that they have had a patient waiting there to see a doctor for over 5 hours. You rush to the medical assessment unit.

Preparation

- Obtain the patient's notes and familiarise yourself with their past medical history and the GP's referral.

Introduction and consultation

- Introduce yourself, establish a rapport with the patient and take a brief history.
- Apologise for the delay and explain that you have been held up on the wards.
- Examine the patient.
- Take the relevant blood samples and arrange the necessary investigations.
- Now contact the consultant's secretary and ask if she can arrange for the consultant to come and see the patient.
  – At this stage the secretary tells you that she is sorry she didn't inform you about the patient.

- This is a difficult situation.
  - Remain calm.
  - Do not point the finger.
  - Avoid attempting to resolve this matter over the phone. Face-to-face conversations are always best, but not in front of the patients or nursing staff.
- Let the senior doctor know about the patient and request his review. In the mean time, go and see the secretary.
- The secretary is extremely apologetic.
  - Explain to her that the mistake she made could have put a patient's life at risk.
  - Ask her to report her mistake to the consultant.
  - Thank her for her honesty and leave.

Ethics and law

End-of-life issues

163 DNAR orders

- The decision not to resuscitate should only be considered if the likelihood of a successful outcome is poor.
- Complete an assessment of the patient's cardiovascular, respiratory, gastrointestinal systems, etc.
- This is a consultant decision.
- Document the order in the medical notes.
- Let all the teams (medical and nursing), the patient (if appropriate) and the family know.
- Include the views of family and staff in the decision-making process.
- The order does not make the decision regarding active treatment (non-invasive ventilation, e.g. continuous positive airway pressure, bilevel positive airway pressure).
- The status should be reviewed in the light of clinical improvement.

164 Withdrawing and withholding life-sustaining treatment

The decision to withdraw or withhold life-sustaining treatment is one of the most difficult decisions we have to make as doctors. The primary goal of medical treatment is to benefit the patient by restoring or maintaining their health as far as possible, maximising benefit and minimising harm. If treatment fails, or no longer gives a net benefit to the patient (or if the patient has competently refused the treatment), the primary goal of medical treatment cannot be realised, and the justification for providing the treatment is removed. This ethical dilemma may be answered by using the Jonsen procedure and the Four Principles.

Jonsen procedure

Four key areas should be addressed:

Medical indications (setting the scene for the decision making)

- What is the patient's diagnosis?
- What further information is required?
- How are you going to obtain this information?
- What treatment options are available?
- What is the patient's prognosis?

Patient's preferences (capacity)

- Is the patient competent (able to understand, retain and weigh the different options available)?
- If yes, what does the patient want?
- If no:
  - Is this temporary or permanent?
  - Did the patient have a living will or advance directive?
  - What is in the patient's best interest?
  - If the patient is a child, what do the parents want?
  - If the patient is a child, what is in the patient's best interest?

Quality of life

- Will treatment improve the patient's quality of life?
- Should the patient be resuscitated in the event of an arrest?
- How can the patient's care be improved?

Associated factors

These include legal, religious or cultural factors that affect the patient's management.

Four principles

- **Autonomy:** Respect the patient's ability to make informed decisions for him- or herself.
- **Beneficence:** Do your best to improve the patient's condition and outcome.
- **Non-maleficence:** Avoid harming the patient.
- **Justice:** Follow the law and respect the patient's rights.

Finally points

- A multi-disciplinary team should conduct the full assessment.
- Ultimately the responsibility for treatment decisions rests with the clinician in charge of the patient's care. However, it is important to involve all members of the medical/surgical team, the patient and their immediate family.
- Good clear communication is essential.
- Follow locally or nationally agreed guidelines.
- Seek advice from colleagues if necessary.
- If the decision to withhold or withdraw life-prolonging treatment is made, it must be clearly documented in the medical notes. The decision must be reviewed to take into account any changes in circumstances. Ensure that there is adequate support for family and friends during and after the decision-making process.

165 Palliative care

Palliative care is a branch of medicine that addresses the dying patient. It involves all areas of the patient's care, including their social, psychological and medical needs. It is important to allow the patient to die symptom free and with dignity.

- Analgesia for pain relief. There are several different routes available (oral, intravenous, patches, subcutaneous pump).
- Consider using a subcutaneous pump for a combination of medications: analgesia (morphine), anti-emetics (cyclizine) and anti-cholinergic agents (hyoscine).
- Anti-emetics for nausea and vomiting.
- Laxatives for constipation.
- Quiet side room.
- Palliative care nurse (Macmillan nursing).
- Family involvement.
- Medical and surgical intervention may have a role (e.g. ERCP and stent insertion to relieve jaundice in cases of pancreatic or gallbladder malignancy, stent inserted into the bronchus or oesophagus in cases of upper gastrointestinal obstruction, defunctioning colostomy for metastatic bowel cancer, fixation of pathological fractures for metastatic bone fractures).
- Routine investigations or blood tests should be avoided except for clinical reasons.

- Consider implementing the Liverpool protocol.
- Consider palliative placement (hospice).

Dealing with death

- Death is a subject that is often neglected by medical students. Their first experience of it comes in the early years, especially through the learning of anatomy.
- The amount of exposure varies. Most experiences of death take place in the final year of medical school or during attachments in geriatric medicine.
- Being able to certify death and write a death certificate is a mandatory skill for newly qualified doctors. Furthermore, breaking the news of the death of a loved one to the relatives or next of kin is a task in itself. Moreover, as we live in a multicultural community we come to appreciate how widely customs vary between the different faiths and denominations.

166 Multicultural aspects of death

Scenario: Jewish autopsy

You are the doctor on call and are asked to speak to Mr Cohen, a practising Jew who has just lost his 16-year-old son after he collapsed on a football pitch. The ambulance brought his son into Accident and Emergency, and the resuscitation team did their best but could not save him. A death certificate could not be written as the cause of death was not known. The coroner has advised you that a post-mortem will be required. Your task is to convey this information to the family.

Preparation

- There are a number of issues that need to be addressed in this scenario.
- First, read the patient's notes and look for any history of pre-existing disease (e.g. epilepsy, congenital heart disease such as hypertrophic obstructive cardiomyopathy (HOCM), or diabetes).

- Secondly, establish from your colleagues the information that has been given to the father about the death. (Assume that he knows his son has passed away.)
- Finally, be aware of Jewish funeral customs.

Introduction and consultation

- Introduce yourself to Mr Cohen and offer your condolences, demonstrating empathy and sympathy.
- Ask him what he knows about the tragedy.
- Tell him that you are unsure about the cause of death and that you have spoken to the coroner. Explain who the coroner is.

The coroner

- Tell Mr Cohen that the coroner has told you a coroner's autopsy will need to be performed. At this stage you may need to explain the differences between a hospital post-mortem and a coroner's post-mortem. Explain that a coroner's post-mortem is conducted in order to establish a cause of death, whereas a hospital post-mortem looks at all the internal organs in a systematic fashion.
- Explain that a coroner's post-mortem:
  - is required by law and cannot be refused
  - is crucial to find out the cause of death, without which knowledge a death certificate cannot be issued.
- Explain that without a death certificate a funeral cannot take place in the UK.
- Relatives have the right to refuse a hospital post-mortem but not a coroner's post-mortem.

Funeral arrangements

- The relatives may tell you that they need to bury the body within 24 hours and ask whether this can be done. This is not hospital policy. Do not offer any time frames or promises. Instead say that you will try to negotiate the earliest possible date with the coroner's office, but it is dependent on how much work the coroner has.
- Reassure the relatives that the post-mortem will be conducted as soon as possible.
- Offer the services of the hospital chaplaincy service that has a Rabbi who can advise them further, and say that you can be present as well.

The relative may say that they want to call their own Rabbi. Offer the use of the hospital phone.

Support and information

- Let Mr Cohen know that the consultant is available should he want to talk to them.
- Offer him a leaflet explaining the coroner's post-mortem, and assess his level of understanding of a post-mortem.
- Ask him if he would like to know what will happen, and reassure him that the body will be dealt with respectfully. The post-mortem will be performed by a histopathologist (a doctor who is an expert in the field), assisted by technicians.
- If Mr Cohen asks about scars and marks on the body, explain that the post-mortem team will try to use existing scars and natural skin folds, and restrict marks to the area around the hairline, and if scars are produced they will be dressed accordingly.
- Reassure him that no organs will be removed or kept, but that some samples of tissue and body fluids may be taken for further analysis and will be returned if appropriate.
- Tell him that the bereavement office is available for further information, and offer him counselling services.
- Ask Mr Cohen if he wants you to talk to any one else on his behalf.

Negotiation and closure

- Ask whether he has any further questions, give him your contact details and bleep number and ask him to call you if he needs to.
- Let him know that you will advise him of the final details of the coroner's post-mortem once these become available.
- Many families also have a preferred undertaker, whom they should call once the coroner's post-mortem has taken place, and who could also keep in contact with the coroner's office.
- Ask Mr Cohen if he would like to view the body in the mean time, and make arrangements for this.
- Thank him for his time.
- Empathise, saying that you know it's a difficult time for him.

Background information

- The Jewish faith is one of the oldest religions in the world. It gains its origins from Christianity through Jesus Christ and is linked to Islam through the Prophet Abraham's son Ishmail.
- Their holy book is the Torah, which is written in Hebrew. The Torah is a collection of books that make up the Old Testament.

Customs at death

- Burial takes place immediately, usually within 24 hours (unless it is the Sabbath), and no more than two nights after death, as the soul needs to return to God.
- The shirt sleeve of next of kin is torn by Rabbi at the funeral (Kria) (left side for parents and right side for others).
- The service starts with a special prayer called Kaddish. This is recited for 30 days for family members and 11 months by the parents.
- All funeral attendees are expected to wash after returning from the funeral, as they believe that evil spirits follow them from the cemetery.
- Many are against post-mortems.
- Embalming is not allowed.
- No parts of the body are to be removed or organs donated.
- There is a 7-day mourning period for seven immediate family members: mother, father and siblings, husband and wife (known as Shiva/Shevah). These members of the family are not allowed to wear leather shoes, shave, have haircuts or bathe.
- Attendance at parties, weddings, etc. is forbidden.
- All mirrors in the house are reversed during mourning.
- Those who marry out of the Jewish faith or commit suicide are buried in a separate part of the cemetery.
- After 1 year a memorial service is held to remember the dead.

Multicultural aspects of death in other cultures and faiths

Islam

- A similar custom is observed by Islam with regard to burial within 24 hours.
- Those who follow Islam are known as Muslims.
- The holy book is known as the Qu'ran.
- Cremation is not permitted.

- A dying patient or those that are buried face Mecca (holy city for Muslims, in Saudi Arabia).
- Mourning involves the expression of emotions, usually crying, and therefore mourners require a quiet room for this. However, you must let them know there are other patients whom they should not disturb.
- The foot of the bed is to face Mecca. The head should be turned towards the right shoulder before rigor mortis begins.
- The body should not be washed, but the hair can be combed and limbs straightened.
- The body is wrapped in two white sheets.
- Organ donation was not allowed in Islamic law until 1982.
- Post-mortem will only be allowed if required by law.
- When relatives come to view the body in the hospital mortuary or chapel of rest, make sure that any religious artefacts relating to other faiths are removed.

Christianity

- The holy book is the Bible. This is believed to be the writings and scriptures. It includes the four accounts of Jesus' life known as the Gospels.
- A number of different denominations exist, but the two main ones are Protestantism (encompassing the Church of England, Methodists and Baptists) and Roman Catholicism.
- Prayers are said at the bedside of the dying.
- The sick patient may receive the Sacrament of the Sick (anointing with oil) and viaticum (Holy Communion for the dying).
- After the death of the patient, the family and friends may stay around the bed and give prayers of thanksgiving for the person's life. If the dying patient is a young child or baby, baptism may also be offered before the patient passes away.
- If the patient is a Roman Catholic, the priest may hear a confession/ anoint the oil and administer viaticum.
- There are no objections to post-mortem or to organ donation.

Hinduism

- Followers are called Hindus.
- This religion developed around the Indian subcontinent.
- Hindus believe in reincarnation.
- The believe that by doing their duties (dharma) and not committing any sins or bad actions (karma) they can be released from the cycle of rebirth and join the ultimate reality (Brahma).
- The three main deities include Brahma (creator), Vishnu (preserver) and Shiva (destroyer), with various other gods and deities that fulfil various duties.
- Hindus believe that they can wash away their sins by washing in the holy waters of the river Ganges in India.
- As the patient is dying, water is placed in the mouth.
- After death the eyes are closed, the limbs are straightened, jewellery and sacred thread are removed.
- The body is wrapped in white sheets.
- The body is washed and dressed before the cremation, and prayers are said by the priest.
- Traditionally the funeral pyre is lit by the eldest son, but in the UK the button for releasing the body into the cremator is pressed by the eldest son. After death the body is always cremated and the ashes are washed away in the rivers, ultimately in the Ganges (if possible).
- Most patients will wish to die at home.
- Post-mortems are allowed if required by law, but all organs must be returned to the body.
- There are no objections to organ donation.
- Similar traditions are held in Buddhism and Sikhism.
- Buddhism was founded by Siddhartha Gautama.
- Buddhists believe in enlightenment by following the Noble Eightfold Path.
- Buddhists believe the consciousness remains for 8–12 hours after death and should be touched or moved.
- The presence of a Buddhist monk is preferred.
- There are no objections to post-mortem or organ donation.

Sikhism

- Sikhism was founded by Guru Nanak.
- The birthplace of the religion is Punjab in India.
- Guru gave spiritual guidance.

- The holy book is known as Guru Granth Sahib.
- The funeral should take place as soon as possible.
- After death the body is washed, wrapped and placed in a coffin.
- Cremation is mandatory, with the ashes scattered in running water.
- There are no objections to post-mortem or donation of organs.

Source: Bereavement Office and Chaplaincy at Conquest Hospital, Hastings and their publication *World Faiths in Hospital*.

167 Confirming death

Introduction

- One of the skills required as a junior doctor is to be able to confirm and certify death.
- You will also be required to identify and check the body (full external) looking for pacemakers, etc., and write a death certificate.
- In the event that a cause of death cannot be established it will be your responsibility to liaise with the coroner.
- The coroner will let you know whether a post-mortem will be required, and if it is you will have to convey this message to the family and next of kin.
- In the event that a cause of death can be established but a further exploration will be beneficial for the existing members of the family (e.g. looking for genetic diseases that could affect them, etc.), a hospital post-mortem will be required, for which consent from the family will be needed.
- A coroner's post-mortem does not require consent from the family, as it is a mandatory requirement by law.

Scenario

You are the doctor on call. At 2am you are called by the sister on a ward to certify the death of 70-year-old Mrs Brown, who was admitted to the ward a few days ago.

- On the ward ask a nurse to accompany you to see the patient.
- Ask her when she found Mrs Brown dead.
- Ascertain:
    - the events leading to admission and preceding death
    - whether the death was expected
    - who found the patient and when.

- Check the identity wrist band of the patient and check this against their notes.
- Review the prescription chart for sedatives or respiratory depressants.
- Shake the patient and call out 'Mrs Brown, can you hear me?' Do this close to the ear.
- Perform a sternal rub.
- Use a pen torch to assess the pupils. Note the pupils to be unreactive, fixed and dilated.
- Using an ophthalmoscope, examine the fundus for rail roading.
- Look, hear and feel for respiratory efforts for 1 minute.
- Auscultate the prechordium for heart sounds for 1 minute, and note absent heart sounds.
- Feel for carotid and femoral pulses for 1 minute, and note the absence of both major pulses.
- The patient may then be pronounced dead.
- Document in the patient's notes the time and place of death, absence of breath sounds, respiratory effort, heart sounds and major pulses. State your name, position and bleep number, date and time, and sign.
- Ask the nurse to make arrangements for removal of the body to the mortuary and inform the patient's next of kin.

168 Death certification

- This is (see figure below) legal documentation that must be filled in by a registered medical practitioner who either saw the body soon after death or had seen the patient during the last illness not more than 2 weeks prior to death.
- However, if you are the doctor who came to verify the death and had no input into the patient's life or treatment during the last stage of the patient's life you are not permitted to fill in the death certificate.
- A death certificate is needed by law to register the death by the Registrar for Births, Deaths and Marriages.
- The funeral undertakers will not remove the body without a death certificate.

Death certficate

- Name of the deceased.
- Place and time of death.

- Age at death.
- Cause of death:
- Parts:
  - 1a: Direct cause of death
  - 1b: Cause leading to 1a
  - 1c: Cause leading to 1b
  - 2: Indirect disease that may have contributed to or accelerated the death process.
- There are a number of causes of death that are not accepted. These include cardiac arrest and any forms of system failure.
- If a system failure is to be put down it needs to be justified.
- If in doubt contact your seniors, staff in the bereavement office are usually helpful, and finally contact the coroner.
- You will also need to tick a box to say whether the cause is directly linked to an industrial disease or poisoning, in which case the coroner will need to be notified.
- Also complete the stump.
- Fill in your details and qualification (e.g. MBBS, MD, MBChB) and the consultant's name and the date.
- In addition you may be required to fill in a cremation form that allows bodies to be cremated. A word of caution on this is that it requires you to view the body and perform a full external examination, looking closely and feeling for any pacemakers, etc.
- In the event that a cause of death cannot be found, the body will need to be sent for a post-mortem which is carried out by the coroner.

169 Deaths that need to be reported to the coroner

These include the following:

- deaths where no doctor satisfies the attendance requirements for being able to certify death
- cause of death is unknown
- sudden, unexpected, suspicious, violent (homicide, suicide, accidental) or unnatural death
- deaths due to alcohol or drugs
- doubtful stillbirth
- deaths related to surgery or anaesthetic
- deaths within 24 hours of admission to hospital
- deaths in prison.

Special cases that need to be reported to the coroner include:

- death from industrial disease, poisoning or accident
- death of a patient in receipt of an industrial or war pension
- death by suicide, poisoning or drugs
- death as a result of an illegal abortion
- death from neglect, want or exposure.

Death certification exercise

- For each of the following case scenarios write down the causes of death using the Part 1a, 1b, 1c and Part 2 system for identifying causes of death.
- Suggested answers are given.
- It is advisable to also photocopy the sample death certificate given and practise filling out these scenarios.

Scenario 1

- Mrs Albert is a 72-year-old woman.
- She was admitted with a 5-day history of dense right hemiplegia and dysphasia.
- Two days ago she developed aspiration pneumonia.
- She deteriorated despite treatment with antibiotics.
- DNAR is signed.
- Past medical history: hypertension and Alzheimer's disease.

Please write down Parts 1a, 1b and 1c and Part 2.
Answer
1a: Aspiration pneumonia.
1b: Cerebrovascular accident.
1c: Hypertension.
2: Alzheimer's dementia.

Scenario 2

- Mr Williams is an 80-year-old man.
- He was admitted 3 days ago for increasing shortness of breath.
- He is known to have carcinoma of the lungs with widespread metastasis.
- He arrested suddenly.
- DNAR order was in place.
- Past medical history of hyperthyroidism and hypertension.

Please write down Parts 1a, 1b and 1c and Part 2.

Answer

1a: Carcinomatosis.

1b: Carcinoma of lung.

2: Hyperthyroidism, hypertension.

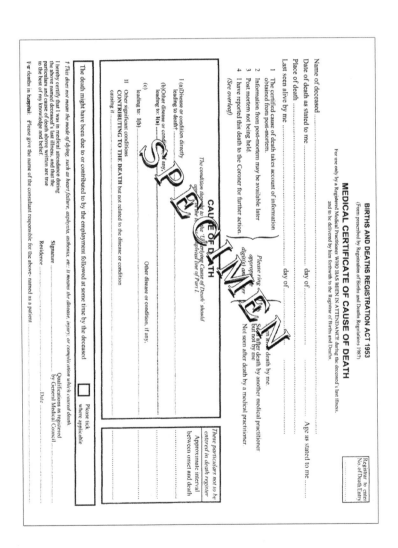

Scenario 3

- Mr Jacobs is a 24-year-old boy.
- He was admitted following his collapse on a football pitch.
- He was brought in by ambulance.
- He arrested and the resuscitation team were unable to revive him.
- He unfortunately died.

Please write down Parts 1a, 1b and 1c and Part 2.
Answer

- Unfortunately the cause of death cannot be established.
- The coroner needs to be notified and a post-mortem needs to take place.
- The coroner will issue a death certificate.

Scenario 4

- Mrs Abbot is a 75-year-old woman.
- She was admitted with a fractured hip.
- The hip had not been fixed due to her increased risk for surgery.
- Ten days later she developed shortness of breath, SVT and cardiac arrest.
- Past medical history: COPD and osteoporosis.

Please write down Parts 1a, 1b and 1c and Part 2.
Answer
1a: Pulmonary embolism.
1b: Deep vein thrombosis.
1c: Fractured hip.
2:   COPD and osteoporosis.

Scenario 5

- Mr Malcolm is a 67-year-old man.
- He was admitted with an upper gastrointestinal bleed.
- He was known to have a duodenal ulcer.
- He was resuscitated and was stable for 5 days.
- Past medical history: COPD, ischaemic heart disease and diabetes.
- On day 6 he complained of abdominal pain and had another episode of gastrointestinal and rectal bleed.
- He arrested and could not be revived.
- Unfortunately he died.

Please write down Parts 1a, 1b and 1c and Part 2.
Answer
1a: Perforated duodenal ulcer.
2: COPD, ischaemic heart disease, diabetes.

170 Brainstem death

Criteria that must be fulfilled before the diagnosis can be made

General	*Specific exclusions*
Irremediable brain damage	Hypothermia ($< 35°C$)
Exclude reversible causes	Metabolic/endocrine abnormalities
Coma dependent on ventilator	Drug intoxication
Known aetiology for the underlying insult	Recent cardiac arrest

Brainstem death testing

- Test performed by two doctors with more than 5 years of clinical practice on two separate occasions (one doctor should be a consultant). No doctor should be a member of the transplant team.
- More than 6 hours after onset of a coma, or more than 24 hours after cardiac arrest.
- Death is pronounced after the first set of tests.
- No pupillary response.
- No corneal reflex.
- No vestibulo-ocular reflex (ensure the tympanic canal is clear of obstruction, ice-cold water inserted into the external auditory meatus, the stimulus should not provoke a response – a normal response is deviation of the eyes towards the syringed ear).
- No facial response to a painful stimulus (no grimacing).
- No gag or cough reflex.
- Apnoea test: Patient is pre-oxygenated with 100% oxygen for 10 minutes. $PaCO_2$ must be recorded in the normal rage (i.e. 4.5–6 kPa). The ventilator is then disconnected while 6 litres/minute are inserted via the ET tube. No ventilator effort is seen and the arterial blood gas is repeated (pCO_2 should be above 6.65 kPa).

Index